AF515218

Nutritional Influences on Bone Health

Connie M. Weaver • Heike Bischoff-Ferrari
Robin M. Daly • Man-Sau Wong
Editors

Nutritional Influences on Bone Health

10th International Symposium

Springer

Editors
Connie M. Weaver
Nutrition and Science
Purdue University
West Lafayette, IN
USA

Heike Bischoff-Ferrari
Geriatrics and Aging Research
University of Zurich
Zurich
Switzerland

Robin M. Daly
Institute for Physical Activity and Nutrition
Deakin University
Melbourne
Victoria
Australia

Man-Sau Wong
Department of Applied Biology
and Chemical Technology
The Hong Kong Polytechnic University
Hung Hom
Hong Kong

ISBN 978-3-319-98463-6 ISBN 978-3-319-98464-3 (eBook)
https://doi.org/10.1007/978-3-319-98464-3

Library of Congress Control Number: 2018957853

© Springer Nature Switzerland AG 2019
This work is subject to copyright. All rights are reserved by the Publisher, whether the whole or part of the material is concerned, specifically the rights of translation, reprinting, reuse of illustrations, recitation, broadcasting, reproduction on microfilms or in any other physical way, and transmission or information storage and retrieval, electronic adaptation, computer software, or by similar or dissimilar methodology now known or hereafter developed.
The use of general descriptive names, registered names, trademarks, service marks, etc. in this publication does not imply, even in the absence of a specific statement, that such names are exempt from the relevant protective laws and regulations and therefore free for general use.
The publisher, the authors, and the editors are safe to assume that the advice and information in this book are believed to be true and accurate at the date of publication. Neither the publisher nor the authors or the editors give a warranty, express or implied, with respect to the material contained herein or for any errors or omissions that may have been made. The publisher remains neutral with regard to jurisdictional claims in published maps and institutional affiliations.

This Springer imprint is published by the registered company Springer Nature Switzerland AG
The registered company address is: Gewerbestrasse 11, 6330 Cham, Switzerland

Preface

The 10th International Symposium on Nutritional Aspects of Osteoporosis in Hong Kong continued the valued opportunity for scientists and students interested in the role of nutrition to optimize bone and muscle health to spend time devoted to this topic exclusively.

Hong Kong brought more participation from the Asian region. The prevalence of fractures in Asia illustrates the urgency of prevention. And what an exciting venue Hong Kong was for the delegates that attended this meeting. Being in such a dynamic city added a great deal of enjoyment to the meeting. We are grateful to Dawn Haan at Purdue University, the staff at the Hong Kong Polytechnic University, and the staff at the Federation of Medical Societies of Hong Kong for their administrative support of this international meeting.

The Proceedings reflect a mixture of reviews, study designs of ongoing major trials, and research presentations that characterized the meeting. The editors hope that the Proceedings make a contribution to the field.

West Lafayette, IN, USA	Connie M. Weaver
Melbourne, VIC, Australia	Robin M. Daly
Hung Hom, Hong Kong	Man-sau Wong
Zurich, Switzerland	Heike Bischoff-Ferrari

Contents

Part I Vitamin D

1 **DO-HEALTH: Vitamin D3-Omega-3-Home Exercise-Healthy Aging and Longevity Trial—Dietary Patterns in Five European Countries** 3
Patricia O. Chocano-Bedoya and Heike A. Bischoff-Ferrari

2 **Vitamin D and Omega-3 Fatty Acid Trial 2017: Addressing Effects on Muscle and Bone** 11
Meryl S. LeBoff, Catherine M. Donlon, Sharon H. Chou, Nancy Cook, Julie Buring, and JoAnn E. Manson

3 **Vitamin D Among Children in Asia** 25
Tsz Ping Lam, Benjamin Hon Kei Yip, Wayne Y. W. Lee, Nelson Leung Sang Tang, Kwong Man Lee, Alec Lik Hang Hung, Bobby Kin Wah Ng, and Jack Chun Yiu Cheng

Part II Micronutrients: Calcium, Sodium, and Potassium

4 **Peak BMC Growth and Calcium Requirements for Children** 37
Michael R. Lawlor, Connie M. Weaver, Bruce A. Craig, Susan J. Whiting, Adam D. G. Baxter-Jones, Hassanali Vatanparast, and George P. McCabe

5 **Integrative Omic Study to Identify Potential Dietary Supplement for Osteoporosis Treatment** 45
Ching-Lung Cheung

6 **Dietary Mineral Intake Ratios and Bone Health in Adults** 53
Andrea J. Lobene, Linda D. McCabe, Michael S. Stone, Joseph M. Kindler, Regan L. Bailey, Alanna J. Moshfegh, Donna G. Rhodes, Joseph D. Goldman, George P. McCabe, and Connie M. Weaver

7 **Dietary Calcium, Lifestyle Factors, and Bone Health in Premenarche Chinese Girls** ... 69
Gordon C. L. Cheung and Yi-Xiang Su

Part III Exercise/Sedentary Behavior

8 **Nutrition and Exercise Approaches to Enhance Muscle, Mobility, and Cognition During Aging** ... 77
Robin M. Daly, Melissa B. Formica, Jamie L. Tait, and Helen Macpherson

9 **Sedentary Behaviors in Children and Adolescents: What Is the Influence on Bone Strength?** ... 95
Simon Higgins, Staci L. Belcher, and Richard D. Lewis

10 **Effects of Low Energy Availability on Bone Health in Exercising Premenopausal Women** ... 109
Nancy I. Williams and Mary Jane De Souza

11 **Lifestyle Intervention to Improve Mobility in Apparently Healthy Chinese Elders: A Hypothesis Generating Study** ... 127
Marie-Noelle Horcajada and Elizabeth A. Offord

Part IV Prebiotics

12 **Diet, Microbiota, and Bone Health** ... 143
René Rizzoli

13 **Therapeutic Targeting of Gut-Bone Signaling to Treat Osteoporosis** ... 169
Laura R. McCabe and Narayanan Parameswaran

14 **Meeting Calcium Needs in Asia and Prebiotic Study Protocol** ... 183
Winnie Chee, Kanimolli Arasu, Chang Chung Yuan, Soon Yee Wong, Ong Shu Hwa, Wai Yew Yang, Megan Chong, Meenal Mavinkurve, and Jia Yuan Khoo

Part V Bioactives/Functional Foods

15 **Effect of Dried Plum on Bone Biomarkers in Men** ... 193
Shirin Hooshmand

16 **Bone-Protective Chinese Herbs: The Story of Fructus Ligustri Lucidi** ... 199
Sisi Cao, Xiao-Li Dong, Yan Zhang, and Man-Sau Wong

Part VI Diet Patterns/Micronutrients

17 The Relationship Between Dietary Fat and Sarcopenia, Skeletal Muscle Loss, Osteoporosis and Risk of Fractures in Aging 211
Ailsa A. Welch and Richard P. G. Hayhoe

18 Dairy Products, Vitamin D, and Bone Health 227
Laura H. van Dongen and S. Sahni

19 Dietary Intake in Chinese Community-Dwelling Older Adults with Sarcopenia: A Focus on Protein 237
Ruth Chan and Liu-Ying Zhu

Part VII Policy and Translation

20 No Relationship Between Serum 25(OH) Vitamin D Concentrations and Perceptions of Vitamin D Dietary Intake Adequacy in US and German Adults Not Using Dietary Supplements. 247
Regan L. Bailey, Sowmyanarayanan V. Thuppal, Katherine D. Sherif, Nigel Denby, Suzanne R. Steinbaum, Bryan Haycock, Alexandra E. Cowan, Jared R. Nieters, and Clemens von Schacky

21 Building and Translating Evidence-Based Nutrition and Bone Research Into Policy and Public Health Messaging 257
Taylor C. Wallace

Index. 269

Part I

Vitamin D

DO-HEALTH: Vitamin D3-Omega-3-Home Exercise-Healthy Aging and Longevity Trial—Dietary Patterns in Five European Countries

1

Patricia O. Chocano-Bedoya and Heike A. Bischoff-Ferrari

Introduction

The increasing number of older adults worldwide poses an important public health challenge [1]. For instance, in the USA, seniors 65 and over grew from 35.0 million in 2000 to 49.2 million in 2016, accounting for 12.4% and 15.2% of the total population, respectively, and they are estimated to represent 20% of the total population by 2040 [2]. The demographic change is even more pronounced in some European countries, where the youngest segment of the population is not expected to grow. For instance, in Switzerland the population segment of adults age 65 years and older is expected to rise from 18.1% in 2015 to 26% in 2045 [3]. Relevant to health care and health economics, the rapid increase in the proportion of older adults will increase the burden of several age-related chronic diseases [4, 5].

Vitamin D may be a promising public health strategy to improve overall health as suggested by prior mechanistic [6] and observational studies [7, 8], as well as by

P. O. Chocano-Bedoya (✉)
Department of Geriatrics and Aging Research, University Hospital and University of Zurich, Zurich, Switzerland

Centre on Aging and Mobility, University Hospital Zurich and Waid City Hospital, Zurich, Switzerland
e-mail: patricia.chocano@waid.zuerich.ch

H. A. Bischoff-Ferrari
Department of Geriatrics and Aging Research, University Hospital and University of Zurich, Zurich, Switzerland

Centre on Aging and Mobility, University Hospital Zurich and Waid City Hospital, Zurich, Switzerland

University Clinic for Acute Geriatric Care, City Hospital Waid, Zurich, Switzerland
e-mail: heike.bischoff@usz.ch

© Springer Nature Switzerland AG 2019

C. M. Weaver et al. (eds.), *Nutritional Influences on Bone Health*,
https://doi.org/10.1007/978-3-319-98464-3_1

a number of randomized clinical trials [9, 10]. While the evidence of a benefit of vitamin D supplementation in the maintenance of bone and muscle health is extensive [11–14], its dosing regimens and desirable blood levels for the prevention of falls and fractures are still being debated [15–17]. Further, the benefit of vitamin D supplementation for other health outcomes including cardiovascular health and cancer prevention has not been established [18, 19]. However, several large ongoing trials, including DO-HEALTH (five countries in Europe), VITAL (USA) [20, 21], FIND (Finland), ViDA (New Zealand), and VIDAL (UK), are addressing the potential non-skeletal benefits of vitamin D. At this point results for DO-HEALTH and VITAL are expected in 2018, and results of the ViDA study have been published recently suggesting that a monthly dose of 100,000 IU vitamin D3 may have no benefit on the incidence of major cardiovascular events [22] and fractures [23].

Beyond individual nutrients such as vitamin D, overall diet is one of the major modifiable risk factors of chronic diseases capable to counteract accelerated aging [24–26] as it benefits multiple systems biological, clinical and social levels [27]. Dietary patterns can be captures by a comprehensive assessment of diet as a whole [28]. Methods to evaluate dietary patterns include *a priori* (based on previous knowledge) and *a posteriori* methods (data-driven) [29]. The *a posteriori* approach is a useful tool for identifying the prevailing dietary habits of a particular study population [30], extracting patterns from the observed dietary data by means of appropriate exploratory statistical methodology, for instance, factor or cluster analysis [31]. Based on these methods, the European EPIC and the SENECA studies have found large differences in dietary patterns between 27 centers (10 European countries), with higher heterogeneity in Western Europe, using standardized 24 h dietary recalls [32], modified diet history assessments [33], and food frequency questionnaires [34]. These variations between countries can also be attributed to differences in aging conditions between countries which should be further investigated and monitored over time.

DO-HEALTH Design

DO-HEALTH in Europe (http://do-health.eu/wordpress/) aims to evaluate the role of two additional interventions (omega-3 fatty acids and a simple home exercise program) next to vitamin D on five primary endpoints including fracture risk, muscle function, cognitive function, rate of infections, and blood pressure. DO-HEALTH has a 2x2x2 factorial trial design to test both the individual and combined benefit of these interventions on the five primary endpoints.

DO-HEALTH was developed with the main objective to enhance healthy aging in European seniors and to reduce health-care costs via the implementation of effective and broadly applicable disease prevention interventions. The study population consists of 2157 healthy seniors 70 years and older living in the community. To represent the pre-frail senior population at risk of institutionalization, 40% of seniors were enrolled based on a fall with or without a fracture in the prior year. The trial was conducted at seven recruitment centers located in five countries: Switzerland (University of Zurich, Basel University Hospital, Geneva University Hospitals),

Table 1.1 Inclusion/exclusion criteria for DO-HEALTH

Inclusion criteria	Exclusion criteria (partial)
• Age ≥70 years • Mini mental state examination score of at least 24 • Living in the community • Sufficiently mobile to reach the study center • Able to walk 10 m with or without a walking aid and get in and out of a chair without help • Able to swallow study capsules • Able and willing to participate, sign informed consent (including consent to analyze all samples until dropout or withdrawal), and cooperate with study procedures	• Consumption of more than 1000 IU vitamin D/day in the 3 months prior to enrollment or unwillingness to reduce to 800 IU/day of vitamin D (current standard of care) for the duration of the trial • Unwilling to limit calcium supplement dose to a maximum of 500 mg per day for the duration of the trial • Taking omega-3 fat supplements in the 3 months prior to recruitment and/or unwilling to refrain from the use of omega-3 supplements for the duration of the trial • Use of any active vitamin D metabolite, PTH treatment, or calcitonin at baseline and unwillingness to forego these treatments during the course of the trial • History of diagnosed cancer (except non-melanoma skin cancer), myocardial infarction, stroke, transient ischemic attack, angina pectoris, or coronary artery intervention in the last 5 years • Others (see clinical trials.gov)

France (University of Toulouse Hospital Centre), Germany (Charité Berlin), Portugal (University of Coimbra), and Austria (Innsbruck Medical University). Inclusion and some exclusion criteria are listed in Table 1.1 (additional exclusion criteria in https://clinicaltrials.gov/ct2/show/NCT01745263).

The three primary treatment comparisons are:

1. 2000 IU vitamin D per day compared to placebo
2. 1 g of omega-3 fatty acids (EPA + DHA, ratio 1:2, from marine algae) compared to placebo
3. Home exercise (HE) program of 30 min three times a week compared to a control exercise program (Flex) 30 min three times a week

DO-HEALTH follows a 2 × 2 × 2 factorial study design. Under the assumption that the three interventions have distinct mechanisms of action and therefore will have an additive effect on the study endpoints, this is the most efficient design. Nevertheless, this RCT is powered with >80% to assess the role of the three interventions on all five primary endpoints, even if interaction between treatments is present. Participants were randomly assigned to 8 groups of 269 participants each including all possible combinations of the study treatments and placebo (Fig. 1.1). All analyses will test the effect of each strategy, while controlling for the others.

DO-HEALTH completed multiple assessments during the 3-year follow-up, including clinical visits at baseline and 12, 24, and 36 months after recruitment and telephone interviews every 3 months between the clinical visits (nine telephone interviews total). During the clinical visits, participants had a full clinical examination and completed several questionnaires regarding demographic and lifestyle information, medical events, as well as adherence to the study interventions and presence of adverse events. At each clinical visit, participants had a DXA scan, and we collected

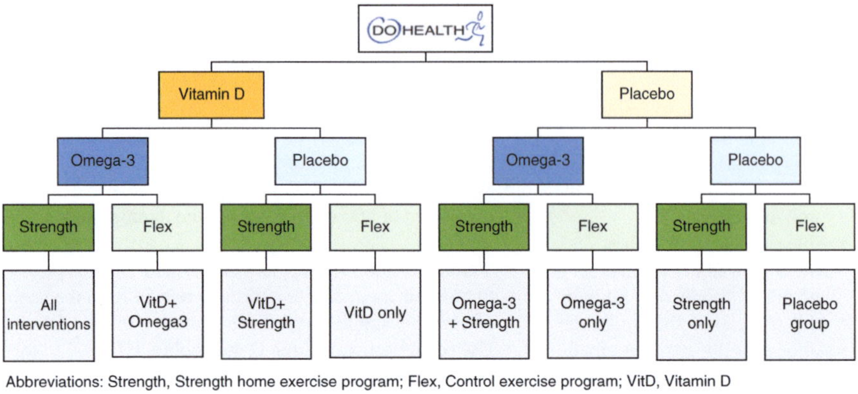

Fig. 1.1 DO-HEALTH clinical trial: 2 × 2 × 2 factorial design including three interventions (vitamin D, omega-3, and a home exercise program). Abbreviations: *Strength* strength home exercise program, *Flex* control exercise program, *VitD* vitamin D

blood and urine samples, which are in the DO-HEALTH biobank. Falls, fractures, and infections as well as other medical events were monitored through phone calls.

Dietary Assessments and Dietary Patterns in Five European Countries

At baseline and at the end of follow-up, DO-HEALTH participants completed a touchscreen food frequency questionnaire (FFQ). This semiquantitative FFQ was based on the one developed by Dr. Willett for the Nurses' Health Study [35] and the Ga2Len FFQ [36] and includes more than 180 food items including 9 options for frequency of usual consumption over the past year.

To estimate a posteriori diet patterns in five DO-HEALTH countries, we used factor analysis with principal components that were based on correlations between predefined food groups. First, we grouped food items into 35 predefined food groups on the basis of similar nutrient compositions and biological origins. Foods that did not fit into any group or that may have represented distinctive dietary behaviors were left as individual categories (e.g., pizza, beer, and tea). To select uncorrelated factors and more realistic diets, we used an orthogonal rotation procedure (varimax).

Overall, we retained three factors (dietary patterns) for the full population based on having an eigenvalue >1 (i.e., the factor explains more of the variance in correlations than is explained by a single variable) and the scree test (Fig. 1.2). The first factor was rich in vegetables, in particular legumes and cruciferous vegetables (factor loadings >0.70); hence, we called it the "vegetable pattern." The second factor included high loadings for red and processed meats (>0.68) but was also high on fish, poultry, and eggs; therefore, we called it the "meat pattern." The third factor was high on cheese, tomatoes, and refined grains ("miscellaneous pattern"). In Table 1.2 we summarize the highest loading food groups and the three selected patterns for the whole population.

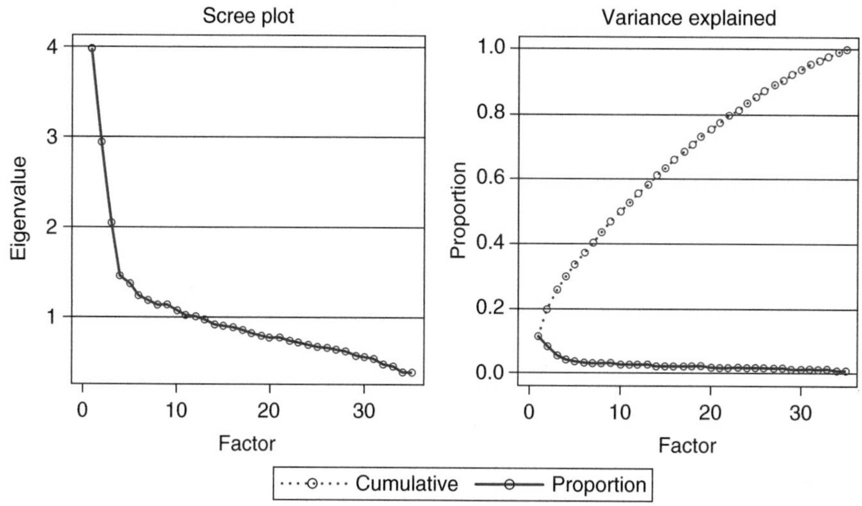

Fig. 1.2 Scree and variance plots for identification of dietary patterns of the overall population of DO-HEALTH by factor analysis. Food intakes (g/day) were aggregated into 35 predefined food groups. Factors considered appropriate for patterns shown in Table 1.2 are the three factors with eigenvalues >2

Table 1.2 Factor loadings for the three rotated factors among all DO-HEALTH participants ($n = 2157$)

Food group	Factor 1 (Vegetable pattern)	Factor 2 (Meat pattern)	Factor 3 (Miscellaneous pattern)
Legumes	0.75		
Cruciferous vegetables	0.70		
Yellow vegetables	0.65		
Vegetable dishes	0.61		
Fish	0.51	0.51	
Other vegetables	0.50		
Olive oil	0.41		
Fruits	0.40		
Red meat		0.70	
Organ meat		0.68	
Processed meat		0.58	
Liquor		0.52	
Poultry	0.42	0.52	
Eggs		0.43	
Cheese			0.55
Tomatoes			0.46
Refined grains			0.44
Nuts			0.43

Values less than ±0.40 are omitted for simplicity

When performing factor analysis by country, we observed that most countries had a "vegetable pattern" and a "meat pattern" except for Coimbra which didn't have a clear "meat pattern" but two "miscellaneous patterns." There was the highest variability between countries for the components of the third factor ("miscellaneous pattern"). For example, in Switzerland it was composed mostly of refined grains and pizza (factor loadings = 0.53 and 0.49, respectively), in Austria it was composed mostly of wine and liquor (factors loadings = 0.68 and 0.51, respectively), and in France it was composed mostly of fruit juice and mayonnaise/sauces (factor loadings = 0.62 and 0.52, respectively). In Coimbra, besides the "vegetable pattern," one pattern was highly loaded with high-fat milk products, organ meat, fruit juice, and poultry and another one with beer, red meat, and wine (factor loadings for these food groups ranged between 0.62 and 0.52).

The working group of the Food and Nutrition Section of the European Public Health Association [37] concluded that despite the economic and geographic differences between European countries, the direction of current dietary patterns seems to be toward a common European diet platform with local and regional variations. In consistency, in our preliminary results, we found similarities between countries for the most common dietary patterns with variations for the food groups of the "miscellaneous food pattern." In the EPIC-Elderly study (European Prospective Investigation into Cancer and Nutrition), a "plant-based" a posteriori pattern similar to the one identified in DO-HEALTH was associated with longer life expectancy [34, 38]. Besides the EPIC group, no previous study has reported yet results for a posteriori dietary patterns using the same FFQ across European countries.

In conclusion, using a single FFQ for all five countries, we were able to identify three unique dietary patterns in this population. Whereas all five countries had a "vegetable pattern" and most countries had a "high meat pattern," most of the differences between countries relied on the last less healthy pattern. The selection of these patterns will allow us to further research associations between dietary patterns based on the populations at hand and several outcomes included in DO-HEALTH, in particular those related to bone, muscle, cardiovascular health, and cognition.

Outlook for DO-HEALTH

The extensive phenotyping of DO-HEALTH participants will allow us to evaluate associations beyond the primary and secondary endpoints including composite scores for several conditions. The last RCT participants were seen for their final 3-year visit in November 2017. Our outlook for this comprehensive dataset is to follow this population in the DO-HEALTH Extension Cohort. This will allow us to study the trajectories of aging and to further evaluate the role of dietary factors, exercise, and vitamin D in several chronic conditions associated with advanced age and to identify prevention strategies to promote healthy aging in Europe.

References

1. Beard JR, Officer AM, Cassels AK. The world report on ageing and health. Gerontologist. 2016;56(Suppl 2):S163–6.
2. Ortman JM, Velkoff VA, Hogan H. An aging nation: the older population in the United States Washington D.C. 2014. Available from: https://www.census.gov/prod/2014pubs/p25-1140.pdf.
3. 2015–2045 scenarios concerning the population development in Switzerland (Szenarien zur Bevölkerungsentwicklung der Schweiz 2015–2045). Swiss Federal Statistical Office, Demography and Migration section. Neuchâtel, Switzerland. 2015.
4. Boucher BJ. The problems of vitamin D insufficiency in older people. Aging Dis. 2012;3(4):313–29.
5. ter Borg S, Verlaan S, Hemsworth J, Mijnarends DM, Schols JM, Luiking YC, et al. Micronutrient intakes and potential inadequacies of community-dwelling older adults: a systematic review. Br J Nutr. 2015;113(8):1195–206.
6. Bouillon R, Bischoff-Ferrari H, Willett W. Vitamin D and health: perspectives from mice and man. J Bone Miner Res. 2008;23(7):974–9.
7. Bischoff-Ferrari HA, Shao A, Dawson-Hughes B, Hathcock J, Giovannucci E, Willett WC. Benefit-risk assessment of vitamin D supplementation. Osteoporos Int. 2010;21(7):1121–32.
8. Chowdhury R, Kunutsor S, Vitezova A, Oliver-Williams C, Chowdhury S, Kiefte-de-Jong JC, et al. Vitamin D and risk of cause specific death: systematic review and meta-analysis of observational cohort and randomised intervention studies. BMJ. 2014;348:g1903.
9. Berridge MJ. Vitamin D deficiency accelerates ageing and age-related diseases: a novel hypothesis. J Physiol. 2017;595(22):6825–36.
10. Bischoff-Ferrari HA, Willett WC, Wong JB, Stuck AE, Staehelin HB, Orav EJ, et al. Prevention of nonvertebral fractures with oral vitamin D and dose dependency: a meta-analysis of randomized controlled trials. Arch Intern Med. 2009;169(6):551–61.
11. Bruyere O, Cavalier E, Reginster JY. Vitamin D and osteosarcopenia: an update from epidemiological studies. Curr Opin Clin Nutr Metab Care. 2017;20(6):498–503.
12. Bischoff-Ferrari HA. Relevance of vitamin D in fall prevention. Geriatr Psychol Neuropsychiatr Vieil. 2017;15(1):e1–7.
13. Rizzoli R, Bischoff-Ferrari H, Dawson-Hughes B, Weaver C. Nutrition and bone health in women after the menopause. Women's Health (Lond Engl). 2014;10(6):599–608.
14. Beaudart C, Buckinx F, Rabenda V, Gillain S, Cavalier E, Slomian J, et al. The effects of vitamin D on skeletal muscle strength, muscle mass, and muscle power: a systematic review and meta-analysis of randomized controlled trials. J Clin Endocrinol Metab. 2014;99(11):4336–45.
15. Bischoff-Ferrari HA, Dawson-Hughes B, Orav EJ, Staehelin HB, Meyer OW, Theiler R, et al. Monthly high-dose vitamin D treatment for the prevention of functional decline: a randomized clinical trial. JAMA Intern Med. 2016;176(2):175–83.
16. Zhao JG, Zeng XT, Wang J, Liu L. Association between calcium or vitamin D supplementation and fracture incidence in community-dwelling older adults: a systematic review and meta-analysis. JAMA. 2017;318(24):2466–82.
17. Holick MF. The vitamin D deficiency pandemic: approaches for diagnosis, treatment and prevention. Rev Endocr Metab Disord. 2017;18(2):153–65.
18. Rejnmark L, Bislev LS, Cashman KD, Eiriksdottir G, Gaksch M, Grubler M, et al. Non-skeletal health effects of vitamin D supplementation: a systematic review on findings from meta-analyses summarizing trial data. PLoS One. 2017;12(7):e0180512.
19. Cianferotti L, Bertoldo F, Bischoff-Ferrari HA, Bruyere O, Cooper C, Cutolo M, et al. Vitamin D supplementation in the prevention and management of major chronic diseases not related to mineral homeostasis in adults: research for evidence and a scientific statement from the European society for clinical and economic aspects of osteoporosis and osteoarthritis (ESCEO). Endocrine. 2017;56(2):245–61.

20. Manson JE, Bassuk SS, Lee IM, Cook NR, Albert MA, Gordon D, et al. The VITamin D and OmegA-3 TriaL (VITAL): rationale and design of a large randomized controlled trial of vitamin D and marine omega-3 fatty acid supplements for the primary prevention of cancer and cardiovascular disease. Contemp Clin Trials. 2012;33(1):159–71.
21. Rautiainen S, Sesso HD, Manson JE. Large-scale randomized clinical trials of bioactives and nutrients in relation to human health and disease prevention—lessons from the VITAL and COSMOS trials. Mol Asp Med. 2017;61:12–7.
22. Scragg R, Stewart AW, Waayer D, Lawes CMM, Toop L, Sluyter J, et al. Effect of monthly high-dose vitamin D supplementation on cardiovascular disease in the vitamin D assessment study: a randomized clinical trial. JAMA Cardiol. 2017;2(6):608–16.
23. Khaw KT, Stewart AW, Waayer D, Lawes CMM, Toop L, Camargo CA Jr, et al. Effect of monthly high-dose vitamin D supplementation on falls and non-vertebral fractures: secondary and post-hoc outcomes from the randomised, double-blind, placebo-controlled ViDA trial. Lancet Diabetes Endocrinol. 2017;5(6):438–47.
24. Chedraui P, Perez-Lopez FR. Nutrition and health during mid-life: searching for solutions and meeting challenges for the aging population. Climacteric. 2013;16(Suppl 1):85–95.
25. Samieri C, Sun Q, Townsend MK, Chiuve SE, Okereke OI, Willett WC, et al. The association between dietary patterns at midlife and health in aging: an observational study. Ann Intern Med. 2013;159(9):584–91.
26. Milte CM, McNaughton SA. Dietary patterns and successful ageing: a systematic review. Eur J Nutr. 2015;55(2):423–50.
27. Malavolta M, Mocchegiani E. Molecular basis of nutrition and aging: a volume in the molecular nutrition series. New York: Elsevier; 2016.
28. Wengreen H, Munger RG, Cutler A, Quach A, Bowles A, Corcoran C, et al. Prospective study of Dietary Approaches to Stop Hypertension- and Mediterranean-style dietary patterns and age-related cognitive change: the Cache County Study on Memory, Health and Aging. Am J Clin Nutr. 2013;98(5):1263–71.
29. Hu FB. Dietary pattern analysis: a new direction in nutritional epidemiology. Curr Opin Lipidol. 2002;13(1):3–9.
30. Jacques PF, Tucker KL. Are dietary patterns useful for understanding the role of diet in chronic disease? Am J Clin Nutr. 2001;73(1):1–2.
31. Newby PK, Tucker KL. Empirically derived eating patterns using factor or cluster analysis: a review. Nutr Rev. 2004;62(5):177–203.
32. Slimani N, Fahey M, Welch AA, Wirfalt E, Stripp C, Bergstrom E, et al. Diversity of dietary patterns observed in the European prospective investigation into Cancer and nutrition (EPIC) project. Public Health Nutr. 2002;5(6b):1311–28.
33. van Staveren WA, de Groot LC, Haveman-Nies A. The SENECA study: potentials and problems in relating diet to survival over 10 years. Public Health Nutr. 2002;5(6a):901–5.
34. Bamia C, Orfanos P, Ferrari P, Overvad K, Hundborg HH, Tjonneland A, et al. Dietary patterns among older Europeans: the EPIC-elderly study. Br J Nutr. 2005;94(1):100–13.
35. Willett W. Nutritional epidemiology. New York: Oxford University Press; 1998.
36. Garcia-Larsen V, Luczynska M, Kowalski ML, Voutilainen H, Ahlstrom M, Haahtela T, et al. Use of a common food frequency questionnaire (FFQ) to assess dietary patterns and their relation to allergy and asthma in Europe: pilot study of the GA2LEN FFQ. Eur J Clin Nutr. 2011;65(6):750–6.
37. Lafranconi A, Birt CA. 'Du bist was du isst': challenges in European nutrition policy. Eur J Pub Health. 2017;27(suppl_4):26–31.
38. Bamia C, Trichopoulos D, Ferrari P, Overvad K, Bjerregaard L, Tjonneland A, et al. Dietary patterns and survival of older Europeans: the EPIC-Elderly Study (European Prospective Investigation into Cancer and Nutrition). Public Health Nutr. 2007;10(6):590–8.

2 Vitamin D and Omega-3 Fatty Acid Trial 2017: Addressing Effects on Muscle and Bone

Meryl S. LeBoff, Catherine M. Donlon, Sharon H. Chou, Nancy Cook, Julie Buring, and JoAnn E. Manson

Rationale

An estimated two million fractures occur each year in the USA, and nine million fractures worldwide are due to osteoporosis [1–3]. Among adults 50 years and older, one out of two women and one out of four men in the USA will suffer an osteoporotic fracture in their remaining lifetime [4]. Hip and other fractures are associated with excess morbidity, mortality, and healthcare expenditures that are projected to reach more than $25.3 billion/year in the USA by 2025 [1, 4, 5]. Primary prevention strategies are needed to reduce the burden of fractures.

Decreased bone density and increased risk of fractures have been associated with low vitamin D levels. Vitamin D deficiency (25-hydroxyvitamin D [25(OH)D] levels <20 ng/ml) is present in 39% of females, 31% of males, and 73% of black adults in North America according to the National Health and Nutrition Examination Survey (NHANES) [6, 7]. More black adults are deficient in vitamin D due to reduced cutaneous vitamin D synthesis and vitamin D intakes [8–13]. In postmenopausal females enrolled in osteoporosis studies and males in the Osteoporotic Fractures in Men Study (MrOS), >50% had 25(OH)D levels <30 ng/ml (75 nmol/L) [14, 15]. Deficient vitamin D levels have also been widely reported among obese adults (due to vitamin D sequestration in fat, increased volume distribution) [16], elders, and those with hip fractures [17–21].

Although vitamin D supplements are widely used to support bone health, systematic reviews and meta-analyses show that there are inconsistent data on the

M. S. LeBoff (✉) · C. M. Donlon · S. H. Chou
Endocrine, Diabetes and Hypertension Division, Brigham and Women's Hospital, Harvard Medical School, Boston, MA, USA
e-mail: MLEBOFF@bwh.harvard.edu

N. Cook · J. Buring · J. E. Manson
Division of Preventative Medicine, Brigham and Women's Hospital, Harvard Medical School, Boston, MA, USA

© Springer Nature Switzerland AG 2019

C. M. Weaver et al. (eds.), *Nutritional Influences on Bone Health*,
https://doi.org/10.1007/978-3-319-98464-3_2

effects of supplemental vitamin D alone on fractures. While the 2011 US Preventive Services Task Force (USPSTF) summary of five RCTs concluded that combined calcium and vitamin D supplementation decreased the risk of fractures by 12% in older adults, vitamin D supplementation *alone* was *not associated* with a reduction in fractures [22]. In a group pooled analysis of seven RCTs from the USA and Europe including 68,500 older adults, the "Vitamin D Individual Patient Analysis of Randomized Trials" (DIPART) found that while vitamin D supplementation alone (400 and 800 IU/day) did not prevent fractures, combined calcium and vitamin D supplementation did reduce hip and total fractures [23] . An updated meta-analysis published in 2016 has also reported beneficial effect of supplemental calcium plus vitamin D on fracture outcomes [24]. In another pooled analysis of 11 RCTs including 31,022 adults (91% females), those assigned to vitamin D had a 7% reduction in non-vertebral fractures, without a significant effect on the risk of hip fractures. However, stratification of the data according to actual intake of vitamin D, rather than supplementation dose, revealed that those in the highest quartile of total, actual vitamin D intake (median 800 IU/day) had a reduction in hip fracture risk by 30% and non-vertebral fracture by 14% [25]. As a result of these conflicting results, a 2014 systematic review for the Agency for Healthcare Research and Quality (AHRQ) concluded that effects of supplemental vitamin D on fracture reduction are inconsistent [26]. Lastly, the extensive review by the Institute of Medicine (IOM) committee emphasized the need for more research from large randomized clinical trials to "test the effects of vitamin D on skeletal and non-skeletal outcomes" and "identify the threshold effects and possible adverse effects where present" [27].

Several new trials are determining the effects of supplemental vitamin D in women and men on a variety of outcomes. The Vitamin D Assessment (ViDA) Study in New Zealand is a double-blind RCT among 5108 healthy men and women aged 50–84 years. Participants were given a monthly bolus dose of 100,000 IU of vitamin D_3 for a mean treatment duration of 3.4 years; it was recently reported that there was no effect on non-vertebral fractures, falls, or cardiovascular disease [28, 29]. Ongoing studies include a RCT, D-Health in Australia, which is studying the effects of monthly bolus doses of 60,000 IU of vitamin D_3 in participants aged 50–84 years with a mean treatment interval of 3.4 years on all-cause mortality and total cancer incidence; however, no baseline blood samples were collected in D-Health [30]. The Vitamin D and Longevity (VIDAL) Trial in the UK is a randomized feasibility study also giving monthly bolus doses of 100,000 IU of vitamin D_3 in 1615 participants aged 64–85 years for a duration of 2 years [31]. DO-Health, a RCT among 2157 participants aged 70 years and older in 7 European cities, is studying the effects of daily supplemental vitamin D_3 (2000 IU) and/or omega-3 fatty acids and/or a home exercise program on a variety of variables including risk of incident non-vertebral fractures, functional decline, and falls for 3 years with a posttreatment follow-up [32]. A recent study in Nebraska among 2303 postmenopausal women studied effects of daily vitamin D_3 (2000 IU) plus calcium (1500 mg) on cancer outcomes and found that supplementation did not lower risk of all-type cancer at 4 years [33]. Most of these new studies used bolus dosing, small sample sizes, or vitamin D plus calcium or had a short duration of treatment and follow-up. Therefore, the VITAL study will provide important new information from a large ancillary study to the large Vitamin D and Omega-3 Fatty Acids Trial (VITAL) in the USA testing whether supplemental vitamin D reduces the risk of incident fractures and/or improves bone and musculoskeletal health.

Design

The *VIT*amin D and Omeg*A*-3 Tria*L* (*VITAL*) is a population-based, double-blind, placebo-controlled primary prevention study among men 50 years of age or older and women 55 years of age or older from 50 states in the USA investigating whether daily supplemental vitamin D_3 (cholecalciferol, 2000 IU) and/or marine omega-3 fatty acids (Omacor® fish oil, a 1 g/day capsule containing EPA [465 mg] + DHA [375 mg]) reduce the risk for developing cancer, heart disease, or stroke in people who do not have a prior history of these illnesses. VITAL's 2 × 2 factorial design randomized participants equally into four intervention groups for a mean treatment length of 5 years: vitamin D and omega-3 fatty acids, vitamin D and placebo, omega-3 fatty acids and placebo, or double placebo.

Eligible participants at study entry had no history of cancer (except non-melanoma skin cancer), myocardial infarction (MI), stroke, transient ischemic attack (TIA), coronary artery bypass graft (CABG), or percutaneous coronary intervention (PCI). Enrollment in VITAL was contingent upon participants: (a) limiting consumption of supplemental vitamin D and calcium to no more than 800 IU/day and 1200 mg/day, respectively, from all sources combined and (b) forgoing use of supplemental fish oil during the trial. Persons were excluded from the study if they had renal failure or dialysis, history of hypercalcemia, hypo- or hyperparathyroidism, severe liver disease (cirrhosis), sarcoidosis or other granulomatous diseases such as active chronic tuberculosis or Wegener's granulomatosis, allergy to soy (in the vitamin D placebo pill) or fish, or other serious illness that would preclude participation. Individuals who met these criteria and demonstrated good pill-taking compliance (taking ≥2/3 of the study pills during the 3-month run-in phase) were randomized into the trial. Among the approximately 40,000 individuals who entered the run-in phase, 25,874 men and women were enrolled between November 2011 and March 2014. A total of 16,953 blood samples were collected at baseline, and an additional ~6000 blood samples will be collected at follow-up. The intervention phase closes on December 31, 2017, and will be followed by an additional 2 years of post-intervention follow-up.

Quality Control

VITAL is using Centers for Disease Control and Prevention (CDC) reference material for quality control (QC), going beyond routine QC procedures. VITAL is also working closely with the CDC to evaluate and calibrate the assays for serum 25(OH)D at Quest Diagnostics (liquid chromatography-tandem mass spectrometry [LC-MS/MS]) and ABBOTT Atherotech Diagnostics (chemiluminescent microparticle immunoassay [CMIA]).

Baseline Characteristics of Parent VITAL Study

The parent VITAL study exceeded the total randomization goal of 20,000 participants by enrolling a total of 25,874 participants. The projected goal for minority enrollment was also surpassed as 5107 (20.2%) African Americans were enrolled into the trial. Among the final cohort enrolled in the parent VITAL study, 38.1% are aged 50–64 years, 49.1% are aged 65–74 years, and 12.8% of participants were aged 75+ at baseline. The mean age at baseline for the overall VITAL cohort was 67.1 ± 7.1 years. VITAL has a broad geographic distribution, with participants enrolled from all 50 states; 27.7% of participants are from the Northeast, 21.4% are from the Midwest region, 22.9% are from the West/Southwest/Mountain region which includes Hawaii and Alaska, and 28.0% are from the Southeast including Puerto Rico [34]. Additional baseline characteristics in the overall VITAL cohort are presented in Table 2.1 [34].

VITAL Bone Health

To comprehensively assess effects of supplemental vitamin D and/or omega-3 fatty acids on bone in terms of fracture risk and bone health outcomes, two concurrent and complementary VITAL bone health ancillary studies are ongoing: *VITAL: Effects on Fractures* and *VITAL: Effects on Bone Structure and Architecture*. There are several mechanisms through which supplemental vitamin D may reduce fracture risk, increase bone mass, and benefit physical performance. These mechanisms include increasing intestinal calcium absorption, improving bone mineralization, decreasing parathyroid hormone (PTH) levels, reducing bone resorption, and enhancing bone structure and architecture and muscle size and/or function (Fig. 2.1)

Table 2.1 Baseline characteristics of overall VITAL cohort [34]

Characteristic	Percent/Mean
Female, %	50.6%
Mean age ± SD, years	67.1 ± 7.1
Age ≥65, %	61.9%
African American, %	20.2%
Current smoker, %	7.2%
Mean body mass index (BMI) ± SD, kg/m^2	28.1 ± 5.7
Obesity (BMI ≥30 kg/m^2), %	28.8%
History of diabetes, %	13.2%
History of hypertension, %	53.6%
Current use of cholesterol-lowering medication, %	37.5%
Current use of multivitamins, %	44.8%
Current use of supplemental vitamin D (≤800 IU/day), %	42.6%
Current use of supplemental calcium (≤1200 mg/day), %	26.4%

[35, 36]. The vitamin D receptor (VDR) is also expressed in muscle cells and is necessary for muscle contractility [37–40]. Vitamin D has also been shown to increase the number and size of type II muscle fibers [41–43]. Additional studies are needed to fully understand the mechanisms through which high doses of daily supplemental vitamin D may affect musculoskeletal health in women and men.

VITAL: Effects on Fractures

Among the overall VITAL cohort of 25,874 participants across the USA, *VITAL: Effects on Fractures* is being conducted to evaluate the effects of supplemental vitamin D and/or omega-3 fatty acids on fracture outcomes. Participants were asked to self-report incident fractures. When a fracture event is self-reported, participants approve the release of medical records, and fractures are adjudicated by study investigators who are blinded to treatment. Hip and pelvic fractures are further adjudicated by review with a musculoskeletal radiologist using X-ray, CT, and MR images. Fractures are either confirmed, disconfirmed (determined not to be a fracture), or unconfirmed (due to lack of/insufficient medical records or assessment by a healthcare provider). Preliminary data of the ongoing VITAL: Effects on Fractures study show, as expected, participants who reported a fracture were more likely to be female, older, and Caucasian, have lower BMI, and, if female, be not currently using hormone replacement therapy. Thus far, the percentage of self-reported fractures that have been confirmed is consistent with prior studies performed in the Women's Health Initiative (WHI) and the Study of Osteoporotic Fractures (SOF) [44, 45]. Verification with data from Centers for Medicare and Medicaid Services (CMS) will help verify unconfirmed fractures and unreported fractures. Overall, the discrepancies in self-reported fractures support the rigorous adjudication of fracture outcomes for clinical studies.

VITAL: Effects on Bone Structure and Architecture

In the second ancillary study titled *VITAL: Effects on Bone Structure and Architecture*, the mechanisms through which supplemental vitamin D and/or omega-3 fatty acids affect musculoskeletal health outcomes are being evaluated in a subcohort of 771 VITAL participants including by dual-energy X-ray absorptiometry (DXA) and peripheral quantitative computed tomography (pQCT) [35]. Participants in the VITAL bone health subcohort are from the New England area and are part of a subgroup of VITAL participants that completed in-person visits at the Harvard Catalyst Clinical and Translational Science Center (CTSC) in Boston. Participants in this subgroup underwent detailed phenotyping (weight, height, and other anthropomorphic measurements), bone health and body composition assessments, as well as physical performance tests at baseline and 2-years post-randomization. High-resolution pQCT (HR-pQCT) was carried out in year 2 post-randomization in a subgroup of participants.

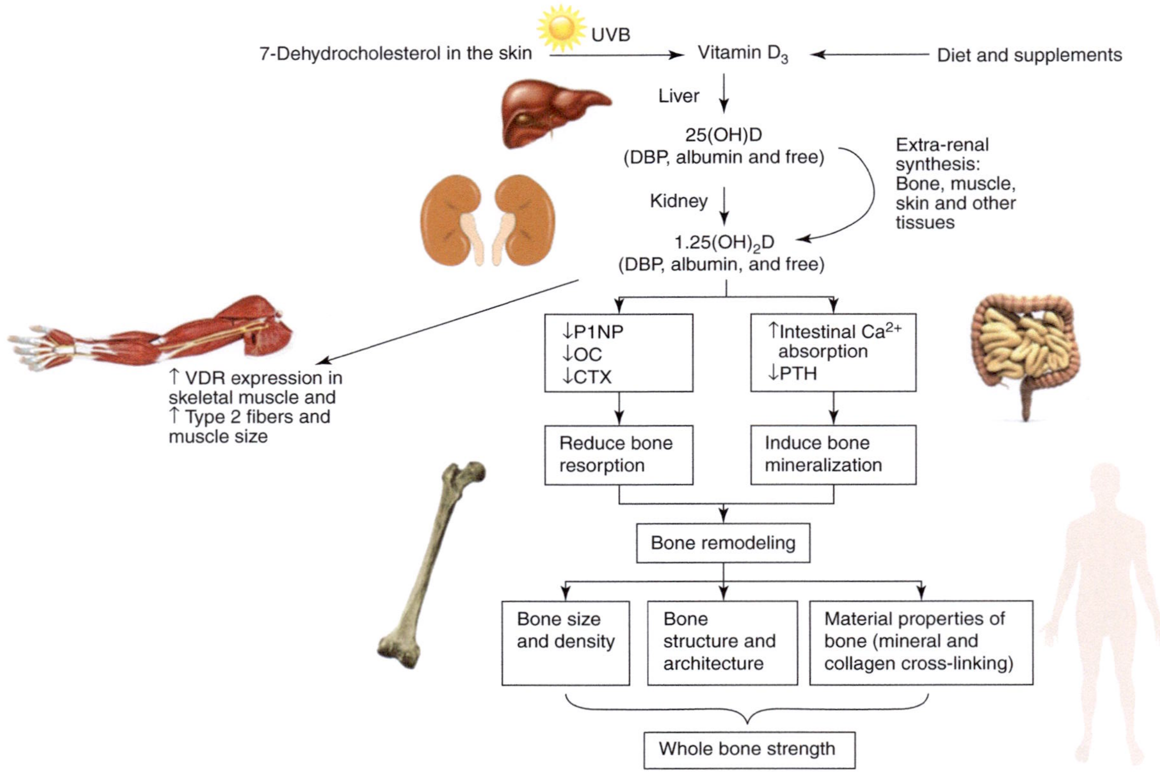

Fig. 2.1 Mechanisms through which high-dose vitamin D may benefit musculoskeletal health. Adapted from "VITAL-Bone Health: Rationale and design of two ancillary studies evaluating the effects of vitamin D and/or omega-3 fatty acid supplements on incident fractures and bone health outcomes in the VITamin D and OmegA-3 TriaL," by M.S. LeBoff et al., 2015, *Contemp Clin Trials, 41*, p. 260

Methods: Bone and Body Composition Imaging Technologies and Physical Performance Tests

A variety of bone imaging technologies are used in the VITAL bone health examinations. DXA measures spine, hip, and total body bone mineral density (BMD) as well as body composition and trabecular bone score (TBS) [35]. TBS predicts fractures risk independent of BMD and can be used to in addition to BMD and the fracture risk assessment tool (FRAX) to improve clinical care. TBS scores decrease with advancing age and have been shown to identify 66–70% of women who had fragility fractures [46, 47]. TBS captures a larger portion of diabetes and obesity-associated fracture risk than does BMD alone [48]. TBS scores are lower in secondary causes of osteoporosis and increase in response to some bone active medications over several years [49–52].

DXA can also distinguish fat and lean tissue and provide measurements of total adiposity including fat mass index (FMI; fat mass/height^2) and total percent body fat as well as regional obesity including visceral adipose tissue (VAT). VAT thresholds (normal 10–100) are associated with metabolic risk factors for coronary heart disease. Additional regional adiposity measurements include truncal and regional fat distribution and muscle mass including lean mass index (LMI; lean mass/height^2) and appendicular (limb) LMI (appendicular lean mass/height^2). Loss of muscle mass, strength, and function is a characteristic of sarcopenia. Recently, the Foundation for the National Institutes of Health (FNIH) Biomarkers Consortium recommended the use of appendicular lean mass adjusted for BMI (ALM/BMI) to determine low lean mass, with ALM/BMI cut points of <0.789 for men and <0.512 for women [53]. The FNIH also uses grip strength cut points of <26 kg for men and <16 kg for women to determine muscle weakness.

Grip strength by hand dynamometer [54, 55] and the short physical performance battery (SPPB) were performed. The SPPB is a composite test consisting of normal walking speed over 6 m; standing balance for three stances including tandem, semi-tandem, and side by side for 10 s each; and timed five repeated chair stands [56, 57]. The timed-up and go (TUG) test was also performed which consists of standing up from a chair, walking 3 m, turning around, and sitting back in the chair [58, 59].

We predict that high-dose supplemental vitamin D will result in (a) reduced risk of total, hip, and non-vertebral fractures; (b) small increases or reduced loss of areal bone mass density (aBMD) in the spine, hip, and total body; (c) reduced bone turnover as assessed by markers of bone resorption (c-telopeptide [CTX]) and formation (amino-terminal propeptide of type 1 collagen [P1NP]); (d) improved vBMD, cortical thickness, and trabecular number; and (e) beneficial effects on body composition and physical function.

Baseline Characteristics of VITAL Bone Health Subcohort

Baseline characteristics were evenly distributed among the four randomized treatment groups. This suggests that unidentified confounders will be similarly distributed. There were 411 men and 360 women who had a mean age of 63.8 ± 6.1 years.

Overall, 57.7% of participants were not taking supplemental vitamin D (≤800 IU/day) at baseline. The mean T-scores at the spine, total hip, and whole body were classified as normal, while the mean T-score at the femoral neck was osteopenic. According to TBS, 35.1% of participants had degraded or partially degraded bone microarchitecture [60]. The mean BMI was 28.31 ± 5.14 kg/m^2; 30% of participants were obese according to BMI criteria, and 38% were obese according to FMI criteria.

Using the FNIH sarcopenia criteria, low muscle mass by ALM/BMI was present in 25.3% of men and 25.6% of women [53]. Muscle weakness, by grip strength, was present in 5.2% of men and 3.7% of women. Low and intermediate physical performance by SPPB score <9 was present in 5.7% of participants [61].

Sex Differences in Baseline Characteristics of VITAL Bone Health Subcohort

There were sex differences among several of the baseline characteristics. Because women were slightly older than men due to enrollment criteria (64.4 vs. 63.3 years), the following variables were adjusted for age. All race, ethnicities, education, and income levels were similarly distributed between men and women except that there were more men who had incomes >$120,000 (35.1% vs. 23.3%). Men were more likely than women to have history of hypertension (50.43% vs. 41.46%) and diabetes (12.41% vs. 7.61%) and use multivitamins (48.20% vs. 38.86%). Women were more likely to use supplemental calcium and consume more servings of milk and vitamin D-fortified foods than men, possibly due to reverse causation.

As expected, women had lower BMD and T-scores at all sites (spine, total hip, femoral neck, and whole body) than men. Women also had lower mean TBS than men (1.31 vs. 1.34). Using FRAX, women had higher major osteoporotic fracture risk than men (10.03 vs. 6.55), but hip FRAX scores were similar between the sexes. More women than men also had a history of a fragility fracture (12.06% vs. 5.30%).

Mean BMI was similar between men and women, but women had a greater body fat percentage (42.4% vs. 31.1%) and a greater FMI (11.98 kg/m^2 vs. 8.79 kg/m^2), as expected. Men had greater VAT area and greater lean mass than women according to LMI, ALM, ALMI, and ALM/BMI.

Physical performance tests were similar between the sexes; however, men had quicker fast walking times than women (1.85 m/s vs. 1.75 m/s), and women had faster TUG test times than men (7.88 s vs. 8.23 s).

Other Hypotheses

Other questions of interest include testing whether these outcomes vary according to BMI, age, and/or race/ethnicity, how adiposity influences vitamin D needs in the population [7], and whether high-dose supplemental vitamin D improves physical performance measures. We are interested in learning the relationship between physical performance, sarcopenia, falls, and bone health/fractures in VITAL as well. Additional assessments will be carried out to investigate the relationship between these outcomes and omega-3 fatty acids. The VITAL study will also make it possible to determine whether supplemental vitamin D and/or omega-3 fatty acids confer other health benefits. There are 18 VITAL ancillary studies, funded by the National Institutes of Health, and 1, funded by the American Heart Association, investigating whether these supplements provide additional benefits such as lowering the risk for diabetes, high blood pressure, asthma, depression, chronic knee pain symptoms, physical disability and falls, autoimmune conditions, and impaired kidney function, among other health conditions. Thus, it will also be possible in VITAL to determine whether there are any associations between bone and a number of medical conditions beyond cancer and cardiovascular health and whether these medical conditions affect fracture risk among older adults. Thus, the VITAL database is an invaluable resource to investigate relationships between vitamin D and omega-3 fatty acids and many outcomes.

Acknowledgments *Endocrinology, Diabetes and Hypertension Division*

Cindy Yu, CBDT (ISCD); Amy Yue, B.A.; Lisa Gao, B.S.; Mary Castro, B.A., CBDT (ISCD).

Preventive Medicine

Joseph Walter; Vadim Bubes, PhD; Gregory Kotler, PhD

Radiology BWH

Bharti Khurana, M.D.

Grant Support

This research is supported by grant R01 AR060574 (PI: LeBoff, MS) and R01 AR59775 (PI: LeBoff, MS) from the National Institute of Arthritis and Musculoskeletal and Skin Diseases (NIAMS/NIH). Its contents are solely the responsibility of the authors and do not necessarily represent the official view of the NIAMS or NIH. The parent VITAL trial is primarily sponsored by grants U01 CA138962 (PI: Manson, JE) and R01 CA138962 (PI: Manson, JE) which include support from the National Cancer Institute; National Heart, Lung, and Blood Institute; Office of Dietary Supplements; National Institute of Neurological Disorders and Stroke; and National Center for Complementary and Integrative Health.

References

1. Burge R, Dawson-Hughes B, Solomon DH, Wong JB, King A, Tosteson A. Incidence and economic burden of osteoporosis-related fractures in the United States, 2005–2025. J Bone Miner Res. 2007;22(3):465–75.
2. Office of the Surgeon General. Bone health and osteoporosis: a report of the Surgeon General. Rockville: U.S. Dept. of Health and Human Services, Public Health Service Office of the Surgeon General; 2004.
3. Johnell O, Kanis JA. An estimate of the worldwide prevalence and disability associated with osteoporotic fractures. Osteoporos Int. 2006;17(12):1726–33. https://doi.org/10.1007/s00198-006-0172-4.
4. Cosman F, de Beur SJ, LeBoff MS, Lewiecki EM, Tanner B, Randall S, Lindsay R. Clinician's guide to prevention and treatment of osteoporosis. Osteoporos Int. 2014;25(10):2359–81. https://doi.org/10.1007/s00198-014-2794-2.
5. Melton LJ 3rd, Eddy DM, Johnston CC Jr. Screening for osteoporosis. Ann Intern Med. 1990;112(7):516–28.

6. Looker AC, Dawson-Hughes B, Tosteson AN, Johansson H, Kanis JA, Melton LJ 3rd. Hip fracture risk in older US adults by treatment eligibility status based on new National Osteoporosis Foundation guidance. Osteoporos Int. 2011;22(2):541–9. https://doi.org/10.1007/s00198-010-1288-0.
7. Looker AC, Johnson CL, Lacher DA, Pfeiffer CM, Schleicher RL, Sempos CT. Vitamin D status: United States, 2001–2006. NCHS Data Brief. 2011;59(59):1–8.
8. Harris SS. Vitamin D and African Americans. J Nutr. 2006;136(4):1126–9.
9. Moore CE, Murphy MM, Holick MF. Vitamin D intakes by children and adults in the United States differ among ethnic groups. J Nutr. 2005;135(10):2478–85.
10. Powe CE, Evans MK, Wenger J, Zonderman AB, Berg AH, Nalls M, Tamez H, Zhang D, Bhan I, Karumanchi SA, Powe NR, Thadhani R. Vitamin D-binding protein and vitamin D status of black Americans and white Americans. N Engl J Med. 2013;369(21):1991–2000. https://doi.org/10.1056/NEJMoa1306357.
11. Aloia J, Mikhail M, Dhaliwal R, Shieh A, Usera G, Stolberg A, Ragolia L, Islam S. Free 25(OH)D and the vitamin D paradox in African Americans. J Clin Endocrinol Metab. 2015;100(9):3356–63. https://doi.org/10.1210/JC.2015-2066.
12. Aloia J, Dhaliwal R, Mikhail M, Shieh A, Stolberg A, Ragolia L, Fazzari M, Abrams SA. Free 25(OH)D and calcium absorption, PTH, and markers of bone turnover. J Clin Endocrinol Metab. 2015;100(11):4140–5. https://doi.org/10.1210/jc.2015-2548.
13. Gallagher CJ, Jindal PS, Smith LM. Vitamin D supplementation in young Caucasian and African American women. J Bone Miner Res. 2013;29(1):173–81. https://doi.org/10.1002/jbmr.2010.
14. Holick MF, Siris ES, Binkley N, Beard MK, Khan A, Katzer JT, Petruschke RA, Chen E, de Papp AE. Prevalence of vitamin D inadequacy among postmenopausal north American women receiving osteoporosis therapy. J Clin Endocrinol Metab. 2005;90(6):3215–24.
15. Orwoll E, Nielson CM, Marshall LM, Lambert L, Holton KF, Hoffman AR, Barrett-Connor E, Shikany JM, Dam T, Cauley JA. Vitamin D deficiency in older men. J Clin Endocrinol Metab. 2009;94(4):1214–22. https://doi.org/10.1210/jc.2008-1784.
16. Wortsman J, Matsuoka LY, Chen TC, Lu Z, Holick MF. Decreased bioavailability of vitamin D in obesity. Am J Clin Nutr. 2000;72(3):690–3.
17. LeBoff MS, Kohlmeier L, Hurwitz S, Franklin J, Wright J, Glowacki J. Occult vitamin D deficiency in postmenopausal US women with acute hip fracture. JAMA. 1999;281(16):1505–11.
18. Chapuy MC, Preziosi P, Maamer M, Arnaud S, Galan P, Hercberg S, Meunier PJ. Prevalence of vitamin D insufficiency in an adult normal population. Osteoporos Int. 1997;7(5):439–43.
19. Chapuy MC, Pamphile R, Paris E, Kempf C, Schlichting M, Arnaud S, Garnero P, Meunier PJ. Combined calcium and vitamin D3 supplementation in elderly women: confirmation of reversal of secondary hyperparathyroidism and hip fracture risk: the Decalyos II study. Osteoporos Int. 2002;13(3):257–64.
20. Leboff MS, Hawkes WG, Glowacki J, Yu-Yahiro J, Hurwitz S, Magaziner J. Vitamin D-deficiency and post-fracture changes in lower extremity function and falls in women with hip fractures. Osteoporos Int. 2008;19(9):1283–90.
21. Bischoff-Ferrari HA, Dawson-Hughes B, Platz A, Orav EJ, Stahelin HB, Willett WC, Can U, Egli A, Mueller NJ, Looser S, Bretscher B, Minder E, Vergopoulos A, Theiler R. Effect of high-dosage cholecalciferol and extended physiotherapy on complications after hip fracture: a randomized controlled trial. Arch Intern Med. 2010;170(9):813–20. https://doi.org/10.1001/archinternmed.2010.67.
22. Chung M, Lee J, Terasawa T, Lau J, Trikalinos TA. Vitamin D with or without calcium supplementation for prevention of cancer and fractures: an updated meta-analysis for the U.S. preventive services task force. Ann Intern Med. 2011;155(12):827–38. https://doi.org/10.7326/0003-4819-155-12-201112200-00005.
23. DIPART. Patient level pooled analysis of 68 500 patients from seven major vitamin D fracture trials in US and Europe. BMJ. 2010;340:b5463. https://doi.org/10.1136/bmj.b5463.
24. Weaver CM, Alexander DD, Boushey CJ, Dawson-Hughes B, Lappe JM, LeBoff MS, Liu S, Looker AC, Wallace TC, Wang DD. Calcium plus vitamin D supplementation and risk of

fractures: an updated meta-analysis from the National Osteoporosis Foundation. Osteoporos Int. 2016;27(1):367–76. https://doi.org/10.1007/s00198-015-3386-5.

25. Bischoff-Ferrari HA, Willett WC, Orav EJ, Lips P, Meunier PJ, Lyons RA, Flicker L, Wark J, Jackson RD, Cauley JA, Meyer HE, Pfeifer M, Sanders KM, Stahelin HB, Theiler R, Dawson-Hughes B. A pooled analysis of vitamin D dose requirements for fracture prevention. N Engl J Med. 2012;367(1):40–9. https://doi.org/10.1056/NEJMoa1109617.
26. Newberry S, Chung M, Shekelle P, Booth MS, Liu J, Maher A, Motala A, Cui M, Perry T, Shanman R, Balk E. Vitamin D and calcium: a systematic review of health outcomes (update). Evidence report/technology assessment. Rockville: Agency for Healthcare Research and Quality; 2014.
27. Ross AC, Manson JE, Abrams SA, Aloia JF, Brannon PM, Clinton SK, Durazo-Arvizu RA, Gallagher JC, Gallo RL, Jones G, Kovacs CS, Mayne ST, Rosen CJ, Shapses SA. The 2011 dietary reference intakes for calcium and vitamin D: what dietetics practitioners need to know. J Am Diet Assoc. 2011;111(4):524–7. https://doi.org/10.1016/j.jada.2011.01.004.
28. Scragg R, Stewart AW, Waayer D, et al. Effect of monthly high-dose vitamin D supplementation on cardiovascular disease in the vitamin D assessment study: a randomized clinical trial. JAMA Cardiol. 2017;2(6):608–16. https://doi.org/10.1001/jamacardio.2017.0175.
29. Khaw KT, Stewart AW, Waayer D, Lawes CMM, Toop L, Camargo CA Jr, Scragg R. Effect of monthly high-dose vitamin D supplementation on falls and non-vertebral fractures: secondary and post-hoc outcomes from the randomised, double-blind, placebo-controlled ViDA trial. Lancet Diabetes Endocrinol. 2017;5(6):438–47. https://doi.org/10.1016/s2213-8587(17)30103-1.
30. Neale RE, Armstrong BK, Baxter C, Duarte Romero B, Ebeling P, English DR, Kimlin MG, McLeod DS, RL OC, van der Pols JC, Venn AJ, Webb PM, Whiteman DC, Wockner L. The D-health trial: a randomized trial of vitamin D for prevention of mortality and cancer. Contemp Clin Trials. 2016;48:83–90. https://doi.org/10.1016/j.cct.2016.04.005.
31. Vitamin D and Longevity (VIDAL) Trial. vidal.lshtm.ac.uk/home/: London School of Hygiene & Tropical Medicine. 2017. [cited 2017].
32. DO-HEALTH Project: Vitamin D3- Omega3- Home Exercise HeALTHy Aging and Longevity Trial. do-health.edu/wordpress/: Bischoff, H. A. 2017. [cited 2017].
33. Lappe J, Watson P, Travers-Gustafson D, et al. Effect of vitamin D and calcium supplementation on cancer incidence in older women: a randomized clinical trial. JAMA. 2017;317(12):1234–43. https://doi.org/10.1001/jama.2017.2115.
34. Bassuk SS, Manson JE, Lee IM, Cook NR, Christen WG, Bubes VY, Gordon DS, Copeland T, Friedenberg G, D'Agostino DM, Ridge CY, MacFadyen JG, Kalan K, Buring JE. Baseline characteristics of participants in the VITamin D and OmegA-3 TriaL (VITAL). Contemp Clin Trials. 2016;47:235–43. https://doi.org/10.1016/j.cct.2015.12.022.
35. LeBoff MS, Yue AY, Copeland T, Cook NR, Buring JE, Manson JE. VITAL-bone health: rationale and design of two ancillary studies evaluating the effects of vitamin D and/or omega-3 fatty acid supplements on incident fractures and bone health outcomes in the VITamin D and OmegA-3 TriaL (VITAL). Contemp Clin Trials. 2015;41C:259–68. https://doi.org/10.1016/j.cct.2015.01.007.
36. Rejnmark L. Effects of vitamin D on muscle function and performance: a review of evidence from randomized controlled trials. Ther Adv Chronic Dis. 2011;2(1):25–37. https://doi.org/10.1177/2040622310381934.
37. Marcinkowska E. A run for a membrane vitamin D receptor. Biol Signals Recept. 2001;10(6):341–9.
38. Bellido T, Boland R. Effects of 1,25-dihydroxy-vitamin D3 on phosphate accumulation by myoblasts. Horm Metab Res. 1991;23(3):113–6.
39. Rodman JS, Baker T. Changes in the kinetics of muscle contraction in vitamin D-depleted rats. Kidney Int. 1978;13(3):189–93.
40. Bischoff-Ferrari HA, Borchers M, Gudat F, Durmuller U, Stahelin HB, Dick W. Vitamin D receptor expression in human muscle tissue decreases with age. J Bone Miner Res. 2004;19(2):265–9. https://doi.org/10.1359/jbmr.2004.19.2.265.

41. Sato Y, Iwamoto J, Kanoko T, Satoh K. Low-dose vitamin D prevents muscular atrophy and reduces falls and hip fractures in women after stroke: a randomized controlled trial. Cerebrovasc Dis. 2005;20(3):187–92. https://doi.org/10.1159/000087203.
42. Boland R. Role of vitamin D in skeletal muscle function. Endocr Rev. 1986;7(4):434–48. https://doi.org/10.1210/edrv-7-4-434.
43. Sorensen OH, Lund B, Saltin B, Andersen RB, Hjorth L, Melsen F, Mosekilde L. Myopathy in bone loss of ageing: improvement by treatment with 1 alpha-hydroxycholecalciferol and calcium. Clin Sci (Lond). 1979;56(2):157–61.
44. Chen Z, Kooperberg C, Pettinger MB, Bassford T, Cauley JA, LaCroix AZ, Lewis CE, Kipersztok S, Borne C, Jackson RD. Validity of self-report for fractures among a multiethnic cohort of postmenopausal women: results from the Women's Health Initiative observational study and clinical trials. Menopause. 2004;11(3):264–74.
45. Nevitt MC, Cummings SR, Browner WS, Seeley DG, Cauley JA, Vogt TM, Black DM. The accuracy of self-report of fractures in elderly women: evidence from a prospective study. Am J Epidemiol. 1992;135(5):490–9.
46. Krueger D, Fidler E, Libber J, Aubry-Rozier B, Hans D, Binkley N. Spine trabecular bone score subsequent to bone mineral density improves fracture discrimination in women. J Clin Densitom. 2013;17(1):60–5. https://doi.org/10.1016/j.jocd.2013.05.001.
47. Hans D, Barthe N, Boutroy S, Pothuaud L, Winzenrieth R, Krieg MA. Correlations between trabecular bone score, measured using anteroposterior dual-energy X-ray absorptiometry acquisition, and 3-dimensional parameters of bone microarchitecture: an experimental study on human cadaver vertebrae. J Clin Densitom. 2011;14(3):302–12. https://doi.org/10.1016/j.jocd.2011.05.005.
48. Roux JP, Wegrzyn J, Boutroy S, Bouxsein ML, Hans D, Chapurlat R. The predictive value of trabecular bone score (TBS) on whole lumbar vertebrae mechanics: an ex vivo study. Osteoporos Int. 2013;24(9):2455–60. https://doi.org/10.1007/s00198-013-2316-7.
49. Popp AW, Guler S, Lamy O, Senn C, Buffat H, Perrelet R, Hans D, Lippuner K. Effects of zoledronate versus placebo on spine bone mineral density and microarchitecture assessed by the trabecular bone score in postmenopausal women with osteoporosis: a three-year study. J Bone Miner Res. 2013;28(3):449–54. https://doi.org/10.1002/jbmr.1775.
50. Silva BC, Leslie WD, Resch H, Lamy O, Lesnyak O, Binkley N, McCloskey EV, Kanis JA, Bilezikian JP. Trabecular bone score: a noninvasive analytical method based upon the DXA image. J Bone Miner Res. 2014;29(3):518–30. https://doi.org/10.1002/jbmr.2176.
51. Krieg MA, Aubry-Rozier B, Hans D, Leslie WD. Effects of anti-resorptive agents on trabecular bone score (TBS) in older women. Osteoporos Int. 2013;24(3):1073–8. https://doi.org/10.1007/s00198-012-2155-y.
52. Kalder M, Hans D, Kyvernitakis I, Lamy O, Bauer M, Hadji P. Effects of exemestane and tamoxifen treatment on bone texture analysis assessed by TBS in comparison with bone mineral density assessed by DXA in women with breast cancer. J Clin Densitom. 2013;17(1):66–71. https://doi.org/10.1016/j.jocd.2013.03.003.
53. Studenski SA, Peters KW, Alley DE, Cawthon PM, McLean RR, Harris TB, Ferrucci L, Guralnik JM, Fragala MS, Kenny AM, Kiel DP, Kritchevsky SB, Shardell MD, Dam TT, Vassileva MT. The FNIH sarcopenia project: rationale, study description, conference recommendations and final estimates. J Gerontol A Biol Sci Med Sci. 2014;69(5):547–58. https://doi.org/10.1093/gerona/glu010.
54. Marino M, Gleim GW. Muscle strength and fiber typing. Clin Sports Med. 1984;3(1):85–100.
55. Ashford RF, Nagelburg S, Adkins R. Sensitivity of the jamar dynamometer in detecting submaximal grip effort. J Hand Surg. 1996;21(3):402–5. https://doi.org/10.1016/S0363-5023(96)80352-2.
56. Guralnik JM, Ferrucci L, Pieper CF, Leveille SG, Markides KS, Ostir GV, Studenski S, Berkman LF, Wallace RB. Lower extremity function and subsequent disability: consistency across studies, predictive models, and value of gait speed alone compared with the short physical performance battery. J Gerontol A Biol Sci Med Sci. 2000;55(4):M221–31.

57. Guralnik JM, Ferrucci L, Simonsick EM, Salive ME, Wallace RB. Lower-extremity function in persons over the age of 70 years as a predictor of subsequent disability. N Engl J Med. 1995;332(9):556–61. https://doi.org/10.1056/nejm199503023320902.
58. Bischoff HA, Sthelin HB, Monsch AU, Iversen MD, Weyh A, von Dechend M, Akos R, Conzelmann M, Dick W, Theiler R. Identifying a cutoff point for normal mobility: a comparison of the timed up and go test in community-dwelling and institutionalised elderly women. Age Ageing. 2003;32(3):315–20. https://doi.org/10.1093/ageing/32.3.315.
59. The timed up and go (TUG) test. www.cdc.gov/steadi/materials/html. Centers for Disease Control and Prevention. 2015. [updated 3/24/2017; cited 2017 9/14/2017]. Available from: www.cdc.gov/steadi/pdf/tug_test-a.pdf.
60. Hans D, Goertzen AL, Krieg MA, Leslie WD. Bone microarchitecture assessed by TBS predicts osteoporotic fractures independent of bone density: the Manitoba study. J Bone Miner Res. 2011;26(11):2762–9. https://doi.org/10.1002/jbmr.499.
61. da Camara SM, Alvarado BE, Guralnik JM, Guerra RO, Maciel AC. Using the short physical performance battery to screen for frailty in young-old adults with distinct socioeconomic conditions. Geriatr Gerontol Int. 2013;13(2):421–8. https://doi.org/10.1111/j.1447-0594.2012.00920.x.

Vitamin D Among Children in Asia

3

"What children get at age 3 determine who they are at 80"

Tsz Ping Lam, Benjamin Hon Kei Yip, Wayne Y. W. Lee, Nelson Leung Sang Tang, Kwong Man Lee, Alec Lik Hang Hung, Bobby Kin Wah Ng, and Jack Chun Yiu Cheng

Introduction

A popular Chinese proverb says "What children get at age 3 determine who they are at 80." The point of essence lies on the belief that childhood is the prime time to lay the foundation for achieving physical, social, and mental well-being as the child grows and matures into adulthood. Notably bone health is no exception. During the 4 years surrounding the peak in bone accretion, 39% of total body bone mineral is acquired; by 4 years following the peak, 95% of adult bone mass has been achieved thus leading to peak bone mass that is key for determining bone health and osteoporosis in late adulthood [1, 2]. From prevention point of view, osteoporosis is therefore not only a geriatric but also a pediatric problem. Putting aside the potential sequela of osteoporosis in late adulthood, the traditional view remains that for a child who is otherwise "healthy," suboptimal bone health will not lead to immediate ailments. In the absence of physical symptoms, bone health and other important lifestyle

T. P. Lam (✉) · W. Y. W. Lee · A. L. H. Hung · B. K. W. Ng · J. C. Y. Cheng
Department of Orthopaedics and Traumatology, Faculty of Medicine, The Chinese University of Hong Kong, Hong Kong, China
e-mail: tplam@cuhk.edu.hk

B. H. K. Yip
Division of Family Medicine and Primary Health Care, Jockey Club School of Public Health and Primary Care, The Chinese University of Hong Kong, Hong Kong, China

N. L. S. Tang
Department of Chemical Pathology, Faculty of Medicine, The Chinese University of Hong Kong, Hong Kong, China

K. M. Lee
Lee Hysan Clinical Research Laboratory, Faculty of Medicine, The Chinese University of Hong Kong, Hong Kong, China

© Springer Nature Switzerland AG 2019
C. M. Weaver et al. (eds.), *Nutritional Influences on Bone Health*,
https://doi.org/10.1007/978-3-319-98464-3_3

factors such as calcium intake and vitamin D status are generally not taken seriously both at clinical settings and at public health levels. This is reflected by prevalence studies on Vit-D insufficiency among children indicating the condition remains highly prevalent worldwide especially in Asian countries. In this chapter, we will give a profile summary of Vit-D status among children in Asia together with a new look at Vit-D insufficiency and related key issues on bone health, pediatric fracture, and measures to address the existing problem of Vit-D insufficiency.

Vit-D Status in Children: The Asian Profile

Cooper et al. made an important scientific projection that the number of hip fractures occurring in the world each year will rise from 1.66 million in 1990 to 6.26 million by 2050 with the majority of cases of 3.25 million occurring in Asia [3]. The Vit-D profile in Asian countries deserves our attention especially for the young population. In "The Asian Audit on Epidemiology, Costs, and Burden of Osteoporosis in Asia 2009" prepared by the International Osteoporosis Foundation (IOF), vitamin D deficiency is prevalent throughout the 14 countries involved in the Audit, particularly in South and Southeast Asia [4]. In spite of the alert call, the situation continued to prevail 4 years later as noted in the "Asia-Pacific Regional Audit on Epidemiology, Costs, and Burden of Osteoporosis in 2013" also prepared by IOF that "vitamin D insufficiency and deficiency are being reported in children and adolescents which suggest that peak bone mass may not be achieved, thus predisposing them to osteoporosis later in life" [5]. As shown in Table 3.1, our young population is not immune from this epidemic of Vit-D insufficiency. Back in 1998, Atiq et al. from Pakistan reported 55% of infants had serum 25(OH)Vit-D < 25 nmol/L [6]. In the subsequent two decades, Vit-D insufficiency remained highly prevalent as reported by studies done in China (Du et al. [7]), the United Arab Emirates (Dawodu et al. [8]), Malaysia (Khor et al. [9]), Korea (Shin et al. [10]), Vietnam (Laillou et al. [11]), Bangladesh (Ahmed et al. [15]), Cyprus (Kolokotroni et al. [12]), Saudi Arabia (Al-Saleh et al. [13]), and India (Chowdhury et al. [16]). In Hong Kong (Table 3.1), our group has reported in 2016 a population-based survey on 333 girls and 230 boys (12–16 years old) with normal health both in summer and winter and noted 64.7% and 11.4% of subjects were insufficient [$25 \leq$ 25(OH) Vit-D ≤ 50 nmol/L] and deficient [25(OH)Vit-D < 25 nmol/L] in Vit-D, respectively. Mean level of serum 25(OH)Vit-D in summer was significantly higher than that in winter (44.7 ± 13.6 and 35.9 ± 12.6 nmol/L, respectively) without obvious gender difference [14].

In Asia, a review of the literature indicates Vit-D insufficiency observes no geographical or national borders with countries at different latitudes being plagued with the same epidemic.

Table 3.1 Serum 25(OH)Vit-D levels in young subjects in Asian countries

Studies	Year	Age group (year)	Location	% <12.5 nmol/L	% <25 nmol/L	% <50 nmol/L
Atiq et al. [6]	1998	Infant	Pakistan		55	
Du et al. [7]	2001	12–14	Beijing (winter)	45.2 (subclinical)		
Du et al. [7]	2001	12–14	Beijing (summer)	6.7 (subclinical)		
Dawodu et al. [8]	2003	Infant	United Arab Emirates		82	
Khor et al. [9]	2011	7–12	Malaysia			72.4
Shin et al. [10]	2012	12–13	Korea			89 in boys 99 in girls
Laillou et al. [11]	2013	<5	Vietnam			57
Kolokotroni et al. [12]	2015	16–17	Cyprus			34.7
Al-Saleh et al. [13]	2015	Mean 15.1	Saudi Arabia			79 in boys 92.5 in girls
Cheung et al. [14]	2016	12–16	Hong Kong			76.1
Ahmed et al. [15]	2017	0.5–2	Bangladesh			45.6
Chowdhury et al. [16]	2017	0.5–2.5	India		34.5	

Cultural and Lifestyle Determinants of Vit-D Status in Asian Population

Within a country, children of both genders from different socioeconomic sectors were affected although to a different extent. While culture-specific lifestyle preference or dressing pattern can lead to Vit-D insufficiency in specific situations, in general, knowledge, attitudes, and lifestyles with respect to vitamin D and sunlight exposure have been widely studied and reported to be important predisposition factors for Vit-D insufficiency that could be of reference values when formulating measures to address the issue of Vit-D insufficiency. Brock et al. reported a cross-sectional study for women and noted the associations with vitamin D deficiency were younger age, higher education, more sun protection behavior, fewer minutes of sun exposure on weekends, low vitamin D and calcium intake through foods or supplements, and less acculturation to Australian lifestyle [17]. Jang et al. investigated East Asian women living in Australia and noted that they expressed preference for fair skin, a tradition of covering skin when outdoors, and no sunbathing culture and that they reported knowledge of the need for sun avoidance due to skin cancer risk and few reported knowledge about the benefits of sun exposure for adequate vitamin D levels [18]. Al-Saleh et al. reported only 45.7% of Saudi school children heard about Vit-D sources in school and 84.6% thought fruits were rich in Vit-D [13]. In Hong Kong, the situation was no better. In the same study by our group in school children mentioned earlier [14], 83.7% did not know what was the function of Vit-D, 75.3% did not know the sources of Vit-D, and 54.8% did not know Vit-D was good for bone health (unpublished data).

Vit-D Insufficiency, Bone Health, and Fractures: A New Look at an Old Problem

For children with serum 25(OH)Vit-D < 25 nmol/L over an extended interval of 1–2 years, adverse outcome in form of rickets will occur severely affecting the musculoskeletal system [19, 20]. In contrast, the condition of Vit-D insufficiency and its phenotypic characteristics are less well defined. The relationship between Vit-D status and areal bone mineral density (aBMD) or bone mineral content (BMC) as reported in the literature for the adolescent population remains inconclusive [21–24]. To assess the bone health status in Vit-D insufficiency, Cashman et al. performed DXA of the non-dominant forearm and dominant heel in adolescent subjects and noted 12–15-year-old girls with high Vit-D level (≧74.1 nmol/L) had significantly greater forearm (but not heel) bone mineral density (BMD). There was no significant relation between Vit-D status and BMD in boys [25]. Nakamura et al. reported a cross-sectional study of 77 healthy women and noted only a weak but significant linear association between 25(OH)Vit-D level and forearm BMC ($R^2 = 0.114$, $p = 0.0052$) but not with BMD [26]. Outila et al. studied 178 healthy female adolescents (aged 14–16 year) and could not demonstrate a clear and significant association between 25(OH)Vit-D level and forearm BMD [27]. Cheng et al. investigated 193 adolescent girls with DXA and pQCT and reported an absence of significant differences between Vit-D status groups in BMC and areal BMD of the total body, femur, or lumbar spine. Neither did linear regression analysis show any association between Vit-D level and BMC or areal BMD. However, they did detect a positive correlation between 25(OH)Vit-D and cortical vBMD of the distal radius [28].

Inconsistent results on the impacts of Vit-D insufficiency on bone health measured by DXA stemmed from limitations with DXA for bone measurements. Firstly, DXA is a two-dimensional (2-D) measurement for a three-dimensional (3-D) structure, and hence the measurement is confounded by bone size and bone geometry [29]. In addition, cortical and trabecular bone cannot be differentiated, and other important information on bone micro-architecture cannot be measured [30]. To better understand the correlation between Vit-D levels and bone health, our group conducted a cross-sectional study using high-resolution peripheral quantitative computed tomography on school children and noted for girls, aBMD and BMC of bilateral femoral necks, cortical area, cortical thickness, total vBMD, and trabecular thickness of non-dominant distal radius were significantly correlated with 25(OH)

Vit-D levels. In boys, aBMD of bilateral femoral necks, BMC of dominant femoral neck, cortical area, cortical thickness, total vBMD, trabecular vBMD, BV/TV, and trabecular separation were significantly correlated with 25(OH)Vit-D levels (Table 3.2) [14].

The correlations between Vit-D status and bone density and bone quality among "healthy" children could carry significant clinical implication. The traditional view among the medical profession is that suboptimal bone health not to the degree of overt rickets in children or osteomalacia in adults probably will not cause immediate ailment. Thus, bone health and related factors of calcium intake and Vit-D status have not received the appropriate attention they deserve until recently when studies reported in the literature began to shed lights on this issue spelling out the need of adopting a new look at an old medical condition of Vit-D insufficiency and related suboptimal bone health in children.

Clark et al. conducted a meta-analysis on eight case-control studies and showed an overall lower bone mass in children with fractures compared with controls (standardized mean difference, −0.26; 95% CI, −0.40 to −0.11; $p < 0.001$) [31]. It was previously

Table 3.2 Correlations between serum 25(OH)D and DXA and HR-pQCT parameters [14]

	Girls ($n = 333$)			Boys ($n = 230$)		
DXA parameters at femoral neck	B	*p*-value	R^2	B	*p*-value	R^2
aBMD						
Non-dominant side	0.0014	**0.003**	0.42	0.0010	**0.021**	0.60
BMC						
Non-dominant side	0.0040	**0.002**	0.57	0.0025	0.101	0.71
HR-pQCT parameters at non-dominant distal radius	($n = 333$)			($n = 229$)		
Bone morphometry						
TotAr	0.018	0.870	0.32	−0.115	0.443	0.33
CtAr	0.116	**0.014**	0.55	0.157	**0.017**	0.56
TbAr	−0.071	0.552	0.27	−0.227	0.158	0.20
CtTh	0.002	**0.020**	0.49	0.003	**0.020**	0.51
CtPm	0.005	0.772	0.30	−0.021	0.375	0.34
vBMD						
Dtot	0.574	**0.022**	0.40	0.698	**0.007**	0.40
Dcort	0.506	0.071	0.53	0.521	0.170	0.45
Dtrab	0.244	0.068	0.07	0.331	**0.038**	0.10
Trabecular bone micro-architecture						
BV/TV	2.1×10^{-4}	0.065	0.07	2.8×10^{-4}	**0.038**	0.10
TbN	5.5×10^{-5}	0.960	0.11	0.002	0.100	0.11
TbTh	1.2×10^{-4}	**0.008**	0.07	6.1×10^{-5}	0.276	0.28
TbSp	-1.9×10^{-4}	0.647	0.07	-9.7×10^{-4}	**0.018**	0.10

Analyzed by multiple linear regression with 25(OH)Vit-D as one of the independent variables, with adjustment for age, sexual maturation stage, body weight, body height, total physical activity level, dietary calcium intake, and season

p-value highlighted in bold figures indicates *p*-value <0.05

suggested that risk and injury-prone behavior contributed to the higher risk of fractures at puberty [32]. More and more evidences showed fractures in childhood can be related to underlying skeletal fragility. Clark et al. further carried out a prospective cohort study measuring total body less head bone mineral density (BMD) with DXA on 6213 children and noted a weak inverse relationship between BMD at 9.9 years and subsequent fracture risk (odds ratio per SD decrease = 1.12; 95% confidence interval 1.02–1.25) [33]. Ryan et al. measured BMD and Vit-D status among African-American children aged 5–9 years with forearm fractures in a case-control study and reported when compared with control subjects, case subjects had lower whole body z scores for BMD (0.62 ± 0.96 vs 0.98 ± 1.09; adjusted odds ratio 0.38 [0.20–0.72]) and were more likely to be vitamin D deficient (47.1% vs 40.8%; adjusted odds ratio 3.46 [1.09–10.94]).

Public Health Measures to Address the Long-Existing Problem of Vit-D Insufficiency

As far as impact on bone health is concerned, Vit-D insufficiency among children may not be as asymptomatic as previously thought. A randomized controlled trial [34, 35] provided strong evidence on the effect of calcium and Vit-D supplementation on improving bone health and preventing disease progression in patients with AIS. Despite more studies being warranted for further confirmation, current evidence supports the notion that Vit-D insufficiency that is correlated with decreased BMD and bone quality among children can also be related to bone fragility resulting in the peak incidence of fracture during adolescence and poor bone health associated with AIS. Remedial measures for Vit-D insufficiency should be considered as primary preventive measures at public health level to improve Vit-D status for our young population. Rizzoli et al. reviewed the literature and noted the efficacy of calcium supplementation and dairy products on improving bone mineral accrual during growth with the view of preventing fracture during adolescence [36]. Winzenberg et al. made a systemic review and noted for the planned subgroup analyses by baseline serum vitamin D level that vitamin D supplementation of deficient children and adolescents could result in clinically useful improvements [37]. For promotion of knowledge and lifestyle for bone health and Vit-D, web-based educational platform (http://bonehealth.ort.cuhk.edu.hk/) or mobile application (https://play.google.com/store/apps/details?id=com.cuhk.vdp) can be cost-effective options to empower subjects on self-care for good bone health. Screening for Vit-D insufficiency has been considered as an active approach for achieving normal Vit-D status and good bone health for the public. Due to the lack of assay standardization and lack of consensus as to what are adequate serum 25(OH)Vit-D values, there is no consensus for routine universal blood sampling screening for Vit-D deficiency in children [38]. McCarthy also mentioned the evidence supporting routine Vit-D screening was insufficient as was also concluded by the US Preventive Services Task Force [39]. Apart from primary prevention, supplementation for treating Vit-D insufficiency should also be considered after fractures have occurred or scoliosis has set in with the objectives of preventing subsequent fracture or controlling curve from progression to bracing or surgical threshold.

Conclusion

Despite early reports on prevalence of Vit-D insufficiency among children in the last century, the condition remains epidemic according to recent reports, especially those from Asia. Vit-D insufficiency deserves attention as it may not be as asymptomatic as previously thought. Pediatric fracture can be related to bone fragility, and there was evidence suggesting Vit-D supplementation can prevent curve progression in scoliosis patients especially for those with Vit-D insufficiency. To promote bone health and alleviate the epidemics of Vit-D insufficiency, remedial measures using supplementation and promoting lifestyle and dietary modification toward good bone health should be considered both at public health levels and with enhanced attention on the issue within the medical profession.

References

1. Weaver CM, Gordon CM, Janz KF, Kalkwarf HJ, Lappe JM, Lewis R, O'Karma M, Wallace TC, Zemel BS. The National Osteoporosis Foundation's position statement on peak bone mass development and lifestyle factors: a systematic review and implementation recommendations. Osteoporos Int. 2016;27(4):1281–386.
2. Baxter-Jones AD, Faulkner RA, Forwood MR, Mirwald RL, Bailey DA. Bone mineral accrual from 8 to 30 years of age: an estimation of peak bone mass. J Bone Miner Res. 2011;26(8):1729–39.
3. Cooper C, Campion G, Melton LJ 3rd. Hip fractures in the elderly: a world-wide projection. Osteoporos Int. 1992;2(6):285–9.
4. Mithal A, Dhingra V, Lau E, editors. The Asian Audit "Epidemiology, costs and burden of osteoporosis in Asia 2009". Nyon: International Osteoporosis Foundation; 2009.
5. Mithal A, Ebeling P, Kyer CS. In: Jagait CK, Misteli L, Pierroz DD, editors. The Asia-Pacific Regional Audit "Epidemiology, costs & burden of osteoporosis in 2013". Nyon: International Osteoporosis Foundation; 2013.
6. Atiq M, Suria A, Nizami SQ, Ahmed I. Vitamin D status of breastfed Pakistani infants. Acta Paediatr. 1998;87(7):737–40.
7. Du X, Greenfield H, Fraser DR, Ge K, Trube A, Wang Y. Vitamin D deficiency and associated factors in adolescent girls in Beijing. Am J Clin Nutr. 2001;74(4):494–500.
8. Dawodu A, Agarwal M, Hossain M, Kochiyil J, Zayed R. Hypovitaminosis D and vitamin D deficiency in exclusively breast-feeding infants and their mothers in summer: a justification for vitamin D supplementation of breast-feeding infants. J Pediatr. 2003;142(2):169–73.
9. Khor GL, Chee WS, Shariff ZM, Poh BK, Arumugam M, Rahman JA, Theobald HE. High prevalence of vitamin D insufficiency and its association with BMI-for-age among primary school children in Kuala Lumpur, Malaysia. BMC Public Health. 2011;11:95.
10. Shin YH, Kim KE, Lee C, Shin HJ, Kang MS, Lee HR, Lee YJ. High prevalence of vitamin D insufficiency or deficiency in young adolescents in Korea. Eur J Pediatr. 2012;171(10):1475–80.
11. Laillou A, Wieringa F, Tran TN, Van PT, Le BM, Fortin S, Le TH, Pfanner RM, Berger J. Hypovitaminosis D and mild hypocalcaemia are highly prevalent among young Vietnamese children and women and related to low dietary intake. PLoS One. 2013;8(5):e63979.
12. Kolokotroni O, Papadopoulou A, Middleton N, Kouta C, Raftopoulos V, Nicolaidou P, Yiallouros PK. Vitamin D levels and status amongst asthmatic and non-asthmatic adolescents in Cyprus: a comparative cross-sectional study. BMC Public Health. 2015;15:48.
13. Al-Saleh Y, Al-Daghri NM, Khan N, Alfawaz H, Al-Othman AM, Alokail MS, Chrousos GP. Vitamin D status in Saudi school children based on knowledge. BMC Pediatr. 2015; 15:53.

14. Cheung TF, Cheuk KY, FW Y, Hung VW, Ho CS, Zhu TY, Ng BK, Lee KM, Qin L, Ho SS, Wong GW, Cheng JC, Lam TP. Prevalence of vitamin D insufficiency among adolescents and its correlation with bone parameters using high-resolution peripheral quantitative computed tomography. Osteoporos Int. 2016;27(8):2477–88.
15. Ahmed AS, Ahmed T, Long KZ, Magalhaes RJS, Hossain MI, Islam MM, Mahfuz M, Gaffar SA, Sharmeen A, Haque R, Guerrant RL, Petri WA, Mamun AA. Prevalence and risk factors of vitamin D insufficiency and deficiency among 6-24-month-old underweight and normal-weight children living in an urban slum of Bangladesh. Public Health Nutr. 2017;20(10):1718–28.
16. Chowdhury R, Taneja S, Bhandari N, Kvestad I, Strand TA, Bhan MK. Vitamin-D status and neurodevelopment and growth in young north Indian children: a secondary data analysis. Nutr J. 2017;16(1):59.
17. Brock KE, Ke L, Tseng M, Clemson L, Koo FK, Jang H, Seibel MJ, Mpofu E, Fraser DR, Mason RS. Vitamin D status is associated with sun exposure, vitamin D and calcium intake, acculturation and attitudes in immigrant East Asian women living in Sydney. J Steroid Biochem Mol Biol. 2013;136:214–7.
18. Jang H, Koo FK, Ke L, Clemson L, Cant R, Fraser DR, Seibel MJ, Tseng M, Mpofu E, Mason RS, Brock K. Culture and sun exposure in immigrant East Asian women living in Australia. Women Health. 2013;53(5):504–18.
19. Food and Nutrition Board. Dietary reference intakes for Calcium, Magnesium, Phosphorus, vitamin D, and fluoride. Washington: National Academy Press, Institute of Medicine; 1997. p. 250–87.
20. Norman AW, Bouillon R. Vitamin D nutritional policy needs a vision for the future. Exp Biol Med. 2010;235(9):1034–45.
21. Mouratidou T, Vicente-Rodriguez G, Gracia-Marco L, Huybrechts I, Sioen I, Widhalm K, Valtuena J, Gonzalez-Gross M, Moreno LA. Associations of dietary calcium, vitamin D, milk intakes, and 25-hydroxyvitamin D with bone mass in Spanish adolescents: the HELENA study. J Clin Densitom. 2013;16(1):110–7.
22. Lee EY, Kim D, Kim KM, Kim KJ, Choi HS, Rhee Y, Lim SK. Age-related bone mineral density patterns in Koreans (KNHANES IV). J Clin Endocrinol Metab. 2012;97(9):3310–8.
23. Pekkinen M, Viljakainen H, Saarnio E, Lamberg-Allardt C, Makitie O. Vitamin D is a major determinant of bone mineral density at school age. PLoS One. 2012;7(7):e40090.
24. Esterle L, Nguyen M, Walrant-Debray O, Sabatier JP, Garabedian M. Adverse interaction of low-calcium diet and low 25(OH)D levels on lumbar spine mineralization in late-pubertal girls. J Bone Miner Res. 2010;25(11):2392–8.
25. Cashman KD, Hill TR, Cotter AA, Boreham CA, Dubitzky W, Murray L, Strain J, Flynn A, Robson PJ, Wallace JM, Kiely M. Low vitamin D status adversely affects bone health parameters in adolescents. Am J Clin Nutr. 2008;87(4):1039–44.
26. Nakamura K, Nashimoto M, Matsuyama S, Yamamoto M. Low serum concentrations of 25-hydroxyvitamin D in young adult Japanese women: a cross sectional study. Nutrition. 2001;17(11–12):921–5.
27. Outila TA, Karkkainen MU, Lamberg-Allardt CJ. Vitamin D status affects serum parathyroid hormone concentrations during winter in female adolescents: associations with forearm bone mineral density. Am J Clin Nutr. 2001;74(2):206–10.
28. Cheng S, Tylavsky F, Kroger H, Karkkainen M, Lyytikainen A, Koistinen A, Mahonen A, Alen M, Halleen J, Vaananen K, Lamberg-Allardt C. Association of low 25-hydroxyvitamin D concentrations with elevated parathyroid hormone concentrations and low cortical bone density in early pubertal and prepubertal Finnish girls. Am J Clin Nutr. 2003;78(3):485–92.
29. Bacchetta J, Boutroy S, Vilayphiou N, Ranchin B, Fouque-Aubert A, Basmaison O, Cochat P. Bone assessment in children with chronic kidney disease: data from two new bone imaging techniques in a single-center pilot study. Pediatr Nephrol. 2011;26(4):587–95.
30. Weber LT, Mehls O. Limitations of dual x-ray absorptiometry in children with chronic kidney disease. Pediatr Nephrol. 2010;25(1):3–5.
31. Clark EM, Tobias JH, Ness AR. Association between bone density and fractures in children: a systematic review and meta-analysis. Pediatrics. 2006;117(2):e291–7.

32. Ma D, Morley R, Jones G. Risk-taking, coordination and upper limb fractures in children: a population based case-control study. Osteoporos Int. 2004;15(8):633–8.
33. Clark EM, Ness AR, Bishop NJ, Tobias JH. Association between bone mass and fractures in children: a prospective cohort study. J Bone Miner Res. 2006;21(9):1489–95.
34. Lam TP, Yip BHK, Tam EMS, Man GCW, Lee WYW, Lee KM, Yu FWP, Qiu Y, Ng BKW, Cheng JCY. Calcium and vitamin D for adolescent idiopathic scoliosis – a further in-depth review using finite element analysis (FEA) for a randomized double-blinded placebo-controlled trial. In: 52nd scoliosis research society annual meeting & course, 2017 Sept 6–9, Philadelphia, PA, USA; 2017.
35. Lam TP, Yip BHK, Tam EMS, Man GCW, Lee WYW, Lee KM, Yu FWP, Ng BKW, Cheng JCY. Preventing curve progression with calcium and vitamin D supplementation in adolescent idiopathic scoliosis (AIS) – a randomized double-blinded Placebo-controlled trial. In: Pediatric orthopaedics society of North America 2016 annual meeting (POSNA), 2016 Apr 27–30, Indianapolis, IN; 2016.
36. Rizzoli R, Bianchi ML, Garabedian M, McKay HA, Moreno LA. Maximizing bone mineral mass gain during growth for the prevention of fractures in the adolescents and the elderly. Bone. 2010;46(2):294–305.
37. Winzenberg T, Powell S, Shaw KA, Jones G. Effects of vitamin D supplementation on bone density in healthy children: systematic review and meta-analysis. BMJ. 2011;342:c7254.
38. Mimouni FB. Vitamin D status in growing children: should we routinely screen for vitamin D adequacy? J Pediatr Gastroenterol Nutr. 2010;51(Suppl 3):S121–2.
39. McCarthy M. Evidence for routine vitamin D screening is insufficient, US panel concludes. BMJ. 2014;348:g4277.

Part II

Micronutrients: Calcium, Sodium, and Potassium

4 Peak BMC Growth and Calcium Requirements for Children

Michael R. Lawlor, Connie M. Weaver, Bruce A. Craig, Susan J. Whiting, Adam D. G. Baxter-Jones, Hassanali Vatanparast, and George P. McCabe

Calcium, Bone, and Growth

Almost all calcium in the human body is in bones. Dual-energy X-ray absorptiometry (DXA) measurements of bone mass are expressed as bone mineral content (BMC). With the assumption that 32% of bone mineral is calcium, we use BMC as a measure of the amount of calcium in the bone [1]. Note that DXA can be used to measure BMC at particular sites in the body, such as the femoral neck or the lumbar spine. Total body bone mineral content (TBBMC) is the BMC for the entire body, including the head.

For adults, calcium is needed to maintain TBBMC, that is, to ensure that the level of bone formation is sufficient to replace the calcium that is lost through bone resorption. For children and adolescents, however, additional calcium is needed for the growth of the skeleton, expressed as bone area in DXA.

By examining the TBBMC growth curve for a healthy growing individual over time, we see how BMC increases during the growth period. The derivative of this growth curve gives us the rate of growth over time for that individual. Through an examination of many individual growth curves, we can assess the variation in growth patterns and the consequent need for calcium.

M. R. Lawlor
Department of Mathematics and Statistics, Oakland University, Rochester, MI, USA

C. M. Weaver
Department of Nutrition Science, Purdue University, West Lafayette, IN, USA

B. A. Craig · G. P. McCabe (✉)
Department of Statistics, Purdue University, West Lafayette, IN, USA
e-mail: mccabe@purdue.edu

S. J. Whiting · H. Vatanparast
College of Pharmacy and Nutrition, University of Saskatchewan, Saskatoon, SK, Canada

A. D. G. Baxter-Jones
College of Kinesiology, University of Saskatchewan, Saskatoon, SK, Canada

© Springer Nature Switzerland AG 2019
C. M. Weaver et al. (eds.), *Nutritional Influences on Bone Health*,
https://doi.org/10.1007/978-3-319-98464-3_4

Dietary Reference Intakes

Dietary Reference Intakes (DRIs) are values of nutrients used to plan and assess nutrient intakes of healthy people. DRIs are specified for females and males of different age groups. Two DRIs that are the focus of this manuscript are the Recommended Daily Allowance (RDA) and the Estimated Average Requirement (EAR) [2].

The RDA is used to assess the adequacy of intake for an individual. Roughly speaking, if the intake for an individual is at or above the RDA, the chance that the individual's intake is adequate is 97.5% or greater. The EAR, on the other hand, is used to assess the prevalence of inadequate intake for a population.

Each of these DRIs is based on the estimated distribution of the amount of the nutrient needed (the requirement) for healthy individuals in the specified sex and chronological age group. When the distribution is normal, $N(\mu, \sigma)$, these DRIs can be expressed in terms of the mean, μ, and the standard deviation, σ. The EAR is μ and RDA is $\mu + 2\sigma$. For cases where a reliable estimate of the standard deviation is not available, a 10% coefficient of variation is assumed. It follows that $\sigma = 0.1\ \mu$, and therefore, the RDA is $\mu + 2\sigma = \mu + 2(0.1\mu) = 1.2\mu$, or 1.2 times the EAR.

Current DRIs for calcium are given in a 2011 report from the Institute of Medicine (IOM) [1]. The EAR was determined using the factorial method, a procedure that takes into account calcium accretion, losses, and estimated absorption. The method does not provide an estimate of the standard deviation nor does it describe the shape of the requirement distribution. Instead, the distribution was assumed to be normal with a 10% coefficient of variation. Although there appeared to be some differences in distribution due to sex and age group, these were judged to be small. As a result, common values for the EAR and the RDA were recommended for boys and girls in both the 9–13-year and the 14–18-year age ranges. These were 1100 mg/day for the EAR and 1300 mg/day for the RDA.

Peak Growth Velocity

The Pediatric Bone Mineral Accrual Study (PBMAS, initiated in 1991), using a mixed longitudinal cohort design, performed DXA scans on subjects over a period of several years [3]. Details regarding the cohorts and the ages at which measurements were taken are given in [4, Table 1]. Several papers describing analyses of these data have been published [4–7].

Of particular relevance for the analysis presented in this paper is the study of peak bone accrual, expressed as change in TBBMC, presented in [8]. The authors quantify the variation in growth patterns among individuals and estimate the ages at peak height velocity and peak BMC velocity for a collection of 60 boys and 53 girls. A key idea is that at a particular age, 14 years, for example, some individuals have not yet entered their rapid growth phase, some are near their rapid growth phase, and some are past their rapid growth phase. Individuals who are near their rapid growth phase will tend to be in the upper tail of the requirement distribution, whereas individuals who have not yet entered their rapid growth phase or who have completed their rapid growth phase will tend to be in the lower tail of the requirement distribution.

A primary finding of this work is that the use of the mean growth velocity as a measure of the need for calcium across age groups, a cross-sectional view, does not sufficiently take into account the need for calcium at the age of peak BMC velocity for individuals, a longitudinal view. They estimate 358 mg/d and 285 mg/d as peak calcium accretion rates for boys and girls, respectively. These rates are substantially higher (27% and 34%) than the cross-sectional rates (282 mg/d and 212 mg/d) that they previously reported based on the same data [8], because cross-sectional-derived average curves blunt the curve as compared with longitudinal-derived individual curves.

Methods

Our analysis uses the TBBMC observations from the PBMAS described in the previous section. We did not consider observations at ages greater than 22 years and included only subjects with at least five remaining observations. This resulted in a data set that had 134 girls, 117 boys, and a total of 1518 TBBMC observations. Plots of TBBMC versus age were examined across subjects. Based on the patterns observed, we chose the following parametric s-shaped function to describe the relationship between TBBMC and age:

$$\text{TBBMC} = \beta_0 \left(1+\exp\left(-\beta_1\left(\text{Age}-\beta_2\right)\right)\right)^{-\gamma}$$

The parameter gamma (γ) is included to account for the asymmetry in the s-shape of the relationship, that is, TBBMC increases more rapidly in the early stages of growth and then slows down after the peak BMC growth. Note that $\gamma = 1$ corresponds to a symmetric function. Preliminary analyses of individual growth curves show very little variation in γ across subjects. Therefore, we set this parameter to a constant, $\gamma = 0.2$, for all of our final analyses. Given a fixed γ, there are three parameters that describe an individual's growth curve. We label this set as

$$\Theta = \left(\beta_0, \beta_1, \beta_2\right)$$

We assume Θ_i is unique for each subject and that the distribution of these parameters is multivariate normal, $N(\Theta, \Sigma)$, where Θ is the mean of the population and Σ is the covariance matrix. Normal quantile plots were used to verify the validity of this assumption. An additional parameter, ν, represents the standard deviation of the observations around the TBBMC curves for individual subjects, that is, the within-person variation. Note that the value of the parameter vector, θ, specifies a curve relating TBBMC to age and vice versa.

SAS PROC NLMIXED was used to estimate the model parameters. This procedure allows us to model the subject-specific nonlinear relationship between TBBMC and age, assuming the multivariate distribution for the Θ_i. It also accounts for the within-subject variation. The iterative approach to compute these estimates requires initial guesses which were determined by a careful analysis of summaries of the relationships for individuals. Here is the model specification of the growth curve for each subject:

$$Y = F(x) = \beta_0 \left(1 + \exp\left(-\beta_1 (x - \beta_2)\right)\right)^{-0.2}$$

where Y is TBBMC and x is age. The within-subject variation of TBBMC around each growth curve is assumed to be normal with variance ν^2, that is, the values of Y are independent with mean $F(x)$ and variance ν^2, $N(F(x), \nu^2)$.

Note that this analytical approach does not compute a curve for each individual and then combine results across individuals; rather, it generates estimates for the model parameters, Θ, Σ, and ν^2, by iteratively solving a system of nonlinear equations.

A particular advantage of the software used is that it is easy to generate the estimates of functions of the model parameters. Standard errors are estimated using the delta method [9]. We are particularly interested in TBBMC growth velocity (TBBMCV), the age at peak BMC velocity, and the peak TBBMC growth velocity (PBMCV).

The TBBMC growth velocity is simply the derivative with respect to age of the curve relating TBBMC to age:

$$\text{TBBMCV} = f(x) = 0.2\,\beta_0\beta_1 \frac{\exp\left(-\beta_1 (x - \beta_2)\right)}{\left(1 + \exp\left(-\beta_1 (x - \beta_2)\right)\right)^{-1.2}}$$

The peak BMC growth velocity is

$$\text{PBMCV} = \beta_0\beta_1 6^{-1.2}$$

And the age at peak BMC growth velocity is

$$\text{Age at PBMCV} = \beta_1^{-1} \log(0.2) + \beta_2$$

Model assumptions regarding the form of the model and the distributions of various quantities were checked using graphical and numerical summaries. No serious violations of the assumptions were detected.

Preliminary analyses were performed using a single model for girls and boys that included terms allowing the model parameters, β_0, β_1, and β_2, to depend on sex. These analyses indicated that β_0 and β_2 depend on sex while β_1 does not. Therefore, our final model assumes a common value of β_1 for both sexes.

Conversion of TBBMC growth velocity (g/y) to the calcium needed for bone growth (mg/d) was performed assuming that 32.3% of bone mass is calcium, 38% of calcium intake is absorbed, and the losses (urinary, endogenous fecal, and sweat) of 273 mg/d and 290 mg/d for girls and boys, respectively [10]. Variability due to the imprecision of these factors and γ has not been taken into account. As a result, there is some underestimation of standard errors.

Results

The estimates of $\Theta = (\beta_0, \beta_1, \beta_2)$ are

$$\Theta_{\text{Boys}} = 2.78, 0.96, 15.41$$

and

$$\Theta_{\text{Girls}} = 2.14, 0.96, 14.03$$

So, the final models for TBBMC are

$$\text{TBBMC}_{\text{Boys}} = 2.78\left(1 + \exp\left(-0.96\left(\text{Age} - 15.41\right)\right)\right)^{-0.2}$$

and

$$\text{TBBMC}_{\text{Girls}} = 2.14\left(1 + \exp\left(-0.96\left(\text{Age} - 14.03\right)\right)\right)^{-0.2}$$

Figure 4.1 shows the average relationship between TBBMC and age for boys and girls with 95% confidence limits for the curves. Note that the graphs are similar initially but then the TBBMC for boys starts to increase and eventually reaches a higher asymptotic value (the parameter β_0, 2.78 kg for boys and 2.14 for girls), reflecting greater average height for boys.

The estimates of the peak BMC velocity, $\beta_0\,\beta_1 6^{-1.2}$, are

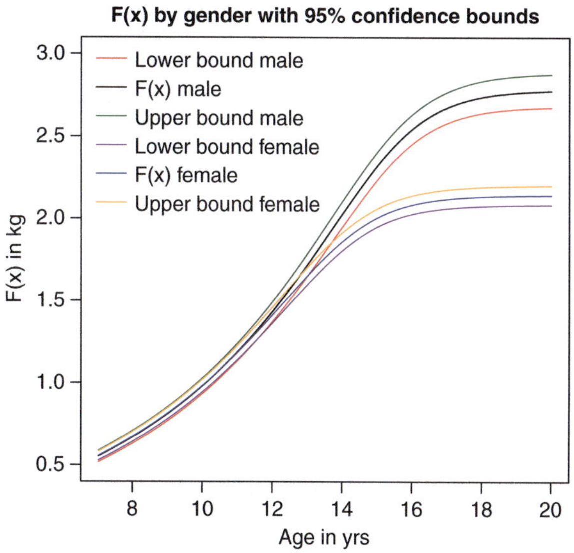

Fig. 4.1 TBBMC versus age for girls and boys with 95% confidence limits for the curves. The curves are similar initially but then the TBBMC for boys continues to increase and reaches a higher asymptotic value

$$\text{PBMCV}_{\text{Boys}} = 310.32\,\text{g}/\text{y}$$

$$\text{PBMCV}_{\text{Girls}} = 236.98\,\text{g}/\text{y}$$

And the estimates of the age at peak BMC velocity, $\beta_1^{-1}\log(0.2)+\beta_2$, are

$$\text{Age at PBMCV}_{\text{Boys}} = 13.74\,\text{y}$$

$$\text{Age at PBMCV}_{\text{Girls}} = 12.35\,\text{y}$$

Figure 4.2 shows the relationship between TBBMC growth velocity and age (the derivative of the function that describes the relationship between TBBMC and age) for girls and boys with 95% confidence limits for the curves. Here, we can see that the curves are similar initially but then diverge with girls peaking at an earlier age and boys reaching a higher peak BMC velocity.

Peak BMC velocity was converted to the amount of calcium needed for BMC growth at age of peak BMC growth. Here are the results.

Calcium needed for bone growth at peak BMC velocity

	Girls	Boys
Mean (mg/d)	1273	1484
SD (mg/d)	105	176
Mean + 2SD (mg/d)	1482	1835

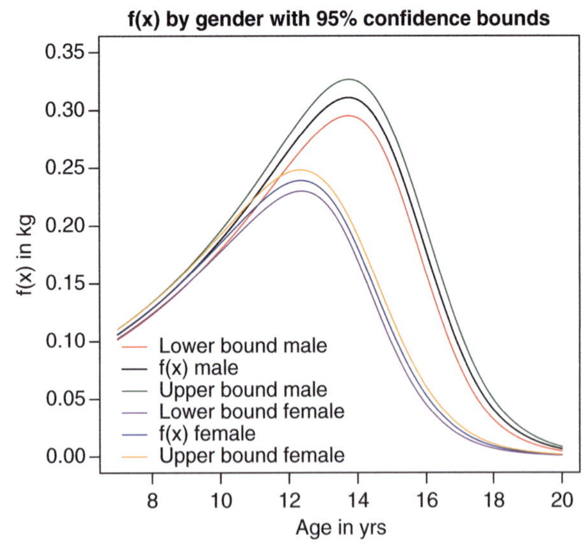

Fig. 4.2 TBBMC growth velocity versus age for girls and boys with 95% confidence limits for the curves. The curves are similar initially but then diverge with girls peaking at an earlier age and boys reaching a higher peak growth velocity

Discussion

The statistical model we developed to analyze the PBMAS data is particularly suited to efficiently estimate a variety of quantities related to the distribution of growth curves. In addition to the estimates described in this paper, the model can be used to estimate other quantities of interest such as the distribution of the change in TBBMC over a range of ages.

The data we used are not particularly diverse. Similar analyses using data that include a variety of races and ethnic groups should be undertaken. Note that the peak BMC velocity results can be converted to estimates to the calcium needed for different subgroups using subpopulation-specific values for the conversion constants [10].

As expected, our estimates of the need for calcium intake to account for bone growth are higher than the current DRI values. They are also higher than estimates of requirements based on maximal retention for girls [11] and for boys [12]. The current EAR of 1100 mg/d is much lower than the means that we calculated at peak BMC velocity, 1274 mg/d for girls and 1484 for boys. Similarly, the RDA of 1300 mg is much lower than our values, 1482 mg/d for girls and 1834 mg/d for boys. To interpret these differences, consider a 14-year-old boy who is at his peak BMC velocity and is consuming the calcium RDA, that is, 1300 mg/d. Using our calculations for the mean and standard deviation of the distribution of his need for calcium, we can calculate a z-score, $z = (1300–1484)/176 = -1.05$. Assuming normality, he is at the 15th percentile of his requirement distribution. Similarly, the calculation for a girl at peak BMC velocity consuming the RDA gives $z = (1300–1273)/105 = 0.26$, corresponding to the 60th percentile. These results suggest that the DRI-assumed CV of 10% used in determining the RDA may not sufficiently take into account the variation in the intake requirement due to the peak BMC velocity.

Note that the current DRIs specify values for children aged 9–18 years, a span much longer than the period of time that an individual child would have a substantial increased need for calcium due to peak BMC velocity. Therefore, DRIs based on peak needs would overestimate the need for calcium for an individual child during much of the 9–18-year age range. Our results suggest that use of the calcium DRIs for children should be qualified by recognizing the increased need for calcium during the period when they are growing rapidly. Note that the age at peak height velocity precedes the age at peak BMC velocity [4] and could serve as a leading indicator of the increased need for calcium.

References

1. IOM (Institute of Medicine). Dietary reference intakes for calcium and vitamin D. Washington: The National Academies Press; 2011.
2. Institute of Medicine (US) Subcommittee on Interpretation and Uses of Dietary Reference Intakes; Institute of Medicine (US) Standing Committee on the Scientific Evaluation of

Dietary Reference Intakes. DRI dietary reference intakes: applications in dietary assessment. Washington: National Academies Press (US); 2000.
3. Bailey DA. The Saskatchewan pediatric bone mineral accrual study. Int J Sports Med. 1997;18:s191–c194.
4. Baxter-Jones ADG, Faulkner RA, Forwood MR, Mirwald RL, Bailey DA. Bone mineral accrual from 8 to 30 years of age: an estimation of peak bone mass. J Bone Miner Res. 2011;26(8):1729–39.
5. Bailey DA, McKay HA, Mirwald RL, Crocker PR, Faulkner RA. A six-year longitudinal study of the relationship of physical activity to bone mineral accrual in growing children: the University of Saskatchewan bone mineral accrual study. J Bone Miner Res. 1999;14:1672–9.
6. Vatanparast H, Bailey DA, Baxter-Jones AD, Whiting SJ. Calcium requirements for bone growth in Canadian boys and girls during adolescence. Br J Nutr. 2010;1-6:57580.
7. Martin AD, Bailey DA, McKay HA, Whiting S. Bone mineral and calcium accretion during puberty. Am J Clin Nutr. 1997;66:611–5.
8. Bailey DA, Martin AD, McKay HA, Whiting S, Mirwald R. Calcium accretion in girls and boys during puberty: a longitudinal analysis. J Bone Miner Res. 2000;15(11):2245–50.
9. Casella G, Berger RL. Statistical inference. 2nd ed. Pacific Grove: Duxbury; 2002.
10. Weaver CM, Lawlor M, McCabe GP. Predicting calcium requirements in children. In: Weaver CM, et al., editors. Nutritional influences in bone health. London: Springer; 2016. https://doi.org/10.1007/978-3-319–32417-316.
11. Jackman LA, Millane SS, Martin BM, Wood O, GP MC, Peacock M, Weaver CM. CAlcium retention in relation to calcium intake and postmenarcheal age in adolescent females. Am J Clin Nutr. 1997;66:327–33.
12. Braun MM, Martin BR, Kern M, McCabe GP, Peacock K, Jiang Z, Weaver CM. Calcium retention in adolescent boys on a range of controlled calcium intakes. Am J Clin Nutr. 2006;84:414–8.

Integrative Omic Study to Identify Potential Dietary Supplement for Osteoporosis Treatment

5

Ching-Lung Cheung

Introduction

Osteoporosis is a common metabolic disease characterized by low bone mass and deterioration in microarchitecture and bone strength and leads to increased risk of fragility fracture. Osteoporosis is a major health issue worldwide. According to the International Osteoporosis Foundation (IOF), osteoporosis is estimated to affect 200 million women worldwide and leads to more than 8.9 fractures annually. In our recent hip fracture projection study, the number of hip fracture in Asia remains high, even though a lot of effort has been paid to prevent hip fracture. Thus, early identification of the onset of osteoporosis is key to fracture prevention by effective intervention. Moreover, it is well established that there is a "crisis in the osteoporosis treatment" worldwide, mainly due to the patients' awareness of the rare side effect of the commonly used anti-osteoporotic medication. Therefore, a novel and effective non-pharmacological intervention may be more acceptable by patients.

The etiology of osteoporosis is multifactorial and complex. It has been established that genetic factors, environmental factors, and their interaction play a major role in disease determination. Using a genome-wide association study (GWAS) approach, more than 66 well-validated loci have been found to be associated with bone mineral density (BMD) variation [1]. A recent GWAS of heel BMD measured by ultrasound in the UK Biobank data has further identified more than 250 susceptibility loci. These GWAS findings have several potential applications, such as

C.-L. Cheung
Department of Medicine, Li Ka Shing Faculty of Medicine, The University of Hong Kong, Hong Kong, China

Department of Pharmacology and Pharmacy, Li Ka Shing Faculty of Medicine, The University of Hong Kong, Hong Kong, China

Centre for Genomic Sciences, Li Ka Shing Faculty of Medicine, The University of Hong Kong, Hong Kong, China
e-mail: lung1212@hku.hk

© Springer Nature Switzerland AG 2019

C. M. Weaver et al. (eds.), *Nutritional Influences on Bone Health*,
https://doi.org/10.1007/978-3-319-98464-3_5

improving the understanding of disease etiology and therapeutic targets for development [2]. Nonetheless, the way in which these genetic variations contribute to BMD variation remains poorly understood.

Metabolites are a group of small molecules that may be metabolic substrates and their products. They represent a range of metabolic pathways and reflect cellular activities. Studies have demonstrated the importance of several metabolic pathways and metabolites in osteoporosis. For example, individuals with cystathionine beta-synthase deficiency, an IEM characterized by elevated serum total homocysteine, are susceptible to osteoporosis; serum homocysteine has been shown to be associated with BMD variation and fracture risk in different populations [3, 4]. Similarly, estrogen metabolism plays a role in BMD determination in both men [5] and women [6, 7] and is affected by genetic variation [7] and diet [6]. These studies demonstrate the importance of metabolites and metabolic pathways in BMD variation and fracture risk.

Metabolites can be detected in cells, tissues, and body fluid. With the burgeoning developments in metabolomic profiling technology, such as mass spectrometry and proton nuclear magnetic resonance (^{1}H-NMR), it is now feasible to study the metabolome in an untargeted fashion. The role of metabolites in common traits can be evaluated systematically to reflect the complexity of the whole system. In this way, serum metabolite levels have been shown to be associated with common diseases, such as chronic kidney disease [8] and diabetes [9]. Nonetheless how a particular serum metabolite is related to osteoporosis remains largely unknown. Only one published study to date has investigated the role of metabolome in BMD variation. In 2014, You et al. [10] performed a metabolomic study of BMD variation in 601 healthy Taiwanese women aged 40–55, including both pre- and postmenopausal women. Serum metabolome was evaluated using ^{1}H-NMR. The participants were classified into two groups: low (BMD at the lumbar spine (LS) < 1.138 g/cm^2) or high BMD (BMD at the LS ≥ 1.138 g/cm^2). In postmenopausal women, elevated glutamine (odds ratio [OR], 5.1) was significantly associated with low BMD at the spine; elevated lactate (OR = 0.55), acetone (OR = 0.51), lipids (OR = 0.04), and very low-density lipoprotein (OR = 0.49) were significantly protective against low BMD. Results were adjusted for age, height, weight, waist circumference, creatinine, exercise, and serum alkaline phosphatase. However, the relationship between metabolome, BMD at the femoral neck (FN), and fracture remains unstudied. In addition, genetic data were unavailable, and the participants were relatively healthy (<1% participants having osteoporosis) [10]. There is thus a need to perform a metabolomic study in a well-powered and characterized cohort to identify the BMD-associated metabolites (metabolites$_{\text{BMD}}$) and their genetic determinants.

Discovery Phase: Metabolomic Study of BMD in the TwinsUK

We conducted a metabolomic study of bone mineral density in the TwinsUK cohort and the Hong Kong Osteoporosis Study (HKOS). The TwinsUK cohort is a nationwide registry of volunteer twins in the UK since 1992, with about 12,000 registered

Table 5.1 Demographic characteristics of the TwinsUK and HKOS cohorts

	TwinsUK	HKOS
N	6055	624
Male:Female	434:5621	112:512
Age, years	53.45 (14.00)	52.05 (14.25)
Body mass index, kg/m^2	26.07 (4.91)	22.83 (3.84)
Height, m	1.62 (0.07)	1.58 (0.08)
Weight, kg	69.24 (13.78)	56.98 (11.26)
Femoral neck BMD, mg/cm^2	786.98 (129.42)	710.62 (167.51)
Total hip BMD, mg/cm^2	926.12 (133.67)	815.12 (176.04)
Lumbar spine BMD, mg/cm^2	985.58 (152.75)	919.03 (203.01)

twins. Details of the cohort have been described elsewhere [11]. The HKOS is a prospective longitudinal cohort study of osteoporosis and fracture that started in 1995. The cohort participants were community-dwelling Southern Chinese men and women of Han descent recruited from public road shows and health fairs held in various districts of Hong Kong from 1995 to 2010; details of the cohort have been described elsewhere [12]. The demographic characteristics of these cohorts are provided in Table 5.1. The metabolomic profiling was conducted in fasting serum sample using a commercially available platform provided by Metabolon (Metabolon Inc., Durham, NC, USA). Details of the platform have been described previously [13]. In total, metabolomic profiling was done in 6055 twins and 631 participants from the TwinsUK and HKOS, respectively. In this study, we analyzed 280 structurally named biochemicals (known metabolites) categorized into the following broad categories: amino acids, lipids, carbohydrates, vitamins, nucleotides, peptides, xenobiotics, and steroids. BMD was measured by Hologic dual-energy X-ray absorptiometry in both cohorts.

In the discovery phase using the data from the TwinsUK, mixed-effects random-intercept models were used to evaluate the metabolite-BMD associations, considering family relatedness and zygosity as random effects variables and age, height, weight, and duration of hormone replacement therapy (HRT; as a continuous variable in units of years) as confounders. In the association analysis, 3 metabolites were associated with femoral neck BMD, 13 metabolites with total hip BMD, and 10 metabolites with lumbar spine BMD (15 metabolites in total, Fig. 5.1); all of these metabolites had a significant p-value after Bonferroni correction for multiple testing ($P < 1.79 \times 10^{-4}$; 0.05 divided by 280, for the number of known metabolites).

Replication in HKOS

To evaluate if these metabolites are also associated with BMD in another ethnic group, a replication study was conducted in the HKOS. A replication study was done using robust regression with adjustment for age, sex, height, and weight. HRT was not adjusted because participants who were on HRT were excluded from

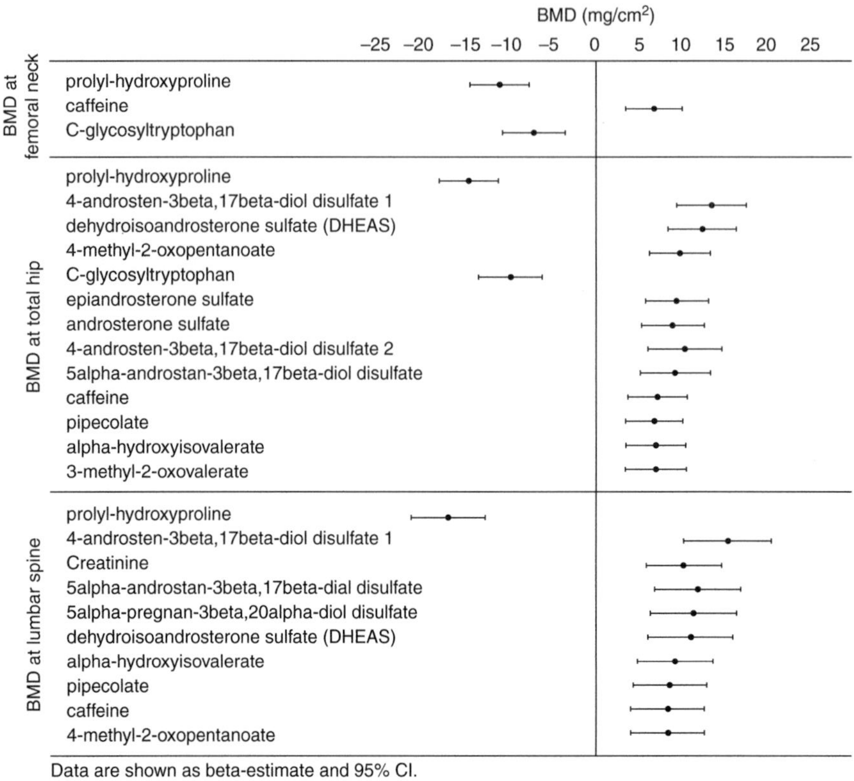

Fig. 5.1 Discovery phase of metabolomic study of BMD in TwinsUK. Data are shown as beta-estimate and 95% CI

the study. Among these 15 metabolites tested, 4 of them were successfully replicated in the HKOS, with the same direction of association (Fig. 5.2). These were 4-androsten-3beta,17beta-diol disulfate 1, epiandrosterone sulfate, androsterone sulfate, and 5alpha-androstan-3beta,17beta-diol disulfate, with beta-estimates ranging from 8.25 to 27.59 mg/cm^2, 7.42 to 20.15 mg/cm^2, and 7.77 to 23.45 mg/cm^2 for BMD at the lumbar spine L1–L4, femoral neck, and total hip, respectively. These metabolites belong to the dehydroepiandrosterone (DHEA) metabolic pathway.

Mendelian Randomization (MR) Study

Observational study cannot infer causality. Thus, it is unknown if these replicated metabolites were causally associated with BMD variation. Thus, a MR analysis was conducted to infer causality. The genetic instrument of androsterone sulfate, epiandrosterone sulfate, and 5alpha-androstan-3beta,17beta-diol disulfate was rs4646450 located on chromosome 7q22.1, whereas the genetic instrument of

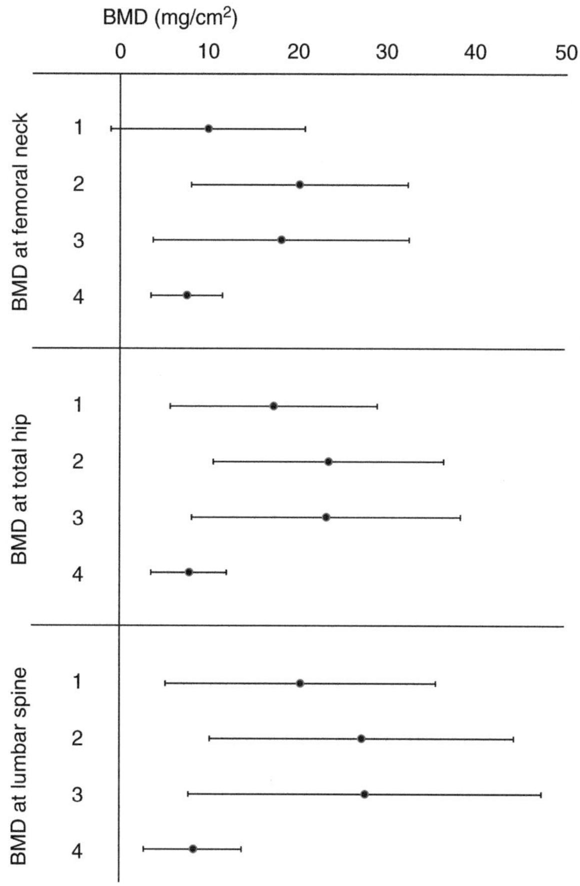

Fig. 5.2 Replication study of the metabolites in the HKOS. Metabolites 1, 2, 3, and 4 correspond to "4-androsten-3beta,17beta-diol disulfate 1," epiandrosterone sulfate, androsterone sulfate, and "5alpha-androstan-3beta,17beta-diol disulfate," respectively. Data are shown as beta-estimate and 95% CI

4-androsten-3beta,17beta-diol disulfate 1 was rs16981893 located on chromosome 19q13.33. Using the direct instrumental variables analysis, all four metabolites showed causal associations with BMD traits (Table 5.2).

Summary

Using integrative omic (metabolomic + genome-wide association) approach, four metabolites related to sulfated adrenal androgens (4-androsten-3beta,17beta-diol disulfate 1, epiandrosterone sulfate, androsterone sulfate, and 5alpha-androstan-3beta,17beta-diol disulfate) were significantly associated with BMD variation, whereas such association was estimated to be causal using MR approach. Given that these metabolites are related to dehydroepiandrosterone (DHEA) metabolism, the current findings are in agreement with the clinical trials showing that DHEA supplementation may improve BMD in human [14, 15]. It is an important observation, because the finding implies that this integrative omic approach can identify novel metabolite that can be used as dietary supplement for treating osteoporosis.

Table 5.2 MR analysis of the replicated metabolites in the TwinsUK study

Metabolite	SNP	EA/ OA	Trait	IV (SNP → metabolite → trait) Beta (SE)	Beta (SE)*	*P*	95% CI (10,000 permutations)
Androsterone sulfate	rs4646450	G/A	FN-BMD	−10.23 (3.5)	25.9 (9.0)	0.0041	(8.2,43.6)
			TH-BMD	−10.25 (3.63)	25.9 (9.2)	0.0049	(7.9,44.0)
			SP-BMD	−11.4 (4.58)	29.1 (11.9)	0.0147	(5.7,52.6)
Epiandrosterone sulfate	rs4646450	G/A	FN-BMD	−10.23 (3.5)	29.6 (10.5)	0.0047	(9.1,50.1)
			TH-BMD	−10.25 (3.63)	29.6 (11)	0.0073	(7.9,51.3)
			SP-BMD	−11.4 (4.58)	33.3 (13.5)	0.0140	(6.7,59.8)
5alpha-androstan-3beta,17beta-diol disulfate	rs4646450	G/A	FN-BMD	−10.23 (3.5)	62.8 (22.8)	0.0059	(18.1107.5)
			TH-BMD	−10.25 (3.63)	56.6 (23.8)	0.0172	(10.0,103.1)
			SP-BMD	−11.4 (4.58)	64.2 (28.7)	0.0256	(7.8120.5)
4-androsten-3beta,17beta-diol disulfate 1	rs16981893	G/A	FN-BMD	5.72 (3.34)	59.7 (28)	0.0329	(4.8114.5)
			TH-BMD	8.33 (3.5)	71.6 (31)	0.0207	(10.9132.2)
			SP-BMD	15.66 (4.34)	110.4 (37)	0.0032	(37.0,183.7)

In the current study, only 280 metabolites were analyzed, whereas the most updated metabolomic platform can identify more than 1000 metabolites in a simple serum sample. Thus, it is expected that future metabolomic study using a larger metabolite set can discover even more new metabolites associating with BMD variation. As aforementioned, there is a "crisis in the osteoporosis treatment" worldwide, mainly due to the patients' awareness of the rare side effect of the commonly used anti-osteoporotic medication. Therefore, the newly identified metabolite may be used as a novel intervention for treating osteoporosis. Since the metabolite is naturally present in human, it is expected that the side effect could be minimal, compared to other pharmacological agent, and therefore it may be more acceptable by patients.

Acknowledgment Metabolomic study in the Hong Kong Osteoporosis Study was funded by Early Career Scheme, Research Grant Council, Hong Kong (HKU: 27100416).

References

1. Hsu YH, Kiel DP. Clinical review: genome-wide association studies of skeletal phenotypes: what we have learned and where we are headed. J Clin Endocrinol Metab. 2012;97:E1958–77.
2. Cheung CL, Xiao SM, Kung AW. Genetic epidemiology of age-related osteoporosis and its clinical applications. Nat Rev Rheumatol. 2010;6:507–17.
3. McLean RR, Jacques PF, Selhub J, Tucker KL, Samelson EJ, Broe KE, Hannan MT, Cupples LA, Kiel DP. Homocysteine as a predictive factor for hip fracture in older persons. N Engl J Med. 2004;350:2042–9.
4. Zhang H, Tao X, Wu J. Association of homocysteine, vitamin B12, and folate with bone mineral density in postmenopausal women: a meta-analysis. Arch Gynecol Obstet. 2014;289:1003–9.
5. Napoli N, Faccio R, Shrestha V, Bucchieri S, Rini GB, Armamento-Villareal R. Estrogen metabolism modulates bone density in men. Calcif Tissue Int. 2007;80:227–32.
6. Napoli N, Thompson J, Civitelli R, Armamento-Villareal RC. Effects of dietary calcium compared with calcium supplements on estrogen metabolism and bone mineral density. Am J Clin Nutr. 2007;85:1428–33.
7. Napoli N, Rini GB, Serber D, Giri T, Yarramaneni J, Bucchieri S, Camarda L, Di Fede G, Camarda MR, Jain S, Mumm S, Armamento-Villareal R. The Val432Leu polymorphism of the CYP1B1 gene is associated with differences in estrogen metabolism and bone density. Bone. 2009;44:442–8.
8. Rhee EP, Clish CB, Ghorbani A, Larson MG, Elmariah S, McCabe E, Yang Q, Cheng S, Pierce K, Deik A, Souza AL, Farrell L, Domos C, Yeh RW, Palacios I, Rosenfield K, Vasan RS, Florez JC, Wang TJ, Fox CS, Gerszten RE. A combined epidemiologic and metabolomic approach improves CKD prediction. J Am Soc Nephrol. 2013;24:1330–8.
9. Wang TJ, Ngo D, Psychogios N, Dejam A, Larson MG, Vasan RS, Ghorbani A, O'Sullivan J, Cheng S, Rhee EP, Sinha S, McCabe E, Fox CS, O'Donnell CJ, Ho JE, Florez JC, Magnusson M, Pierce KA, Souza AL, Yu Y, Carter C, Light PE, Melander O, Clish CB, Gerszten RE. 2-Aminoadipic acid is a biomarker for diabetes risk. J Clin Investig. 2013;123:4309–17.
10. You YS, Lin CY, Liang HJ, Lee SH, Tsai KS, Chiou JM, Chen YC, Tsao CK, Chen JH. Association between the metabolome and low bone mineral density in Taiwanese women determined by (1)H NMR spectroscopy. J Bone Miner Res. 2014;29:212–22.
11. Spector TD, Williams FM. The UK adult twin registry (TwinsUK). Twin Res Hum Genet. 2006;9:899–906.
12. Cheung CL, Tan KC, Kung AW. Cohort profile: the Hong Kong osteoporosis study and the follow-up study. Int J Epidemiol. 2018;47:397–398f. https://doi.org/10.1093/ije/dyx172.
13. Menni C, Kastenmuller G, Petersen AK, Bell JT, Psatha M, Tsai PC, Gieger C, Schulz H, Erte I, John S, Brosnan MJ, Wilson SG, Tsaprouni L, Lim EM, Stuckey B, Deloukas P, Mohney R, Suhre K, Spector TD, Valdes AM. Metabolomic markers reveal novel pathways of ageing and early development in human populations. Int J Epidemiol. 2013;42:1111–9.
14. von Muhlen D, Laughlin GA, Kritz-Silverstein D, Bergstrom J, Bettencourt R. Effect of dehydroepiandrosterone supplementation on bone mineral density, bone markers, and body composition in older adults: the DAWN trial. Osteoporos Int. 2008;19:699–707.
15. Jankowski CM, Gozansky WS, Schwartz RS, Dahl DJ, Kittelson JM, Scott SM, Van Pelt RE, Kohrt WM. Effects of dehydroepiandrosterone replacement therapy on bone mineral density in older adults: a randomized, controlled trial. J Clin Endocrinol Metab. 2006;91:2986–93.

Dietary Mineral Intake Ratios and Bone Health in Adults

6

Andrea J. Lobene, Linda D. McCabe, Michael S. Stone, Joseph M. Kindler, Regan L. Bailey, Alanna J. Moshfegh, Donna G. Rhodes, Joseph D. Goldman, George P. McCabe, and Connie M. Weaver

Introduction

Dairy products are rich in minerals including calcium, potassium, and magnesium and have long been considered advantageous for bone health. For example, dairy intake was shown to be significantly related to BMD at the total hip and femoral neck in elderly white and black women, though not men [1]. In addition, a diet abundant in fruits and vegetables has been regarded for many years as not only optimal for overall general health but for bone health as well. Fruits and vegetables are rich in the minerals that are required for the development and maintenance of healthy bone (e.g., calcium, potassium, magnesium) and may also provide various bioactive constituents (e.g., phytochemicals, polyphenols) that help to further promote favorable bone outcomes [2, 3]. Cross-sectional, observational studies have consistently supported a benefit of fruit and vegetable intakes on bone health in adolescent boys and girls [4–7], pre- and postmenopausal women [6, 8], and elderly men and women [4, 9].

Several mechanisms may explain the relationships between mineral intake, especially potassium, and bone health. Alkaline potassium salts, which are derived from fruits and vegetables and are present in potassium supplements (potassium bicarbonate or citrate), are thought to protect against bone resorption and maintain pH homeostasis (~7.35–7.45). The impact of excess systemic acid on bone may also be mediated directly via cell based mechanisms (e.g., upregulation of bone resorbing cell [osteoclast] activity) [10]. Although evidence for the interaction between systemic acid-base balance and bone health-related outcomes is

A. J. Lobene · L. D. McCabe · M. S. Stone · J. M. Kindler · R. L. Bailey · C. M. Weaver (✉)
Department of Nutrition Science, Purdue University, West Lafayette, IN, USA
e-mail: weavercm@purdue.edu

A. J. Moshfegh · D. G. Rhodes · J. D. Goldman
Food Surveys Research Group, USDA, ARS, Beltsville, MD, USA

G. P. McCabe
Department of Statistics, Purdue University, West Lafayette, IN, USA

© Springer Nature Switzerland AG 2019

C. M. Weaver et al. (eds.), *Nutritional Influences on Bone Health*,
https://doi.org/10.1007/978-3-319-98464-3_6

conflicting [11, 12], higher potassium intakes have been associated with reduced urinary calcium excretion and improvement in overall calcium balance [13, 14]. In women who participated in the Aberdeen Prospective Osteoporosis Screening Study (APOSS) (45–49 years of age, $n = 994$), low fruit and vegetable intakes during early adulthood were associated with lower lumbar spine (LS) and trochanteric bone mineral density (BMD) ($P < 0.01$). Additionally, potassium consumption was associated with greater LS, femoral neck (FN), and trochanteric BMD, and this relationship remained significant after adjustment for confounding variables, including age, weight, height, physical activity, socioeconomic status, and smoking ($P < 0.05$) [8]. In a second study by the same group in a similar population, women aged 45–55 years with lower intakes of fruits and vegetables had lower forearm BMD and higher bone resorption, with potassium intake accounting for 7.4% of the variation in forearm BMD [15]. Collectively, these results support a potential positive influence of fruit and vegetable intake on bone health, which might be attributed to potassium intake.

While dietary intervention studies assessing the impact of specific nutrients are sparse, the DASH trial and implementation of the DASH diet show a link between a higher potassium intake and improved bone health. In an ancillary study to the DASH trial, Lin et al. found that the DASH diet significantly reduced bone turnover (osteocalcin by 8–11% and CTX by 16–18%) in men and women ages 23–76 years [16]. Findings from supplement trials generally show a persistent hypocalciuria in both men and women provided potassium supplements [13, 17]. In a recent randomized, double-blind, placebo-controlled study, men and women ($n = 52$) randomly assigned to 6 months of 60 or 90 mmol/day of potassium citrate supplementation had decreases in urinary calcium and net acid excretion resulting in positive calcium balance on the highest dose, compared to control (0 mmol/day) [14]. Serum CTX, a marker of bone turnover, also decreased significantly in both potassium groups. Further, Jehle et al. showed that 24 months of 60 mEQ potassium citrate/day versus placebo resulted in favorable changes in spine areal BMD (aBMD), trabecular bone microarchitecture, and FRAX index score in older adults (ages >65 years) [18]. While limited, findings suggest the importance of potassium form and dose in any potential benefit for bone.

In contrast to potassium, sodium intake appears to be detrimental to bone health. In a controlled feeding study in postmenopausal women, urinary calcium increased, and calcium balance became more negative on high salt intakes [19]. Reductions in sodium have also been shown to benefit bone. For example, in the DASH-sodium trial, reductions in sodium intake decreased calcium excretion for both control and DASH diet groups [16]. In addition, no bone loss was observed in a 2-year longitudinal study of 124 postmenopausal women if urinary sodium levels were below 2100 mg/day (92 mmol/day) [20]. Given the interactions between sodium (Na) and potassium (K) in the body, it may be more important to consider the intake of both minerals concurrently when exploring the relationship between intake and disease risk. Indeed, a recent cross-sectional study in Chinese adults found an inverse association between Na/K and BMD, but no association with either mineral by itself [21]. We know that other minerals, including calcium and magnesium, are also important for bone health, but no studies have explored the association between other mineral intake ratios and bone outcomes. Therefore, the relationship between mineral intake ratios and bone health remains uncertain.

Study Aims

The aim of this study was to assess the relationship between sodium, potassium, calcium, and magnesium intake and their ratios and aBMD and fracture incidence in a representative sample of US adults.

Methods

Study Participants and Demographic Data

This analysis was completed using data from the National Health and Nutrition Examination Survey (NHANES), 2013–2014. NHANES is a nationally representative, cross-sectional health examination survey that is planned and conducted by the US Centers for Disease Control and Prevention and National Center for Health Statistics (NCHS). Non-institutionalized, civilian US residents are sampled using a complex, stratified, multistage probability cluster sampling design. The NHANES survey protocol was approved by the National Center for Health Statistics research ethics review board. Written informed consent was obtained from all participants, and data were collected through an in-home interview and a visit to a mobile exam center (MEC).

For this analysis, we included adult men and women ≥40 years of age, who were not pregnant or lactating, with complete and plausible data. The final analytical sample was $n = 2617$. Demographic data, including sex, age, and race/ethnicity, were collected by a computer-assisted personal interview in the participants' homes. The self-reported race/ethnic groups are defined by NHANES as non-Hispanic white, non-Hispanic black, Hispanic and Mexican American, non-Hispanic Asian, and "other" (referred to hereafter as white, black, Hispanic, and Asian). The "other" group is represented in the estimates for the total sample, but per the NCHS guidelines, it is not presented separately in this analysis. Tobacco smoking status was categorized as yes or no based on self-report. Height and weight were measured in the MEC and were used to calculate BMI as kg/m^2.

Dietary Data

Dietary data in NHANES were collected as part of the What We Eat in America (WWEIA) survey (USDA, 2014) using the USDA's automated multiple-pass method (AMPM) [22, 23]. Two 24-h dietary recalls were collected that capture all foods, beverages, and dietary supplements consumed within the previous 24 h. The first 24-h recall was collected in the MEC, and the second was collected 3–10 days later via telephone. The AMPM methodology used for the 24-h dietary recall has been validated for sodium and potassium; reporting accuracy, calculated as the ratio of reported sodium intake to that estimated from the urinary biomarker, was 0.93 (95% CI, 0.89–0.97) for males and 0.90 (95% CI, 0.87–0.94) for females on average [24]. Recovery biomarkers do not exist to estimate the magnitude of misreporting for calcium and magnesium. To determine dietary intake, we used the average of the two 24-h recalls. The USDA Food and Nutrient Database for Dietary Studies was used to convert foods and beverages as reported into gram amounts and to determine their respective energy and nutrient content [25]. In addition to dietary intake, comprehensive information on use of all types of prescription and non-prescription dietary supplements were collected during the household interview; detailed collection procedures have been described elsewhere [26]. Briefly, trained interviewers asked participants to provide supplement product containers if they were available; containers were available for >80% of the reported supplements. Information regarding product type, name, frequency/duration of use, and dosage were recorded for each supplement reported during the interview. During the 24-h recall, trained interviewers asked participants if they used the products reported in the home and collected detailed information on any new products added since the home interview. Average daily intake of nutrients from all supplements and medications that may contain nutrients was calculated for individuals by the National Center for Health Statistics using the information provided by the participant.

Nutrient content from foods, beverages, and dietary supplements were combined and used to estimate intake of sodium, potassium, magnesium, and calcium as well as the mineral intake ratios sodium/potassium (Na/K), sodium/calcium (Na/Ca), sodium/magnesium (Na/Mg), and calcium/magnesium (Ca/Mg). The targeted values for these ratios were determined based on Dietary Reference Intakes for each individual nutrient, which are as follows: <2300 mg/day (100 mmol/day) for sodium, 4700 mg/day (120 mmol/day) for potassium, 1000 mg/day (25 mmol/day) for calcium, and 320 mg/day (13.2 mmol/day) for magnesium for women aged >31 years and 420 mg/day (17.3 mmol/day) for men >31 years, [27–29]. The RDA for calcium increases to 1200 mg/day in older adults, but we considered this increase to be trivial and used the RDA of 1000 mg/day to calculate the target mineral intake ratios. Based on intake recommendations in mg/day, the calculated target mineral intake ratios were as follows: 0.49 for Na/K, 2.3 for Na/Ca, 7.19 for Na/Mg for women and 5.48 for men, and 3.13 for Ca/Mg for women and 2.38 for men. Based on intake recommendations in mmol/day, the calculated mineral intake ratios were as follows: 0.83 for Na/K, 4.04 for Na/Ca, 7.60 for Na/Mg for women and 5.78 for men, and 1.90 for Ca/Mg for women and 1.44 for men.

Bone Outcomes

Dual-energy X-ray absorptiometry (DXA) scans of the proximal femur were performed in the MEC. Scans were acquired on Hologic QDR-4500A fan-beam densitometers (Hologic, Inc., Bedford, Massachusetts) using Apex software version 3.2 and were analyzed using APEX software version 4.0. The left hip was routinely scanned unless the participant self-reported a fractured left hip, a left hip replacement, or a pin in the left hip, in which case the right hip was scanned. Participants were excluded from the femur scan if they had fractured both hips, had replacement of both hips, or had pins in both hips. Femur scans provided bone measurements of aBMD for the total femur and femoral neck. Self-report of previous fracture after age 20 years was determined using a computer-assisted personal interview in the participants' homes. The questionnaire asked about incidence of hip fracture, wrist fracture, spine fracture, or other fractures. The responses to these four items were summarized into a single "previous self-reported fracture" item and were categorized as either yes or no.

Statistical Analyses

All statistical analyses were performed using SAS software (Version 9.4, SAS Institute Inc.) and SAS-callable Sudan software (Version 11.0; RTI International). NHANES sample weights were used to account for differential non-response and/or non-coverage, to adjust for planned oversampling of some groups, and to adjust the dietary data for uneven representation of days of the week. Since intakes of sodium, potassium, calcium, and magnesium were strongly skewed to the right, all analyses were performed using logs of these variables and their ratios. Extreme outliers of protein and calorie intake were Winsorized to reduce their influence.

Regression models were used to examine the association of individual minerals and their ratios with total femur aBMD, femoral neck aBMD, and fracture incidence controlled for known covariates. Parallel analyses were performed for total femur aBMD, femoral neck aBMD, and fracture incidence, and men and women were analyzed separately. A model for predicting bone outcomes was developed using the following explanatory variables: age, race, height, weight, and a binary indicator of current smoking status. Effects of individual mineral intakes and their ratios separately were assessed by adding each of these terms to the basic model. Subsets of these mineral variables were also examined. Statistical significance was set at $P \leq 0.05$.

Results

Subject characteristics and usual mineral intakes for the 1302 men and 1315 women who met our inclusion criteria are given in Table 6.1. Usual intakes of sodium were higher than the recommended 2300 mg/day, usual intakes of potassium and magnesium were below the recommendations, and usual intakes of calcium were at the recommended level. In addition, mineral intakes were highly correlated, with correlation coefficients ranging from $r = 0.59$ to $r = 0.87$. Figure 6.1 shows the distribution of usual mineral intake ratios relative to the recommended

Table 6.1 Participant characteristics

Characteristic	Women (n = 1315)	Men (n = 1302)
Age, year	57.95 ± 11.71	58.60 ± 11.78
Height, cm	160.16 ± 6.92	173.94 ± 7.73
Weight, kg	75.28 ± 18.91	86.61 ± 19.15
Body mass index, kg/m^2	29.29 ± 6.87	28.52 ± 5.40
Race/ethnicity, %		
Non-Hispanic white	72%	73%
Non-Hispanic black	10%	10%
Hispanic	11%	11%
Non-Hispanic Asian	5%	4%
Current smoker, %		
Yes	16%	17%
No	84%	83%
Areal bone mineral density (g/cm^2)		
Total femur	0.81 ± 0.16	0.91 ± 0.16
Femoral neck	0.65 ± 0.14	0.75 ± 0.16
Fracture since age 20 years, %		
Yes	31%	20%
No	69%	80%
Usual mineral intake, mg		
Sodium	2851 ± 1155	3823 ± 1607
Potassium	2328 ± 872	2926 ± 1100
Calcium	1055 ± 596	1063 ± 571
Magnesium	267 ± 104	329 ± 136

Values represent the mean ± SD unless otherwise indicated

mineral intake ratios, based on intake recommendations expressed in mmol, for men and women. Less than 1% of women and men (0.88% and 0.23%, respectively) achieved the desired Na/K intake ratio. In addition, 14.15% of women and 2.28% of men achieved the desired Na/Mg ratio, 13.0% of women and 6.82% of men achieved the desired Na/Ca ratio, and 53.52% of women and 30.53% of men achieved the desired Ca/Mg ratio.

Table 6.2 outlines the factors that were predictive of bone mineral density in men and women. Weight explained more than 15% of the variation in total femur and femoral neck aBMD in both men and women. Age accounted for about 20% of the variation in total femur and femoral neck aBMD in women, but less than 6% of the variation in men. Race accounted for 3–7% of the variation in aBMD in both men and women, with blacks exhibiting greater aBMD than other races. In our sample of nearly 3000 individuals, 365 women and 368 men reported having a previous fracture. Table 6.3 shows the factors that were predictive of fracture incidence in men and women. In women, race was significantly positively associated with fracture incidence, with whites having greater fracture incidence than any other race. Age was also significantly positively associated with fracture incidence in women, with age and race each accounting for approximately 3% of the variation in fracture incidence. Weight was a significant positive predictor of fracture in women, though it

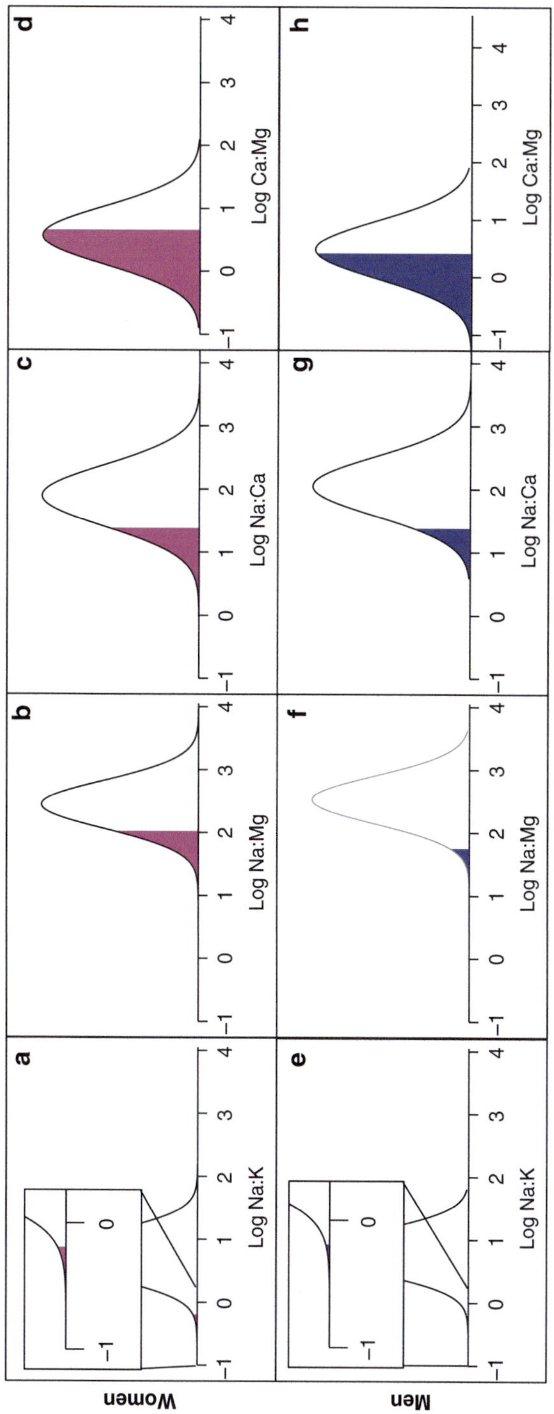

Fig. 6.1 Usual mineral intake ratio distributions in adult women (**a–d**) and men (**e–h**). Shaded areas represent the percent below the recommended intake ratio, indicating they achieved the desired mineral intake ratio. Ratios are based on mineral intake recommendations expressed in mmol. Percentages displayed in figure represent the percent of women and men, respectively, that meet the desired mineral intake ratio

Table 6.2 Predictors of bone mineral density in the US National Health and Nutrition Examination Survey, 2013–2014

	Femoral neck aBMD		Total Femur aBMD	
	Women	Men	Women	Men
Age, year	$R^2 = 0.20$** Negative coefficient	$R^2 = 0.06$** Negative coefficient	$R^2 = 0.17$** Negative coefficient	$R^2 = 0.02$** Negative coefficient
Height	$R^2 = 0.09$** Positive coefficient	$R^2 = 0.04$** Positive coefficient	$R^2 = 0.06$** Positive coefficient	$R^2 = 0.03$** Positive coefficient
Weight	$R^2 = 0.22$** Positive coefficient	$R^2 = 0.15$** Positive coefficient	$R^2 = 0.29$** Positive coefficient	$R^2 = 0.21$** Positive coefficient
Smoking	$R^2 = 0.003$* No>yes	$R^2 = 0.003$	$R^2 = 0.008$* No>yes	$R^2 = 0.009$* No>yes
Race/ethnicity[a]	$R^2 = 0.07$** B > H > W, A	$R^2 = 0.06$** B > H > W, A	$R^2 = 0.04$** B,H > W,A	$R^2 = 0.03$** B > W,A
Total model	$R^2 = 0.41$	$R^2 = 0.24$	$R^2 = 0.42$	$R^2 = 0.25$

B black, *A* Asian, *W* white, *H* Hispanic, *aBMD* areal bone mineral density
*$p < 0.05$
**$p < 0.001$
[a]There are ten comparisons. The adjusted p value requirement for each comparison is 0.005 based on a Bonferroni correction

Table 6.3 Predictors of fracture incidence in the US National Health and Nutrition Examination Survey, 2013–2014

	Women	Men
Age, year	$R^2 = 0.03$** Positive coefficient	$R^2 = 0.003$
Height	$R^2 = 0.001$	$R^2 = 0.0004$
Weight	$R^2 = 0.003$* Positive coefficient	$R^2 = 0.0001$
Smoking	$R^2 = 0.003$	$R^2 = 0.01$* Yes>no
Race/ethnicity[a]	$R^2 = 0.03$** W > B,H,A	$R^2 = 0.02$* W > B,A
Total model	$R^2 = 0.06$	$R^2 = 0.04$

B black, *A* Asian, *W* white, *H* Hispanic
*$p < 0.05$
**$p < 0.001$
[a]There are ten comparisons. The adjusted p value requirement for each comparison is 0.005 based on a Bonferroni correction

explained only a fraction of the variance in fracture incidence. In men, race accounted for 2% of the variation in fracture incidence, with whites being greater than other races. The final model used to predict bone outcomes included age, race, height, weight, and smoking status. Final models for women resulted in $R^2 = 0.25$ for predicting total femur aBMD, $R^2 = 0.24$ for predicting femoral neck aBMD, and

$R^2 = 0.06$ for predicting fracture incidence. Final models for men resulted in $R^2 = 0.25$ for predicting total femur aBMD, $R^2 = 0.24$ for predicting femoral neck aBMD, and $R^2 = 0.04$ for predicting fracture incidence.

Mineral intakes and mineral intake ratios were added individually to the original model for predicting femoral neck and total femur aBMD. Dietary mineral and mineral ratio predictors of aBMD are given in Table 6.4. The R^2 values shown in the table represent the R^2 for the original prediction model (including age, height, weight, race, and smoking status) plus the mineral or mineral ratio of interest. Mineral intakes and mineral intake ratios each explained <2% of the variation in femoral neck and total femur aBMD in both men and women, as shown by the negligible increases in the model R^2 values. After adjusting for age, height, weight, race, and smoking status, log sodium ($p = 0.02$), log potassium ($p = 0.04$), and log calcium ($p = 0.04$) were significant positive predictors of total femur aBMD in men. Similarly, log sodium ($p < 0.01$), log potassium ($p = 0.03$), and log calcium ($p < 0.01$) were significant positive predictors of femoral neck aBMD in men. Log magnesium was a positive predictor of femoral neck aBMD ($p = 0.02$) in men, and appeared to be a positive predictor of total femur aBMD, though the relationship did not reach statistical significance ($p = 0.06$). Log

Table 6.4 Dietary mineral and mineral ratio predictors of bone mineral density in the US National Health and Nutrition Examination Survey, 2013–2014

	Femoral neck aBMD		Total femur aBMD	
Prediction model with age, height, weight, race, and smoking	Women	Men	Women	Men
	$R^2 = 0.41$	$R^2 = 0.24$	$R^2 = 0.42$	$R^2 = 0.25$
Mineral intake (log)[a]				
Sodium	$R^2 = 0.41$	$R^2 = 0.25$* Positive coefficient	$R^2 = 0.43$	$R^2 = 0.25$* Positive coefficient
Potassium	$R^2 = 0.41$	$R^2 = 0.25$* Positive coefficient	$R^2 = 0.42$	$R^2 = 0.26$* Positive coefficient
Calcium	$R^2 = 0.41$	$R^2 = 0.25$* Positive coefficient	$R^2 = 0.42$	$R^2 = 0.25$* Positive coefficient
Magnesium	$R^2 = 0.41$	$R^2 = 0.25$* Positive coefficient	$R^2 = 0.42$	$R^2 = 0.26$
Mineral intake ratios (log)[a]				
Na/K	$R^2 = 0.41$	$R^2 = 0.25$	$R^2 = 0.42$	$R^2 = 0.25$
Na/Ca	$R^2 = 0.41$	$R^2 = 0.25$	$R^2 = 0.42$	$R^2 = 0.25$
Na/Mg	$R^2 = 0.41$	$R^2 = 0.25$	$R^2 = 0.42$	$R^2 = 0.25$
Ca/Mg	$R^2 = 0.41$	$R^2 = 0.24$	$R^2 = 0.42$	$R^2 = 0.25$

aBMD areal bone mineral density

*$p < 0.05$

[a]Mineral intake and mineral intake ratios were added one at a time to the original prediction model including age, height, weight, race, and smoking; R^2 values represent R^2 of original model plus each individual mineral or mineral ratio

Table 6.5 Dietary mineral and mineral ratio predictors of fracture incidence in the US National Health and Nutrition Examination Survey, 2013–2014

Prediction model with age, height, weight, race, and smoking	Women	Men
	$R^2 = 0.06$	$R^2 = 0.04$
Mineral intake (log)[a]		
Sodium	$R^2 = 0.07$	$R^2 = 0.04$* Negative coefficient
Potassium	$R^2 = 0.06$	$R^2 = 0.04$
Calcium	$R^2 = 0.06$	$R^2 = 0.04$
Magnesium	$R^2 = 0.07$	$R^2 = 0.04$
Mineral intake ratios (log)[a]		
Sodium/potassium	$R^2 = 0.06$	$R^2 = 0.04$
Sodium/calcium	$R^2 = 0.06$	$R^2 = 0.04$
Sodium/magnesium	$R^2 = 0.06$	$R^2 = 0.04$
Calcium/magnesium	$R^2 = 0.06$	$R^2 = 0.04$

*$p = 0.053$
[a]Mineral intake and mineral intake ratios were added one at a time to the original prediction model including age, height, weight, race, and smoking; R^2 values represent R^2 of original model plus each individual mineral or mineral ratio

sodium appeared to be a positive predictor of total femur aBMD after adjusting for the same factors in women, though the relationship did not reach statistical significance ($p = 0.05$). Mineral intake ratios were not significant predictors of total femur or femoral neck aBMD in men nor in women. Similarly, mineral intakes and mineral intake ratios were added individually to the original model for predicting fracture incidence. Table 6.5 shows the dietary mineral and mineral ratio predictors of fracture incidence in men and women. The R^2 values shown in the table represent the R^2 for the original prediction model (including age, height, weight, race, and smoking status) plus the mineral or mineral ratio of interest. Mineral intakes and mineral intake ratios each explained <2% of the variation in fracture incidence in both men and women, as shown by the negligible increases in the model R^2 values. Log sodium appeared to be a negative predictor of fracture risk in men ($p = 0.03$), but after adjusting for age, height, weight, race, and smoking status, the relationship was no longer significant ($p = 0.053$). No other relationships between mineral intake and mineral ratios and fracture incidence in men were observed, and no relationships between minerals and mineral ratios and fracture were observed in women.

To further examine the relationship between minerals and bone, separate log regression analyses were conducted on a subsample who fell within the lower quartile of total femur and femoral neck aBMD, with separate analyses conducted in men and women. We observed 327 women and 322 men in the lower quartile of femoral neck aBMD and 322 of each sex in the lower quartile of total femur aBMD. After adjusting for age, height, weight, race, and smoking status, log calcium and logCa/Mg were significant negative predictors of femoral neck aBMD ($p = 0.048$ and $p = 0.03$, respectively), whereas logNa/Ca was a significant positive predictor of femoral neck aBMD (0.03) in men. Minerals and mineral ratios were not predictive of femoral neck aBMD in women in the lower quartile of aBMD. In addition, mineral intake and mineral ratios were not predictive of total femur aBMD in this subsample.

Discussion

In our nationally representative sample of US adults, we found that age, weight, and race explained most of the variation in bone outcomes. Sodium, potassium, calcium, and magnesium intake were positive predictors of aBMD in men, but not in women. Though previous studies have reported the Na/K ratio is inversely related to aBMD in adults [21], mineral intake ratios were not predictive of aBMD in the current study. These conflicting results may be due to different methods of analyzing sodium and potassium intake. Because the current study found positive associations of individual mineral intakes and bone outcomes, but no associations with mineral ratios, this may suggest that the minerals assessed have an effect on bone that is independent of their interaction with other minerals. Interestingly, mineral intake was not predictive of fracture incidence in men or women, though this may be due to our relatively small sample that reported having a previous fracture.

The positive relationship between sodium intake and aBMD conflicts with previous literature suggesting that sodium has a negative effect on bone [19, 30]. The largest sources of dietary sodium in our sample were mixed dishes and protein foods, so we suspected the positive relationship between sodium and bone may be driven by a correlation between sodium and protein intake, as protein is known to be beneficial for bone [31]. However, when we added protein to our model, our results did not change. We also suspected that those who consume more energy per day may incidentally be consuming more minerals. We added energy intake to our model, but this also did not change our findings. Therefore, neither protein nor calorie intake was included in our final prediction models. In an effort to tease out the relationship between mineral intake and aBMD in those who could be at highest risk for fracture, we performed subgroup analyses on those who fell in the lower quartile of femoral neck aBMD. We found that log calcium and log Ca/Mg were significant negative predictors of femoral neck aBMD, whereas logNa/Ca was a significant positive predictor of femoral neck aBMD in men. While this seems to indicate that a lower calcium intake is linked to higher aBMD, it is more likely that for individuals in the lower quartile of aBMD, additional factors (e.g., genetics, lack of exercise) are negatively affecting aBMD that could not be controlled for.

Most Americans failed to meet the desired mineral intake ratios. These poor mineral intake ratios were driven by a high sodium intake combined with a low intake of potassium and magnesium. When considering the ratios involving calcium (i.e., Na/Ca and Ca/Mg), we chose to use the RDA of 1000 mg/day for calcium and disregard the increase to 1200 mg/day for women over age 50 years and men over age 70 years when calculating the ratios. If we recalculate the target Na/Ca and Ca/Mg ratios for older adults, more adults meet the desired target ratio for Ca/Mg, but fewer meet the desired target ratio for Na/Ca. Looking at the intake of all of these minerals in combination rather than individually is important because micronutrients are rarely consumed separately and often have interacting effects in the body. Our findings do not support a link between mineral ratios and bone outcomes. However, previous studies suggest that mineral intake ratios, especially Na/K, are important in considering risk factors for other chronic diseases. For instance, Na/K has been identified as a negative predictor of blood pressure, cardiovascular disease, and mortality [32, 33]. Further research is needed to confirm the utility of mineral intake ratios with respect to bone health.

Strengths of this study include the use of a large, nationally representative cohort of adults. This study also has limitations. One such limitation is that mineral intake was determined by self-report. The questionable reliability of self-reported sodium intake, especially in women and obese individuals [24], might have contributed to our inconclusive results. Fracture history was assessed via self-report, but fractures were not confirmed by radiological assessment. This approach might have introduced unwanted error in assessing fracture incidence. Furthermore, our cross-sectional design limits our ability to make any causal conclusions regarding the relationships between mineral intake, bone density, and skeletal fracture. Prospective observational studies and randomized controlled trials will help enhance our understanding of these processes.

Translational Implications: Achieving a Desirable Na to K Ratio

As outlined above, it is well established that sodium and potassium have contrasting effects on various aspects of human health. With respect to bone health, high sodium intake increases calcium excretion, and high potassium intake improves calcium balance as a result of modulations in bone turnover. Healthy individuals are recommended to consume a Na/K <1.0 [34]; however it has been noted that only about one in ten US adults meet this recommended intake balance [35]. Nonetheless, Yang et al. showed that consuming a Na/K < 1.0 was associated with more favorable cardiovascular health and a reduced risk of all-cause mortality [34]. Despite these and other findings that highlight the importance of considering sodium and potassium in conjunction while elucidating their roles in human health, practical and efficacious strategies to optimize the ratio of sodium and potassium intake are few and far between.

Simply, the Na/K can be improved by either reducing sodium or increasing potassium consumption. However, practically speaking, it is difficult to manipulate only a single nutrient in the diet. Bailey et al. examined food group contributors to sodium and potassium intake in individuals who consumed a Na/K less than or greater than 1.0 using data from NHANES [35]. These authors showed that mixed dishes such as sandwiches, soups, etc. and protein foods were the dominant contributors to sodium intake and that fruit/vegetables, dairy, and nonalcoholic beverages were the major sources of potassium for those who consumed a Na/K < 1.0. Therefore, these might be ideal target food groups to optimize the Na/K. Certain diet patterns such as the

Mediterranean diet and DASH diet have inherently favorable mineral ratios, including Na/K. With respect to DASH, this dietary pattern is associated with an optimal Na/K, as both potassium and sodium intake are fixed values and meet, or nearly meet, the DRIs (4700 mg and 3000 mg, respectively) [36]. This dietary pattern is high in fruits, vegetables, low-fat milk, whole grains, fish, poultry, nuts, and seeds, and has been linked to cardiovascular disease and type 2 diabetes risk reduction [37], likely due to beneficial effects on blood pressure, serum lipids, glucose metabolism, and systemic inflammation [36–38], as well as promotes favorable changes in bone turnover [16]. Therefore, adopting such dietary patterns may be useful for optimizing overall health, thereby reducing the risk for cardiometabolic disease and orthopedic complications such as skeletal fracture and osteoporosis later in life.

Conclusion

In summary, intakes of sodium, potassium, calcium, and magnesium individually were positive predictors of aBMD in men, but not in women. In addition, mineral intake ratios were not predictive of aBMD, which may suggest that the minerals assessed have an effect on bone that is independent of their interaction with other minerals. In the future, randomized, controlled, full-feeding studies should be conducted to determine the effect of consuming these minerals from food as well as the ratio of their intakes on bone outcomes. Such findings would have important implications for making dietary recommendations and designing dietary interventions for improving bone health.

Acknowledgments Author contributions: Drs. Weaver and G. McCabe had full access to all of the data in the study and take responsibility for the integrity of the data and the accuracy of the data analysis. Study concept and design: Weaver, Bailey, and G. McCabe. Acquisition, analysis, or interpretation of data: All authors. Drafting of the manuscript: Lobene, Kindler, Stone, and Weaver. Critical revision of the manuscript for important intellectual content: All authors. Statistical analysis: L. McCabe and G McCabe. Conflict of interest disclosures: Weaver is a scientific advisor for Pharmavite and Pfizer and is on the Board of the International Life Sciences Institute. Funding/support: The present work was supported by International Life Sciences Institute-North America. The funder had no role in the conduct of the study; collection, management, analysis, and interpretation of the data; preparation, review, or approval of the manuscript; and decision to submit the manuscript for publication.

References

1. McCabe LD, Martin BR, McCabe GP, Johnston CC, Weaver CM, Peacock M. Dairy intakes affect bone density in the elderly. Am J Clin Nutr. 2004;80(4):1066–74.
2. Weaver CM. Potassium and health. Adv Nutr. 2013;4(3):368s–77s. https://doi.org/10.3945/an.112.003533.
3. Muhlbauer RC, Lozano A, Reinli A. Onion and a mixture of vegetables, salads, and herbs affect bone resorption in the rat by a mechanism independent of their base excess. J Bone Miner Res. 2002;17(7):1230–6. https://doi.org/10.1359/jbmr.2002.17.7.1230.
4. Prynne CJ, Mishra GD, O'Connell MA, Muniz G, Laskey MA, Yan L, Prentice A, Ginty F. Fruit and vegetable intakes and bone mineral status: a cross sectional study in 5 age and sex cohorts. Am J Clin Nutr. 2006;83(6):1420–8.

5. Tylavsky FA, Holliday K, Danish R, Womack C, Norwood J, Carbone L. Fruit and vegetable intakes are an independent predictor of bone size in early pubertal children. Am J Clin Nutr. 2004;79(2):311–7.
6. Li JJ, Huang ZW, Wang RQ, Ma XM, Zhang ZQ, Liu Z, Chen YM, Su YX. Fruit and vegetable intake and bone mass in Chinese adolescents, young and postmenopausal women. Public Health Nutr. 2013;16(1):78–86. https://doi.org/10.1017/s1368980012001127.
7. Vatanparast H, Baxter-Jones A, Faulkner RA, Bailey DA, Whiting SJ. Positive effects of vegetable and fruit consumption and calcium intake on bone mineral accrual in boys during growth from childhood to adolescence: the University of Saskatchewan Pediatric Bone Mineral Accrual Study. Am J Clin Nutr. 2005;82(3):700–6.
8. New SA, Bolton-Smith C, Grubb DA, Reid DM. Nutritional influences on bone mineral density: a cross-sectional study in premenopausal women. Am J Clin Nutr. 1997;65(6):1831–9.
9. Tucker KL, Hannan MT, Chen H, Cupples LA, Wilson PW, Kiel DP. Potassium, magnesium, and fruit and vegetable intakes are associated with greater bone mineral density in elderly men and women. Am J Clin Nutr. 1999;69(4):727–36.
10. Brandao-Burch A, Utting JC, Orriss IR, Arnett TR. Acidosis inhibits bone formation by osteoblasts in vitro by preventing mineralization. Calcif Tissue Int. 2005;77(3):167–74. https://doi.org/10.1007/s00223-004-0285-8.
11. Hanley DA, Whiting SJ. Does a high dietary acid content cause bone loss, and can bone loss be prevented with an alkaline diet? J Clin Densitom. 2013;16(4):420–5. https://doi.org/10.1016/j.jocd.2013.08.014.
12. Lemann J Jr, Bushinsky DA, Hamm LL. Bone buffering of acid and base in humans. Am J Physiol Renal Physiol. 2003;285(5):F811–32. https://doi.org/10.1152/ajprenal.00115.2003.
13. Frassetto L, Morris RC Jr, Sebastian A. Long-term persistence of the urine calcium-lowering effect of potassium bicarbonate in postmenopausal women. J Clin Endocrinol Metab. 2005;90(2):831–4. https://doi.org/10.1210/jc.2004-1350.
14. Moseley KF, Weaver CM, Appel L, Sebastian A, Sellmeyer DE. Potassium citrate supplementation results in sustained improvement in calcium balance in older men and women. J Bone Miner Res. 2013;28(3):497–504. https://doi.org/10.1002/jbmr.1764.
15. New SA, Robins SP, Campbell MK, Martin JC, Garton MJ, Bolton-Smith C, Grubb DA, Lee SJ, Reid DM. Dietary influences on bone mass and bone metabolism: further evidence of a positive link between fruit and vegetable consumption and bone health? Am J Clin Nutr. 2000;71(1):142–51.
16. Lin PH, Ginty F, Appel LJ, Aickin M, Bohannon A, Garnero P, Barclay D, Svetkey LP. The DASH diet and sodium reduction improve markers of bone turnover and calcium metabolism in adults. J Nutr. 2003;133(10):3130–6.
17. Lemann J Jr, Gray RW, Pleuss JA. Potassium bicarbonate, but not sodium bicarbonate, reduces urinary calcium excretion and improves calcium balance in healthy men. Kidney Int. 1989;35(2):688–95.
18. Jehle S, Hulter HN, Krapf R. Effect of potassium citrate on bone density, microarchitecture, and fracture risk in healthy older adults without osteoporosis: a randomized controlled trial. J Clin Endocrinol Metab. 2013;98(1):207–17. https://doi.org/10.1210/jc.2012-3099.
19. Teucher B, Dainty JR, Spinks CA, Majsak-Newman G, Berry DJ, Hoogewerff JA, Foxall RJ, Jakobsen J, Cashman KD, Flynn A, et al. Sodium and bone health: impact of moderately high and low salt intakes on calcium metabolism in postmenopausal women. J Bone Miner Res. 2008;23(9):1477–85. https://doi.org/10.1359/jbmr.080408.
20. Devine A, Criddle RA, Dick IM, Kerr DA, Prince RL. A longitudinal study of the effect of sodium and calcium intakes on regional bone density in postmenopausal women. Am J Clin Nutr. 1995;62(4):740–5.
21. Cao WT, He J, Chen GD, Wang C, Qiu R, Chen YM. The association between urinary sodium to potassium ratio and bone density in middle-aged Chinese adults. Osteoporos Int. 2017;28(3):1077–86. https://doi.org/10.1007/s00198-016-3835-9.
22. Blanton CA, Moshfegh AJ, Baer DJ, Kretsch MJ. The USDA Automated Multiple-Pass Method accurately estimates group total energy and nutrient intake. J Nutr. 2006;136(10):2594–9.

23. Moshfegh AJ, Rhodes DG, Baer DJ, Murayi T, Clemens JC, Rumpler WV, Paul DR, Sebastian RS, Kuczynski KJ, Ingwersen LA, et al. The US Department of Agriculture Automated Multiple-Pass Method reduces bias in the collection of energy intakes. Am J Clin Nutr. 2008;88(2):324–32.
24. Rhodes DG, Murayi T, Clemens JC, Baer DJ, Sebastian RS, Moshfegh AJ. The USDA Automated Multiple-Pass Method accurately assesses population sodium intakes. Am J Clin Nutr. 2013;97(5):958–64. https://doi.org/10.3945/ajcn.112.044982.
25. United States Department of Agriculture ARS. Internet: https://www.ars.usda.gov/northeast-area/beltsville-md/beltsville-human-nutrition-research-center/food-surveys-research-group/docs/fndds-download-databases/.
26. Bailey RL, Gahche JJ, Miller PE, Thomas PR, Dwyer JT. Why US adults use dietary supplements. JAMA Intern Med. 2013;173(5):355–61. https://doi.org/10.1001/jamainternmed.2013.2299.
27. IOM (Institute of Medicine). Dietary reference intakes for calcium and vitamin D. Washington, DC: National Academies Press; 2011.
28. IOM (Institute of Medicine). Dietary reference intakes for calcium, phosphorus, magnesium, vitamin D, and fluoride. Washington, DC: National Academies Press; 1997.
29. IOM (Institute of Medicine). Dietary reference intakes for water, potassium, sodium, chloride, and sulfate. Washington, DC: National Academies Press; 2005.
30. Park SM, Joung JY, Cho YY, Sohn SY, Hur KY, Kim JH, Kim SW, Chung JH, Lee MK, Min YK. Effect of high dietary sodium on bone turnover markers and urinary calcium excretion in Korean postmenopausal women with low bone mass. Eur J Clin Nutr. 2015;69(3):361–6. https://doi.org/10.1038/ejcn.2014.284.
31. Cao JJ. High dietary protein intake and protein-related acid load on bone health. Curr Osteoporos Rep. 2017;15(6):571–6. https://doi.org/10.1007/s11914-017-0408-6.
32. Okayama A, Okuda N, Miura K, Okamura T, Hayakawa T, Akasaka H, Ohnishi H, Saitoh S, Arai Y, Kiyohara Y, et al. Dietary sodium-to-potassium ratio as a risk factor for stroke, cardiovascular disease and all-cause mortality in Japan: the NIPPON DATA 80 cohort study. BMJ Open. 2016;6(7):e011632. https://doi.org/10.1136/bmjopen-2016-011632.
33. Perez V, Chang ET. Sodium-to-potassium ratio and blood pressure, hypertension, and related factors. Adv Nutr. 2014;5(6):712–41. https://doi.org/10.3945/an.114.006783.
34. Yang Q, Liu T, Kuklina EV, Flanders WD, Hong Y, Gillespie C, Chang MH, Gwinn M, Dowling N, Khoury MJ, et al. Sodium and potassium intake and mortality among US adults: prospective data from the Third National Health and Nutrition Examination Survey. Arch Intern Med. 2011;171(13):1183–91. https://doi.org/10.1001/archinternmed.2011.257.
35. Bailey RL, Parker EA, Rhodes DG, Goldman JD, Clemens JC, Moshfegh AJ, Thuppal SV, Weaver CM. Estimating sodium and potassium intakes and their ratio in the American diet: data from the 2011-2012 NHANES. J Nutr. 2016. https://doi.org/10.3945/jn.115.221184.
36. Appel LJ, Moore TJ, Obarzanek E, Vollmer WM, Svetkey LP, Sacks FM, Bray GA, Vogt TM, Cutler JA, Windhauser MM, et al. A clinical trial of the effects of dietary patterns on blood pressure. DASH Collaborative Research Group. N Engl J Med. 1997;336(16):1117–24. https://doi.org/10.1056/nejm199704173361601.
37. Schwingshackl L, Bogensberger B, Hoffmann G. Diet quality as assessed by the healthy eating index, alternate healthy eating index, dietary approaches to stop hypertension score, and health outcomes: an updated systematic review and meta-analysis of cohort studies. J Acad Nutr Diet. 2018;118(1):74–100.e11. https://doi.org/10.1016/j.jand.2017.08.024.
38. Shirani F, Salehi-Abargouei A, Azadbakht L. Effects of Dietary Approaches to Stop Hypertension (DASH) diet on some risk for developing type 2 diabetes: a systematic review and meta-analysis on controlled clinical trials. Nutrition. 2013;29(7–8):939–47. https://doi.org/10.1016/j.nut.2012.12.021.

Dietary Calcium, Lifestyle Factors, and Bone Health in Premenarche Chinese Girls

7

Gordon C. L. Cheung and Yi-Xiang Su

Introduction

Osteoporosis and associated frailty receive much attention in the era of longevity and aging population globally, with special attention to the Asian countries due to the low dairy consumption. The median dietary calcium intake for the adult Asian population is approximately 450 mg/day, which might be considered at a level with potential detrimental impact on bone health [1]. Dietary calcium intake of most Asian countries is far below the FAO/WHO recommendations of between 1000 and 1300 mg/day. It was projected that more than about 50% of all osteoporotic hip fractures will occur in Asia by the year 2050 [2, 3].

Osteoporosis affects almost 70 million Chinese over the age of 50 and causes 687,000 hip fractures in China each year [4], with rising trends in the prevalence of osteoporosis and the incidence of hip fractures. A meta-analysis indicated a significant increase in the prevalence of osteoporosis in China from 2003 to 2015 [5], and the incidence of hip fractures in Beijing increased by 34% in women and 33% in men from 1988 to 1992 [6]. As with other Asian ethic groups, the calcium intake in a typical Chinese diet would be considered to be low. Population-wide data indicate that the average population dietary calcium intakes of Mainland China and Hong Kong were 389 mg and 430 mg, respectively [7, 8].

Peak bone mass (PBM) is one of the most significant predictors of postmenopausal osteoporosis [9, 10], and factors such as genetic factors, body weight, soft tissue composition, endocrine factors, nutrient intake, and physical activity would influence PBM. Studies in Australia and Finland showed that the premenarcheal

G. C. L. Cheung (✉)
Department of Applied Biology and Chemical Technology, The Hong Kong Polytechnic University, Hong Kong, China
e-mail: gordon.cl.cheung@polyu.edu.hk

Y.-X. Su
Faculty of Nutrition, School of Public Health, Sun Yat-Sen University, Guangzhou, China

© Springer Nature Switzerland AG 2019

C. M. Weaver et al. (eds.), *Nutritional Influences on Bone Health*,
https://doi.org/10.1007/978-3-319-98464-3_7

period is a critical window for bone mineral acquisition [11–13]. Ethnic-specific evidence on the dietary and lifestyle factors affecting bone mass accretion in the premenarcheal period of Chinese girls is needed in order to formulate tailored public health strategies to prevent osteoporosis in the Chinese population. The focus of this chapter is to provide a review of the evidence summarizing (1) the degree of association among dietary calcium intake, physical activity, and bone mass in premenarche Chinese girls, (2) the calcium metabolism in premenarche Chinese girls as reflected by calcium balance studies, (3) the effects of calcium supplementation on bone mass accretion of prepuberty girls, and (4) the interaction of the polymorphism of bone-related genes with calcium and physical activity in Chinese girls.

Diet, Physical Activity, and Bone Mass of Chinese Girls

A cross-sectional study was conducted to investigate the association of calcium intake and physical activity and bone mass [14, 15]. A total of 194 premenarche Chinese girls were recruited, and data on the bone mineral content (BMC) and bone mineral density (BMD) of four body sites, dietary intake, and types and duration of physical activity were collected. More than half of the participants were in Tanner stage II, the mean daily calcium intake was 620 + 277 mg/day and the mean 321 kcal/day and energy expenditure from physical activity [14, 15]. Both calcium intake and overall and weight-bearing physical activity have significant impact on the bone health of premenarche Chinese girls. BMC and BMD of whole body, femoral neck, Ward's triangle, and lumbar spine were significantly correlated with daily calcium intake ($p < 0.01$ except whole body BMD $p < 0.05$) [14], and the rise in daily calcium intake from 257 mg/day to 759 kcal/day increased the BMC and BMD at different sites by 13–22% and 3.6–16%, respectively [14]. For the impact of physical activity on bone health, the study showed that BMC and BMD of whole body, femoral neck, Ward's triangle, and lumbar spine were significantly correlated with both overall and weight-bearing physical activity ($p < 0.01$) [15]. The increase in weight-bearing physical activity expenditure from 227 kcal/day to 415 kcal/day elevated BMC and BMD at different sites by 17.5–29% and 8.8–17.1%, respectively [15].

Apart from calcium intake and physical activity levels, body composition also played a vital role in the bone health of the Chinese girls. A similar study in Beijing recruited 373 premenarche Chinese girls with mean age of 10.1 years old [16]. Multiple regression analysis showed that bone mineral-free lean (BMFL) and fat mass together explained 6.3 and 51.6% of the variation in total body BMC and BMD, respectively. BMFL mass contributed to a substantial proportion of the variation in forearm BMC and BMD. Calcium intake, height, age, and physical activity score also identified as minor but significant predictors of total body bone mass.

Calcium Metabolism of Chinese Girls

The characteristics of calcium metabolism in premenarche Chinese girls with different calcium intake levels were studied in a small intervention trial with 45 girls from 9 to 11.5 years old [17]. The subjects would be randomized into either of the four intervention groups with different designated calcium intake level for 6 days, and the urine, stool, and the duplicated food samples of the last 3 days of the intervention period were collected to assess calcium retention. The calcium absorption rate ranged from 52% to 55% and showed no significant difference across different intervention groups. Without any significant difference in the mean intake of protein and phosphorous, calcium retention was significantly correlated with the calcium-to-phosphorus ratio and calcium-to-protein ratio ($p < 0.01$), and the calcium absorption rate was also correlated with calcium-to-phosphorus ratio ($p < 0.01$). Nonlinear curve fit of calcium intake and predicted calcium retention indicated that calcium intake of premenarche Chinese girls at about 1100 mg would achieve the maximum calcium retention.

Effects of Calcium Supplementation on Chinese Girls

To further confirm the effective dose of calcium intake on bone mass accretion of prepuberty girls, a 2-year randomized controlled trial including 241 healthy prepuberty girls aged 10.0 ± 0.7 years was conducted in the southern part of China [18]. Subjects were randomized to one of three groups: (1) habitual diet (450 ± 100mg/day calcium), (2) habitual intake plus 250 ml cow milk (800 ± 100mg/day calcium), and (3) habitual intake plus 250 ml cow milk and calcium supplement with 300 mg calcium (1100 ± 100mg calcium), and the data on dietary intake, physical activity, and the bone mineral content and density were collected regularly during the study period. Positive correlation between the average daily calcium intake and the total body BMC or BMD was found among the subjects. The accretion of the total body BMC of Group 2 and Group 3 with mean calcium intake more than 864 mg was higher than those in Group 1 (mean calcium intake of 552 mg/day) (Table 7.1). This study also revealed that the accretion of BMC and BMD at femoral neck and BMD

Table 7.1 Accrual of BMC (g) after the intervention period

	Group I ($n = 57$)	Group II ($n = 58$)	Group III ($n = 59$)	*P*-value
Total body	257.4 ± 86.2	317.1 ± 99.2	357.7 ± 94.8	<0.001
Lumbar spine	7.95 ± 4.73	9.96 ± 4.84	12.30 ± 3.78	<0.001
Total hip	4.14 ± 2.06	4.49 ± 2.10	5.45 ± 2.29	0.006
Femoral neck	0.38 ± 0.29	0.43 ± 0.26	0.59 ± 0.27	0.001
Ward's	0.03 ± 0.13	0.06 ± 0.16	0.09 ± 0.16	0.089
Trochanter	1.11 ± 0.69	1.33 ± 0.71	1.30 ± 0.98	0.360
Intertrochanter	2.65 ± 1.53	2.72 ± 1.62	3.54 ± 1.90	0.009

Table 7.2 Accrual of BMD (g cm^{-2}) after the intervention period

	Group I (n = 57)	Group II (n = 58)	Group III (n = 59)	P-value
Total body	0.036 ± 0.032	0.059 ± 0.038	0.079 ± 0.034	<0.001
Lumbar spine	0.083 ± 0.054	0.103 ± 0.057	0.129 ± 0.055	0.003
Total hip	0.054 ± 0.048	0.064 ± 0.045	0.090 ± 0.049	<0.001
Femoral neck	0.052 ± 0.042	0.056 ± 0.044	0.087 ± 0.050	<0.001
Ward's	0.017 ± 0.085	0.032 ± 0.098	0.068 ± 0.102	0.010
Trochanter	0.049 ± 0.043	0.054 ± 0.040	0.075 ± 0.050	0.004
Intertrochanter	0.060 ± 0.056	0.079 ± 0.054	0.099 ± 0.054	0.010

at lumbar spine was significantly higher in the in Group 3 (Tables 7.1 and 7.2), indicating the calcium needs for prepubertal girls to achieve maximum bone accretion would be about 1200 mg/day.

Bone-Related Polymorphism in Chinese Population

Apart from the environmental factors, bone mineral density is also influenced by multiple genetic factors, with estimated heritability of 0.5–0.9 [19]. A list of candidate genes have been identified in the genetic epidemiology studies, including interleukin-6 (IL-6) genes, estrogen receptor genes, parathyroid hormone (PTH) genes, osteoprotegerin (OPG) gene, calcium-sensing receptor (CASR) genes, and vitamin D receptor (VDR) genes [20].

Studies confirmed that the premenarche Chinese girls with T alleles at the promotor region A163G, T245G, and T950C polymorphism of IL-6 gene or H alleles of OC gene polymorphism had significantly lower BMD [21, 22].

A study on IL-6 gene polymorphisms indicated that IL-6-634C/G polymorphism was significantly associated with BMD, and the impact of calcium intake and physical activity on the BMC and BMD was significantly different between the CC and G allele carriers [23]. The PTH BstB I polymorphism was found to have significant interaction with calcium intake on bone accretion in Chinese girls, with a better gain in bone accretion by high calcium intake in the BB genotype than those with b allele [24]. The IL-6-634C/G and ER-α PvuII polymorphism were also found to have an interactional effect on BMD accrual in Chinese adolescent girls [25]. The Fok I polymorphism of VDR gene had significant interaction with physical activity on bone mass accrual, and high physical activity level would be beneficial to the girls with FF genotype [26].

Conclusions

Early intervention should be started from prepuberty in Chinese population to prevent osteoporosis. Calcium intake at about 1100–1200 mg per day would be recommended for the prepubertal Chinese girls to maximize the calcium retention and to optimize bone accretion. High weight-bearing physical activity level would also enhance bone accretion substantially. A number of specific genotypes might deserve attention in the future for tailoring the intervention strategy to increase the peak bone mass.

References

1. International Osteoporosis Foundation. The Asian audit: epidemiology, costs and burden of osteoporosis in Asia 2009. London: IOF; 2009. www.iofbonehealth.org.
2. Gullberg B, Johnell O, Kanis JA. World-wide projections for hip fracture. Osteoporos Int. 1997;7:407.
3. Cooper C, Campion G, Melton LJ 3rd. Hip fractures in the elderly: a world-wide projection. Osteoporos Int. 1992;2:285.
4. China Health Promotion Foundation. White paper China 2008, Osteoporosis a Summary Statement of China. 2008.
5. Chen P, Li Z, Hu Y. Prevalence of osteoporosis in China: a meta-analysis and systematic review. BMC Public Health. 2016;16:1039.
6. Xu L, Lu A, Zhao X, et al. Very low rates of hip fracture in Beijing, People's Republic of China the Beijing Osteoporosis Project. Am J Epidemiol. 1996;144:901.
7. Wang LD. Chinese National Nutrition and health survey one: synthesis report 2002 (Chinese edition). Beijing: People's Medical Publishing House; 2005.
8. FEHD. The first Hong Kong Total diet study: minerals. Hong Kong: FEHD; 2014. http://www.cfs.gov.hk/english/programme/programme_firm/files/Report_on_the_1st_HK_Total_Diet_Study_Minerals_e.pdf.
9. Hui SL, Slemenda CW, Johnston CC. The contribution of bone loss of postmenopausal osteoporosis. Osteoporos Int. 1990;1:30–4.
10. Seeman E. Reduced bone density in women with fractures: contribution of low peak bone density and rapid bone loss. Osteoporos Int. 1994;4(suppl 1):15–25.
11. Kannus P, Haapasalo H, Sankelo M, Sievanen H, Pasanen M, Heinonen A, Oja P, Vuori I. Effect of starting age of physical activity on bone mass in the dominant arm of tennis and squash players. Ann Intern Med. 1995;123:27–31.
12. Khan KM, Bennell KL, Hopper JL, Flicker L, Nowson CA, Sherwin AJ, Crichton KJ, Harcourt PR, Wark JD. Self-reported ballet classes undertaken at age 10–12 years and hip bone mineral density in later life. Osteoporos Int. 1998;8:165–73.
13. Bass S, Pearce G, Bradney M, Hendrich E, Delmas PD, Harding A, Seeman E. Exercise before puberty may confer residual benefits in bone density in adulthood: studies in active prepubertal and retired female gymnasts. J Bone Miner Res. 1998;13:500–7.
14. Wang L, Chen YM, He GP, Xiao XC, Su YX. Association of habitual calcium intake with bone mass in premenarche Chinese girl. Acta Nutr Sin. 2007;29(1):239–41. 245.
15. Wang L, Chen YM, Xiao XC, Su YX. Association of physical activity with bone mass in premenarche Chinese girls. Chin J Prev Med. 2007;41(5):396–8.
16. Zhu K, Du XQ, Greenfield H, Zhang Q, Ma GS, Hu XQ, Fraser DR. Bone mass in Chinese premenarcheal girls: the roles of body composition, calcium intake and physical activity. Br J Nutr. 2004;92:985–93.
17. Luo XL, Xiao XC, Lai XH, Feng X, Su YX. Study on calcium absorption rate in premenarche Chinese girls aged 9–11.5 years. J Hygiene Res. 2005;34(4):445–8.
18. Liu Z, Li X, Xiao XC, He GP, Chen YM, Su YX. Effect of calcium intakes on bone mass accretion of prepuberty girls - a two-year randomized controlled trial. Acta Nutr Sin. 2009;31(3):241–5.
19. Liu YZ, Liu YJ, Recker RR, Deng HW. Molecular studies of identification of genes for osteoporosis: the 2002 update. J Endocrinol. 2003;177:147–96.
20. Ho NC, Jia L, Driscoll CC, Gutter EM, Francomano CA. A skeletal gene database. J Bone Miner Res. 2000;15:2095–122.
21. He GP, Chan YM, Li X, Su YX. Effect of osteoprotegerin gene polymorphism on bone mass in premenarche girls. Acta Nutr Sin. 2007;29(4):359–63.
22. Xiao XC, Su YX, Luo XL. Association of osteocalcin gene polymorphism with bone mass in Chinese premenarche girls. Acta Nutr Sin. 2006;28(6):479–82.

23. Li X, He GP, Zhnag B, Chen YM, Su YX. Interactions of interleukin-6 gene polymorphisms with calcium intake and physical activity on bone mass in pre-menarche Chinese girls. Osteoporos Int. 2008;19:1629–37.
24. Li X, He GP, Su YX. Interaction of parathyroid hormone gene polymorphism with calcium intake on bone mass accretion in Chinese adolescent girls. Acta Nutr Sin. 2007;29(6):556–60.
25. Li X, He GP, Chen YM, Su YX. Interaction of interleukin-6 and estrogen receptor gene polymorphisms on bone mass accrual in Chinese adolescent girls. J Bone Miner Metab. 2008;26:493–8.
26. Li X, GP HE, Su YX. Interaction of the polymorphism of vitamin D receptor gene start codon with physical activity on bone mass accrual in Chinese adolescent girls. Chin J Prev Med. 2008;42(4):238–43.

Part III

Exercise/Sedentary Behavior

Nutrition and Exercise Approaches to Enhance Muscle, Mobility, and Cognition During Aging

8

Robin M. Daly, Melissa B. Formica, Jamie L. Tait, and Helen Macpherson

Introduction

The 2015 World Health Organization (WHO) report on aging and health reported that "the health of older people is not keeping up with increasing longevity" and outlined a framework for action around the concept of functional ability to foster healthy aging [1]. By definition, functional ability is comprised of an individual's intrinsic capacity, both physical and mental, as well as relevant environmental characteristics and their interactions [1]. It is well established that aging is associated with a loss in muscle mass, strength, power, and function, which has been linked to multiple chronic diseases as well as an increased risk for falls, frailty, disability, loss of independence, and reduced quality of life [2–4]. There is also evidence that dementia and related cognitive deficits that can occur with advancing age, particularly deficits in executive function including the ability to concentrate, attend selectively, multi-task, plan, and strategize, are key risk factors for falls [5]. Other cognitive abilities commonly shown to experience an age-related deterioration include working memory, episodic memory, processing speed, and attention, but the age of onset for the decline in these measures varies. Conversely, crystallized abilities and faculties acquired over a lifetime such as vocabulary, visuospatial ability, and procedural memory tend to display greater stability with aging [6]. With the exception of cognitive assessments designed to aid in the diagnosis of cognitive impairment related to dementia and other neurological conditions, there is currently no "gold standard" or standardized measures of cognitive function for use in research. Studies focused on exercise or dietary interventions tend to include a range of measures of individual cognitive domains (e.g., executive function,

R. M. Daly (✉) · M. B. Formica · J. L. Tait · H. Macpherson
Institute for Physical Activity and Nutrition Research, School of Exercise and Nutrition Sciences, Deakin University, Melbourne, VIC, Australia
e-mail: rmdaly@deakin.edu.au

© Springer Nature Switzerland AG 2019

C. M. Weaver et al. (eds.), *Nutritional Influences on Bone Health*,
https://doi.org/10.1007/978-3-319-98464-3_8

memory, attention), and it is recommended that a composite of individual measures be used to provide an index of global cognitive function [7].

Several overlapping mechanisms are currently proposed to contribute to both cognitive and functional impairments, which can lead to an increased risk for falls and frailty. For instance, chronic inflammation, insulin resistance, vascular risk factors, and hormonal changes are all relevant to both declines to brain health and physical function [8]. Recent data also indicate that low muscle mass and strength and accelerated losses in muscle mass are associated with cognitive impairment [9–12] and brain atrophy [13]. Similarly, poor gait performance and a decline in gait speed over time have been shown to be predictive of incident dementia [14, 15]. Collectively, these findings provide evidence to support a link between cognition and muscle mass and function, but questions still remain as to the direction of this relationship. It is possible that there is a bidirectional relationship: factors causing muscle or functional losses may contribute to impaired cognitive function, or factors leading to cognitive impairment may contribute to a decline in muscle health and function. Despite this, there is growing interest in identifying strategies that can simultaneously improve muscle and cognitive health to ensure that older people maintain their physical and cognitive functions in order to live an independent and relatively disease- and disability-free life.

Regular exercise and adequate nutrition are widely promoted as two key modifiable lifestyle factors that can optimize physical, functional, and cognitive health into old age. To date, the vast majority of research has focused on the independent effects of exercise and various nutritional factors on physical or cognitive function. Whether combining these two health-related behaviors can result in additive or synergistic health benefits to both muscle and cognitive functions remains uncertain. However, as illustrated in Fig. 8.1 and discussed throughout this chapter, there is a sound rationale to support the role of exercise and nutrition for improving both cognitive- and muscle-related outcomes. This chapter will provide a brief overview of the evidence related to the role of exercise and nutrition for optimizing muscle, mobility, and cognition in older adults, followed by a discussion on the latest research into whether various nutritional factors can enhance the effects of exercise on muscle health, functional ability, and cognitive function. The aim is not to provide a complete review of all the available literature and the underlying mechanisms but to provide an update on more recent randomized controlled trials (RCTs) in older adults which included both muscle and functional measures with cognition as outcomes.

Exercise to Optimize Muscle Health and Mobility in Older Adults

Regular exercise and physical activity have been consistently shown to have beneficial effects on a broad range of physical, functional, and cognitive measures in older people [16–18]. However, not all forms of exercise are equally effective, with the benefits being modality and intensity-dependent and reliant on adequate nutrition.

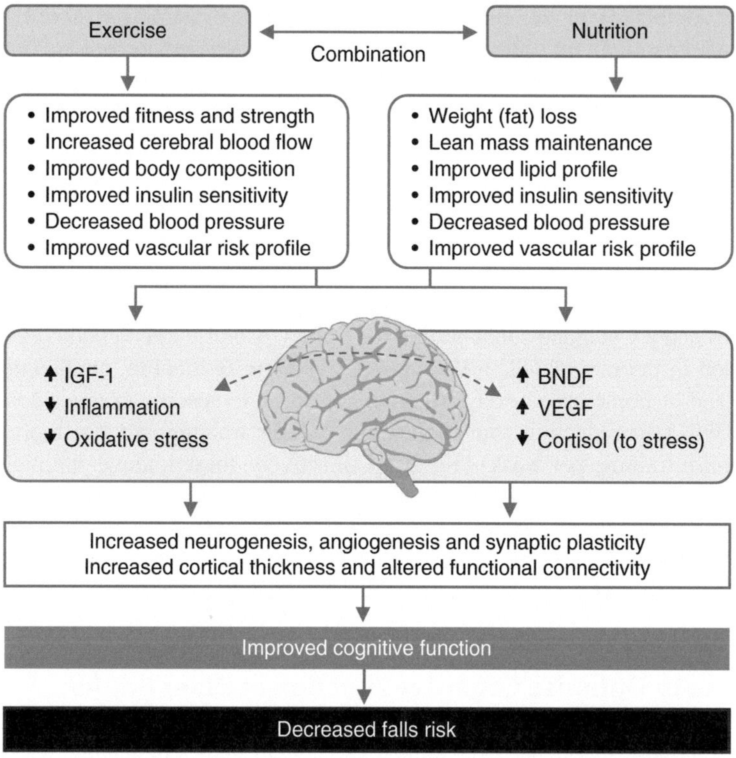

Fig. 8.1 Theoretical model of the mechanisms by which exercise and nutritional factors may influence both cognitive and functional outcomes. IGF-1, insulin-like growth factor (IGF)-1; BDNF, brain-derived neurotrophic factor; VEGF, vascular endothelial growth factor

For instance, progressive resistance training (PRT) has been shown to be effective for improving muscle mass, size, and strength in older adults and the frail elderly [19, 20], but there remains considerable uncertainty with regard to the effect of this mode of training on functional ability (e.g., balance, mobility, gait speed) and reducing falls in older people [17, 21]. This is likely related in part to the lack of training specificity, that is, most resistance training programs focus on slow and controlled movements to maximize muscle strength and not the ability to generate force quickly (termed *muscle power*) which is often needed for a rapid coordinated and dynamic response specific to many functional tasks (e.g., stepping quickly in response to a trip). Indeed, there is evidence that many common tasks of daily living are more strongly related to muscle power than muscle mass or maximal muscle strength [22]. Thus, targeted programs that are designed to optimize neuromuscular function and which are specific to tasks of daily living are likely to provide the greatest benefits.

High-velocity PRT or functional power training, which is characterized by rapid concentric movements or muscle contractions, is an alternative approach that has been shown to improve movement speed, muscle power, and functional performance in older adults [23]. In fact, there is evidence this mode of training is more effective than traditional PRT for improving physical performance [18], as well as "real-life" functional ability (e.g., car braking speed) in the elderly [24]. While the long-term effects of high-velocity training on falls remain unknown, the findings from a meta-analysis of seven RCTs indicated that volitional and reactive step training interventions involving quick, multidirectional stepping movements and weight transfers, which incorporate elements of functional muscle power, improved functional ability and reduced the rate of falls by 52% [rate ratio 0.48 (95% CI, 0.36–0.65)] in older people [17, 25]. It is noteworthy that the magnitude of the reduction in falls following step training interventions is greater than that reported in previous meta-analyses and a Cochrane collaboration for general exercise interventions (21–32% reduction in the rate of falls following general exercise training, multicomponent group and/or home-based exercise training) and more specific exercise combinations (39% falls reduction with challenging balance training and 3 or more hours of exercise training per week) [17, 26]. Collectively, these findings highlight that targeted multicomponent exercise programs incorporating high-velocity PRT, functional activities relevant to everyday tasks, and challenging balance activities are likely to provide the greatest benefits in terms of optimizing muscle mass, strength, power, and functional capacity and reducing falls risk in older people.

Exercise to Optimize Cognitive Function in Older Adults

There is mounting evidence from animal and human studies indicating that regular exercise can induce a cascade of neural and vascular adaptations which can improve brain structure, function, and/or neural connectivity through the promotion of neurogenesis, angiogenesis, and synaptic plasticity, the release of various growth and neurotrophic factors [e.g., insulin-like growth factor-1 (IGF-1) and brain-derived neurotrophic factor (BDNF)], and the modulation of systemic inflammation and oxidative stress (Fig. 8.1). While more detailed information is provided in several reviews [27, 28], additional mechanisms include exercise-related benefits to cardiovascular health and insulin sensitivity, which can have long-term effects on brain health and dementia risk later in life [29]. For instance, a study of over 3000 individuals above the age of 60 from the Framingham Study found that those within the lowest category of physical activity had a 1.5-fold increased 10-year risk of dementia incidence compared to those with higher levels of physical activity [30]. While these findings suggest that exercise might exert a neuroprotective effect on the aging brain, questions still remain as to whether there is an optimal type and dose of exercise that is needed to elicit cognitive benefits and/or prevent the progression to dementia. To date, a larger body of research has focused on aerobic training benefits to cognition than PRT or multicomponent programs. However, a systematic review and meta-analysis of 36 RCTs in community-dwelling adults aged 50 years and older reported that aerobic training, PRT, and the combination all had significant and similar effects on cognitive function (effect size, 0.24, 0.29, and 0.33, respectively), regardless of cognitive status [16]. However, moderator analysis revealed that moderate- to high-intensity (but not low intensity) training and a duration of at least 45 minutes were most effective [16].

There is also emerging data that functional training programs designed to prevent falls, including step training interventions [25] and dual-task cognitive-motor programs [31], whereby cognitive or motor tasks are performed sequentially or simultaneously with exercise training, can improve measures of cognitive function, including executive function, attention, and short-term memory. Moreover, the performance of functional tasks (e.g., stepping) and/or exercise in combination with a secondary task may be innately cognitively demanding as they require the engagement of executive processes (e.g., inhibition, planning, and execution of a rapid motor response in response to an external cue) and attentional aspects (e.g., distribution of attention between movement components). At present, the neurophysiological mechanisms underlying any cognitive improvements following combined cognitive and exercise training remain uncertain, but cognitive and exercise training may stimulate similar neurobiological processes which could produce a synergistic response (refer to Tait et al. [31] for a more detailed review). In this regard, a combination of physical exercise, sensorimotor stimulation, and cognitive engagement may also facilitate neurophysiological changes that contribute to wider cognitive benefits which may translate into physical or functional benefits. In part support of this notion, a 2017 review that included 19 studies found that interventions that adopted physical-cognitive training or multimodal programs were most effective for improving a range of physical, motor, and cognitive outcomes in older adults than single intervention programs [32]. Collectively, these findings suggests that exercise programs designed to optimize muscle mass and function and prevent falls in the elderly may also simultaneously improve cognitive health, but further study is needed to define whether there is an optimal type (or combination) and dose.

Nutritional Approaches to Optimize Muscle Health and Mobility in Older Adults

In a comprehensive review of the role of nutrition for the prevention and management of sarcopenia, Robinson et al. [33] highlighted that many epidemiologic and prospective cohort studies have shown that various nutritional factors (protein, vitamin D, antioxidant nutrients, omega-3 fatty acids), whole foods (dairy products), and dietary patterns (Mediterranean diet) can play a role in attenuating age-related losses in muscle mass and to a lesser extent muscle strength and/or function. However, the findings from several systematic reviews and meta-analyses of RCTs have shown that the effects of specific nutrients or supplements alone (without exercise) on muscle and functional outcomes in older adults are equivocal [34–37], with the exception of perhaps vitamin D that appears to have a small positive effect on muscle strength and function in older adults, particularly in those with low basal levels [38, 39]. While it has been suggested that the lack of any marked effects of various nutritional factors on muscle or mobility-related outcomes may be related to the low number of studies, short-term follow-up periods, and heterogeneous study designs [33], it is also likely that some of these trials were biologically flawed. For instance, many recruited healthy older people who were not functionally impaired, already had adequate intakes, and/or failed to provide a sufficient dose of a given nutrient to markedly increase levels above baseline or relative to controls. As a result of these limitations, many trials lacked the ability to detect any marked effects and were essentially designed to fail. In part support of this notion, a recent meta-analysis of RCTs in adults aged ≥ 55 years found no overall effect of dairy-based protein supplementation and vitamin D on muscle or functional measures, but there was a trend for a positive effect on lean body mass when supplemental doses of protein were ≥ 20 g per day or when given to (pre)frail or inactive older adults [40].

Nutritional Approaches to Optimize Cognitive Function in Older Adults

Several review articles have concluded that, based on evidence from epidemiologic studies and a limited number of RCTs, that certain dietary patterns or nutrients, including but not limited to the Mediterranean diet, omega-3 fatty acids, vitamin D, antioxidants, creatine, and B-vitamins, may be protective against cognitive decline and even the risk of incident dementia [41–43]. Albeit limited, there is also evidence that dietary protein and its constituent amino acids, particularly tryptophan and tyrosine, may provide some cognitive benefits [44]. Despite these findings, a meta-analysis of 24 nutritional RCTs (six using omega-3 fatty acids, seven using B-vitamins, three using vitamin E, eight using other interventions) in non-demented middle-aged and older adults [45] and a systematic review of randomized, double-blinded controlled trials of nutraceuticals and dietary supplements of at least 1-year duration and with at least 100 participants aged ≥65 years [46] both reported no consistent evidence to support any beneficial effects of nutrition on cognition. This may be related to a number of factors, including the health status of participants and the lack of sensitivity of certain cognitive measures to detect subtle changes over time. While it is clear that further long-term and adequately powered RCTs in suitable populations are still needed, given that multiple lifestyle factors (as well as environment and genetic factors) have been implicated with cognitive related disorders, it is likely that the greatest benefits on cognition (and muscle health and functional ability) will occur with a targeted exercise program combined with a nutritional intervention.

Effect of Nutrition Combined with Exercise on Muscle, Mobility, and Cognition in Older Adults

As illustrated in Fig. 8.1, from a mechanistic perspective, there is a sound rationale to support an interactive effect of exercise and nutrition on both muscle and cognitive functions. For instance, animal and human studies have reported that both exercise and various nutritional factors can influence various growth and neurotrophic factors [e.g., IGF-1, BDNF, and vascular endothelial growth factors (VEGF)] as well as modulate various inflammatory markers, all of which have been implicated with muscle and cognitive/brain health [27, 28]. A more comprehensive review of the potential underlying mechanisms by which exercise and nutrition may enhance cognitive function is provided in several excellent reviews [28, 47, 48]. The focus of this chapter is to briefly review the latest evidence from RCTs addressing whether various nutritional factors, specifically protein and dairy-based supplementation, vitamin D, fish oil, and omega-3 fatty acids, creatine, antioxidant nutrients, and multi-nutrient supplements, can enhance the effects of exercise on muscle health and/or function and cognition in older adults.

Protein or Dairy Supplementation with Exercise

Over the past decade, there have been equivocal findings from many intervention trials and meta-analyses of RCTs investigating the combined effects of exercise with different types of protein, essential amino acids, β-hydroxy-β-methylbutyrate (HMB), or dairy food supplements, on muscle mass, strength, and function in older adults. This is highlighted in a 2017 systematic review of combined exercise and nutrition interventions in adults aged 60 years and over which reported that only 25% (3/12) of protein supplementation (including dairy, whey, meat, collagen peptide) trials and 0 (0/3) to 33% (1/3) of essential amino acids or HMB trials detected a significant additive effect on muscle mass or strength; none of the trials observed an added benefit on physical performance [49] (Table 8.1). The lack of a consistent effect may be due to a range of factors, including differences in the type and dose of protein/dairy prescribed; differences in the timing of consumption, compliance, spread, and/or pattern of intake; as well as heterogeneity in the cohorts studied (age, physical and nutritional status, current activity levels), study duration, and the type and dose of exercise prescribed [50]. Nevertheless, it is likely that the greatest benefits will be apparent in high-risk individuals (e.g., frail or sarcopenic) who have inadequate dietary intakes (e.g., protein intake below the recommended level of 0.8–1.0 g/kg/d).

Table 8.1 Summary of the proportion of randomized controlled trials that have reported a significant additive effect of nutrition on exercise-induced changes in muscle mass, strength, and function

Exercise with	Muscle mass	Muscle strength	Physical function
Protein	3/12 (25%)	3/12 (25%)	0/9 (0%)
Essential amino acids	0/3 (0%)	0/3 (0%)	0/2 (0%)
HMB	1/3 (33%)	0/3 (0%)	0/2 (0%)
Multi-nutrients	0/4 (0%)	1/5 (20%)	0/4 (0%)
Creatine	4/5 (80%)	4/5 (80%)	1/4 (25%)
Vitamin D	0/1 (0%)	0/2 (0%)	1/2 (50%)
Other[a]	0/6 (0%)	0/5 (0%)	2/5 (50%)
Summary	*8/34 (23%)*	*8/35 (23%)*	*4/28 (14%)*

Adapted from Beaudart et al. [49]

HMB β-hydroxy-β-methylbutyrate (HMB)

[a]Other included green tea, tea catechin, magnesium oxide, milk fat globule membrane, soy isoflavones, and vitamin- and mineral-enhanced dairy and fruit products

With regard to whether additional protein can enhance the effects of exercise on cognitive function in older adults, we are aware of only two published trials [51, 52]. In a 24-week RCT in 62 frail elderly people aged 65 years and over, neither twice weekly PRT alone nor with protein supplementation (2 × 15 g milk protein concentrate per day) improved cognitive function [assessed via the Mini-Mental State Examination (MMSE)], despite a greater gain in lean mass in the PRT plus protein group [51]. The same group then combined the findings from the above study with a parallel run protein (2 × 15 g/d milk protein concentrate) versus placebo supplementation trial in frail and pre-frail adults and reported that there were no exercise-protein interactions on a larger battery of cognitive tests [51, 52]. However, they did find that PRT plus protein improved information processing speed compared to protein supplementation alone, but surprisingly protein supplementation improved verbal fluency compared to exercise plus protein. Given that cognition was a secondary outcome in both these trials and neither was adequately powered to detect an interactive effect, these findings must be interpreted with caution and highlight the need for further well-designed, long-term trials.

Vitamin D Supplementation with Exercise

Exercise and vitamin D supplementation have been independently shown to improve muscle strength and function, and thus it has been hypothesized that there might be an additive effect when combining these two approaches. However, the findings from a meta-analysis of seven trials (792 participants aged ≥65 years) reported that there were no additive benefits of combined exercise (predominantly PRT) and vitamin D (this included studies using vitamin D and calcium supplementation or fortified milk) on muscle function in older adults, but there was a trend for a greater improvement in muscle strength [53]. The lack of a consistent additive effect is likely related to the marked heterogeneity with regard to the study durations (12 weeks to 24 months), dose of vitamin D prescribed (400–1920 IU/d), basal serum 25(OH)D concentrations, differences in the exercise regimens, and/or study methodology (e.g., functional measures) [53]. To our knowledge, there are no published intervention trials which have investigated whether exercise combined with vitamin D supplementation alone can improve cognitive function in older people. However, in a 2-year factorial design RCT in healthy older women aged 70–80 years which was designed to examine the independent and combined effects of exercise (functional balance and weight-bearing exercise and resistance training) and vitamin D (800 IU/d) supplementation on falls and muscle function, Uusi-Rasi et al. reported that there was no effect of the intervention on cognitive function [assessed by the Mini-Mental State Examination (MMSE), a brief screening measure for cognitive impairment] (personal communication). This is likely due to the inclusion of healthy women with adequate basal vitamin D levels [mean 25(OH)D ~67 nmol/L] who were cognitively intact (mean baseline MMSE scores were at the upper range, 28/30) and the use of the MMSE tool which may not be sensitive to subtle changes that can occur across specific cognitive domains [54].

Fish Oil and Omega-3 Supplementation with Exercise

Several short-term trials have reported that fish oil and omega-3 fatty acid supplementation may enhance the effects of PRT on muscle mass and strength in older adults [55, 56]. For instance, a study in 45 women (mean age 64 years) randomized to PRT alone for 90 days or PRT plus fish oil supplementation (2 g/d for 90 days or 2/d for 60 days before training followed by 2 g/d for 90 days) found that there were additive benefits on lower limb muscle strength (peak torque and chair rising time), but not muscle function; neither muscle mass nor cognition were assessed [56]. Several observational studies have indicated that a low omega-3 to omega-6 polyunsaturated fatty acid (PUFA) ratio may be protective against cognitive decline and dementia [57] and predict better cognitive function in healthy older people [58]. However, excess consumption of omega-6 PUFA, which is common among a Western dietary pattern, may adversely impact cognition by depleting docosahexaenoic acid (DHA), the omega-3 PUFA most prevalent in the brain [59]. Despite the rationale for increasing omega-3 intake, data from the 3-year randomized, placebo-controlled Multi-domain Alzheimer Prevention Trial (MAPT) in 1680 community-dwelling, non-demented adults aged 70+ years with either memory complaints, limitations with one instrumental activities of daily living, or slow gait speed reported that there were no significant effects of omega-3 fatty acid supplementation [800 mg/d (DHA) and 250 mg/d eicosapentaenoic acid (EPA)] and a multi-domain intervention (cognitive training, physical activity and nutrition advice, and three preventative consultations), alone or in combination, compared with placebo on cognitive (primary outcome) and physical (secondary outcome) function [short physical performance battery (SPPB)] [60] (Fig. 8.2). However, the combination of omega-3 fatty acids and the multi-domain intervention was found to enhance cognitive performance on a secondary measure of cognitive function. The lack of an

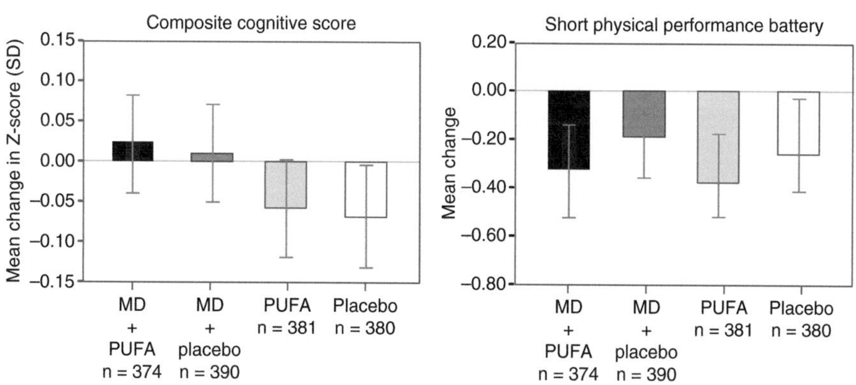

Fig. 8.2 Mean changes (with 95% confidence intervals) after 3 years in global cognitive function and the short physical performance battery in participants (aged 70 years and older) enrolled in the Multi-domain Alzheimer Preventive Trial (MAPT) who were randomized to the multi-domain (MD) and polyunsaturated fatty acid supplementation (PUFA) group alone or in combination or placebo [60]. Error bar represents 95% confidence intervals

effect, particularly on physical function, may be related in part to the fact that participants only received generic physical activity advice to be more active (e.g., walk 30 min per day) and not a targeted program designed to enhance functional capacity. Furthermore, exploratory subgroup analyses showed that the combined intervention arms or the multi-domain intervention alone may help to slow cognitive decline in those most at risk (e.g., those with an increased dementia risk score and those with evidence of brain amyloid pathology), but there was no evidence of any beneficial effects on functional capacity with the per protocol analysis (excluding non-compliers). Based on the above findings, it appears that omega-3 fatty acids do not enhance the effects of exercise on functional ability in healthy older people or those with impaired function, but there may be some added benefits to muscle mass and strength and cognitive function.

Creatine Supplementation with Exercise

As highlighted in Table 8.1, there are a number of RCTs which have shown that creatine supplementation is an effective approach to enhance the effects of exercise on muscle mass and strength (4/5 studies showed improvements) in older adults and to a lesser extent muscle function (only one of four studies reported an additive effect on physical performance) [49]. Further to its anabolic skeletal muscle effects, there is some evidence that creatine supplementation may improve cognitive function [61]. However, to our knowledge there is only one trial which has investigated whether creatine can enhance the effects of exercise on measures of cognition and muscle strength [62]. In a 24-week factorial design, double-blind, placebo-controlled RCT in 56 healthy older women aged 60–80 years, Alves et al. [62] reported that neither twice weekly PRT nor creatine supplementation (4 × 5 g/d for 5 days followed by 5 g/d) alone or in combination improved any measure of cognitive function, and there was no additive benefit of creatine on muscle strength. However, given the small sample size and the inclusion of healthy older women in this study, these findings must be interpreted with caution and highlight the need for further adequately powered trials in at-risk cohorts (e.g., those with cognitive and/or functional impairment).

Antioxidant Nutrients with Exercise

Aging is associated with a steady increase in oxidative stress (free radical production that can induce cell damage) that has been implicated in many chronic diseases, including sarcopenia and cognitive impairment. While regular exercise and various antioxidant nutrients (e.g., vitamins A, C, and E, selenium, and carotenoids) are reported to protect older people from oxidative stress, whether single antioxidant supplements or a combination can prevent muscle and cognitive decline remains uncertain [33]. At present, there are also conflicting findings from the limited trials available on the combined effects of antioxidant supplementation with exercise on muscle mass, strength, and/or function. For instance, a 6-month factorial design RCT in 57 healthy adults aged 59–73 years found that high-intensity PRT combined with vitamin C (1000 mg/d) and E (600 mg/d) supplementation significantly increased muscle mass (fat-free mass), but not muscle strength, in older adults [63]. In contrast, 6 months of vitamin E supplementation (900 IU/d) had no additive effects beyond aerobic training (walking) on physical function in 57 sedentary older adults [64]. Moreover, a 12-week trial in 34 elderly men aged 60–81 years found that vitamin C (1000 mg/d) and E (235 mg/d) supplementation attenuated PRT-induced gains in total lean mass and leg muscle thickness, but not muscle strength [65]. This suggests that antioxidants may blunt the anabolic skeletal muscle effects of PRT, but given the small sample size and short-term nature of this trial, further studies are needed to investigate this intriguing finding.

With regard to the effects of exercise and antioxidant supplementation on brain/cognitive health, we were unable to identify any long-term human RCTs that had been conducted in older adults. However, a narrative review on the effects of exercise with antioxidant supplementation (specifically vitamin C and E) on brain and/or cognitive function and related biomarkers highlighted that there are contrasting results from the limited number of animal and human studies that have been conducted [66]. For instance, some studies have reported an additive beneficial effect, while others reported no effects or a negative response in which antioxidants may block the beneficial effects of exercise [66]. Clearly this is an area that requires further study.

Multi-nutrient Supplements with Exercise

Since a number of different nutrients have been associated with exercise-induced gains in muscle health and/or cognitive function, there has been interest in whether multi-nutrient supplements (e.g., various combinations of protein, amino acids, vitamin D, calcium, creatine, omega-3 fatty acids, and/or other vitamins and/or minerals) can provide additive benefits to exercise on muscle and to a lesser extent cognitive function. Of the trials included in the systematic review by Beaudart et al. [49], there was little evidence of any additive benefits with multi-nutrient supplementation on muscle mass (0 of 4 trials), muscle strength (1 of 5 trials), or physical performance (0 of 4 trials) (Table 8.1). While the authors acknowledged that the majority of studies were poor quality (graded on the Jadad scale), a number of more recent well-designed trials have observed conflicting findings with regard to the combined effects of exercise with multi-nutrient supplements on muscle outcomes in older adults (mean age ≥65 years) [67–70]. For instance, 12 weeks of a daily nutritional supplement (whey protein, essential amino acids, vitamin D, and other minerals) with exercise (5/week of muscle strengthening and balance training) led to greater gains in fat-free mass, handgrip strength, and physical functioning compared to exercise alone in sarcopenic older men and women [70]. The positive findings in this study are likely due in part to the fact that participants were screened from hospitalized patients with evidence of malnutrition. In contrast to these findings, the provision of a daily multi-nutrient drink (whey protein, vitamin D, calcium, and an assortment of other vitamins and minerals) for 24 weeks did not enhance the effects of exercise (3/week of walking, lower limb strength, balance, and flexibility exercises) on physical function (400 m walk or SPPB), muscle strength, or power in 149 adults aged 70 years and over with mobility limitations (SPPB ≤9) and low vitamin D status (25OHD ≥9 and ≤24 ng/ml) [68, 71]. However, nutritional supplementation was associated with a greater reduction in thigh intermuscular fat, which is important given that increased muscle fat infiltration has been associated with both metabolic and muscular dysfunctions [72]. While many of the above trials did include a measure of cognition (e.g., MMSE) as part of the baseline assessment, changes in response to the intervention were not assessed (or reported), but given that most studies included cognitively intact older adults and were relatively short-term (12 weeks to 6 months), it is likely that any potential benefits on cognition would be modest.

There have been a number of recent multi-domain intervention trials incorporating exercise training, nutritional supplementation, cognitive training, medication review, and/or vascular risk monitoring, which have quantified changes in both cognitive and physical functions in older adults [73, 74]. In a 12-week multi-domain intervention involving twice weekly strength/balance training with a daily protein nutritional supplement for 6 weeks, twice weekly memory workshops for 6 weeks, and medication review in 352 pre-frail/frail elderly people (mean age 77 years), Romera-Liebana et al. [73] reported that there were significant improvements in both functional and cognitive performance measures relative to usual care controls, despite relatively poor adherence to both the exercise and memory training sessions (mean adherence 54%). Furthermore, many of the functional and cognitive benefits were maintained up to 18 months, despite the intervention ceasing after 3 months. While it is difficult to explain these findings given the short-term nature (6 weeks) and modest adherence to the intervention, it is possible that the positive findings are related to the inclusion of a high-risk cohort of elderly people (e.g., 75% were classified as frail).

To our knowledge, the 2-year Finnish Geriatric Intervention Study (FINGER) is the largest multi-domain intervention trial in older adults with cognition as the primary outcome and functional performance as a secondary outcome. In this study, 1260 community-dwelling older people aged 60–77 with risk factors for dementia were randomized to an intensive multi-domain intervention (described below) or regular health advice (oral and written information regarding strategies to maintain a healthy diet, physical and social activities, and management of vascular factors and disability prevention) [74]. The multi-domain intervention incorporated four components: (1) individual and group nutrition sessions in which participants were advised to consume a diet with 10–20% of daily energy from proteins, 25–35% from fat [<10% from saturated plus trans-fatty acids, 10–20% from monounsaturated fatty acids, 5–10% from polyunsaturated fatty acids (including 2.5–3.0 g/day omega-3 fatty acids)], 45–55% from carbohydrates (<10% refined sugar), 25–35 g/day dietary fiber, <5 g/day salt, and < 5% from alcohol, (2) individually tailored PRT (one to three times a week) in combination with aerobic training (two to five times a week) and postural exercises, (3) group and individual computer-based cognitive training, and (4) social interactions (group meetings). The main finding from this trial was that the multi-domain intervention was associated with significantly greater improvements to global cognitive function, executive function, and processing speed compared to regular health advice. Improvements to cognition were in the magnitude of 25–150% greater than the control group. In contrast, there was no effect of the intervention on physical performance (assessed via SPPB) [74]. It is difficult to explain this latter finding given that 76–83% of participants reported completing the resistance or aerobic exercise one or more times per week and the programs did include exercises to improve postural balance. One possible explanation for the lack of any functional benefits is that the participants included were not functionally impaired and were relatively active (e.g., >70% reported being active two or more times per week). Based on these findings, further trials are needed to explore the optimal multi-domain approach that can improve both cognitive and physical performance measures in older adults and whether this ultimately translates into a reduction in the incidence of dementia, sarcopenia, and falls.

Conclusion

In summary, there is strong evidence that targeted and progressive exercise programs, particularly multicomponent interventions incorporating resistance training, functional activities relevant to everyday tasks (e.g., rapid stepping), and challenging balance training, can improve muscle mass, strength, power, and function and reduce falls risk in older people. Whether this translates into a reduction in fracture risk remains unknown. While there is also emerging evidence that the above modes of training, along with aerobic exercise, can improve measures of cognitive function, questions still remain with regard to the optimal dose (intensity, duration, and frequency). In contrast, there is little evidence from RCTs to support the role of individual or a combination of nutrients as an effective approach to improve muscle health, functional performance, or cognition in healthy older adults. There is, however, some evidence showing that various nutritional factors can improve muscle mass and/or strength in the elderly at risk (e.g., those with functional impairment, frailty, sarcopenia, or malnutrition), but the greatest benefits are likely to be achieved with exercise. Currently, however, the vast majority of intervention trials which have investigated whether individual nutrients or multi-nutrient supplements can enhance the effects of exercise on measures of muscle mass, strength, and function and/or cognition have produced negative findings. While this is likely due to the fact that most studies included relatively healthy older adults who did not present with nutritional deficiency, many of these studies were also not designed nor powered to detect improvements in muscle, functional, and cognitive measures. Given the emerging link between muscle mass, strength, and function with brain health and cognitive function and subsequent disease risk (e.g., dementia and falls), there is a need for further long-term, well-designed, and appropriately powered intervention trials to evaluate the combined effects of exercise and nutrition, including dietary approaches (e.g., Mediterranean diet), on muscle, mind, and mobility outcomes in the elderly.

References

1. World Health Organisation. World report on ageing and health. Geneva; 2015.
2. Cruz-Jentoft AJ, Baeyens JP, Bauer JM, Boirie Y, Cederholm T, Landi F, Martin FC, Michel JP, Rolland Y, Schneider SM, et al. Sarcopenia: European consensus on definition and diagnosis: report of the European working group on sarcopenia in older people. Age Ageing. 2010;39(4):412–23.
3. Fielding RA, Vellas B, Evans WJ, Bhasin S, Morley JE, Newman AB, Abellan van Kan G, Andrieu S, Bauer J, Breuille D, et al. Sarcopenia: an undiagnosed condition in older adults. Current consensus definition: prevalence, etiology, and consequences. International working group on sarcopenia. J Am Med Dir Assoc. 2011;12(4):249–56.
4. Scott D, Daly RM, Sanders KM, Ebeling PR. Fall and fracture risk in sarcopenia and dynapenia with and without obesity: the role of lifestyle interventions. Curr Osteoporos Rep. 2015;13(4):235–44.
5. Hsu CL, Nagamatsu LS, Davis JC, Liu-Ambrose T. Examining the relationship between specific cognitive processes and falls risk in older adults: a systematic review. Osteoporos Int. 2012;23(10):2409–24.
6. Harada CN, Natelson Love MC, Triebel KL. Normal cognitive aging. Clin Geriatr Med. 2013;29(4):737–52.
7. Posner H, Curiel R, Edgar C, Hendrix S, Liu E, Loewenstein DA, Morrison G, Shinobu L, Wesnes K, Harvey PD. Outcomes assessment in clinical trials of Alzheimer's disease and its precursors: readying for short-term and long-term clinical trial needs. Innov Clin Neurosci. 2017;14(1–2):22–9.
8. Halil M, Cemal Kizilarslanoglu M, Emin Kuyumcu M, Yesil Y, Cruz Jentoft AJ. Cognitive aspects of frailty: mechanisms behind the link between frailty and cognitive impairment. J Nutr Health Aging. 2015;19(3):276–83.
9. Boyle PA, Buchman AS, Wilson RS, Leurgans SE, Bennett DA. Association of muscle strength with the risk of Alzheimer disease and the rate of cognitive decline in community-dwelling older persons. Arch Neurol. 2009;66(11):1339–44.
10. Hsu YH, Liang CK, Chou MY, Liao MC, Lin YT, Chen LK, Lo YK. Association of cognitive impairment, depressive symptoms and sarcopenia among healthy older men in the veterans retirement community in southern Taiwan: a cross-sectional study. Geriatr Gerontol Int. 2014;14(Suppl 1):102–8.
11. Nourhashemi F, Andrieu S, Gillette-Guyonnet S, Reynish E, Albarede JL, Grandjean H, Vellas B. Is there a relationship between fat-free soft tissue mass and low cognitive function? Results from a study of 7,105 women. J Am Geriatr Soc. 2002;50(11):1796–801.
12. Tolea MI, Galvin JE. Sarcopenia and impairment in cognitive and physical performance. Clin Interv Aging. 2015;10:663–71.
13. Burns JM, Johnson DK, Watts A, Swerdlow RH, Brooks WM. Reduced lean mass in early Alzheimer disease and its association with brain atrophy. Arch Neurol. 2010;67(4):428–33.
14. Beauchet O, Annweiler C, Callisaya ML, De Cock AM, Helbostad JL, Kressig RW, Srikanth V, Steinmetz JP, Blumen HM, Verghese J, et al. Poor gait performance and prediction of dementia: results from a meta-analysis. J Am Med Dir Assoc. 2016;17(6):482–90.
15. Dumurgier J, Artaud F, Touraine C, Rouaud O, Tavernier B, Dufouil C, Singh-Manoux A, Tzourio C, Elbaz A. Gait speed and decline in gait speed as predictors of incident dementia. J Gerontol A Biol Sci Med Sci. 2017;72(5):655–61.
16. Northey JM, Cherbuin N, Pumpa KL, Smee DJ, Rattray B. Exercise interventions for cognitive function in adults older than 50: a systematic review with meta-analysis. Br J Sports Med. 2018;52(3):154–60.
17. Sherrington C, Michaleff ZA, Fairhall N, Paul SS, Tiedemann A, Whitney J, Cumming RG, Herbert RD, Close JCT, Lord SR. Exercise to prevent falls in older adults: an updated systematic review and meta-analysis. Br J Sports Med. 2017;51(24):1750–8.

18. Steib S, Schoene D, Pfeifer K. Dose-response relationship of resistance training in older adults: a meta-analysis. Med Sci Sports Exerc. 2010;42(5):902–14.
19. Borde R, Hortobagyi T, Granacher U. Dose-response relationships of resistance training in healthy old adults: a systematic review and meta-analysis. Sports Med. 2015;45(12):1693–720.
20. Stewart VH, Saunders DH, Greig CA. Responsiveness of muscle size and strength to physical training in very elderly people: a systematic review. Scand J Med Sci Sports. 2014;24(1):e1–10.
21. Latham NK, Bennett DA, Stretton CM, Anderson CS. Systematic review of progressive resistance strength training in older adults. J Gerontol A Biol Sci Med Sci. 2004;59(1):48–61.
22. Bean JF, Kiely DK, Herman S, Leveille SG, Mizer K, Frontera WR, Fielding RA. The relationship between leg power and physical performance in mobility-limited older people. J Am Geriatr Soc. 2002;50(3):461–7.
23. Reid KF, Fielding RA. Skeletal muscle power: a critical determinant of physical functioning in older adults. Exerc Sport Sci Rev. 2012;40(1):4–12.
24. Sayers SP, Gibson K. Effects of high-speed power training on muscle performance and braking speed in older adults. J Aging Res. 2012;2012:426278.
25. Okubo Y, Schoene D, Lord SR. Step training improves reaction time, gait and balance and reduces falls in older people: a systematic review and meta-analysis. Br J Sports Med. 2017;51(7):586–93.
26. Gillespie LD, Robertson MC, Gillespie WJ, Sherrington C, Gates S, Clemson LM, Lamb SE. Interventions for preventing falls in older people living in the community. Cochrane Database Syst Rev. 2012;9:CD007146.
27. Cotman CW, Berchtold NC, Christie LA. Exercise builds brain health: key roles of growth factor cascades and inflammation. Trends Neurosci. 2007;30(9):464–72.
28. Meeusen R. Exercise, nutrition and the brain. Sports Med. 2014;44(Suppl 1):S47–56.
29. Kennedy G, Hardman RJ, Macpherson H, Scholey AB, Pipingas A. How does exercise reduce the rate of age-associated cognitive decline? A review of potential mechanisms. J Alzheimers Dis. 2017;55(1):1–18.
30. Tan ZS, Spartano NL, Beiser AS, DeCarli C, Auerbach SH, Vasan RS, Seshadri S. Physical activity, brain volume, and dementia risk: the Framingham study. J Gerontol A Biol Sci Med Sci. 2017;72(6):789–95.
31. Tait JL, Duckham RL, Milte CM, Main LC, Daly RM. Influence of sequential vs. simultaneous dual-task exercise training on cognitive function in older adults. Front Aging Neurosci. 2017;9:368.
32. Levin O, Netz Y, Ziv G. The beneficial effects of different types of exercise interventions on motor and cognitive functions in older age: a systematic review. Eur Rev Aging Phys Act. 2017;14:20.
33. Robinson SM, Reginster JY, Rizzoli R, Shaw SC, Kanis JA, Bautmans I, Bischoff-Ferrari H, Bruyere O, Cesari M, Dawson-Hughes B, et al. Does nutrition play a role in the prevention and management of sarcopenia? Clin Nutr. 2017;37(4):1121–32. pii: S0261-5614(17)30299-6.
34. Beaudart C, Rabenda V, Simmons M, Geerinck A, Araujo De Carvalho I, Reginster JY, Amuthavalli Thiyagarajan J, Bruyere O. Effects of protein, essential amino acids, B-Hydroxy B-Methylbutyrate, creatine, dehydroepiandrosterone and fatty acid supplementation on muscle mass, muscle strength and physical performance in older people aged 60 years and over. A systematic review on the literature. J Nutr Health Aging. 2018;22(1):117–30.
35. Cruz-Jentoft AJ, Landi F, Schneider SM, Zuniga C, Arai H, Boirie Y, Chen LK, Fielding RA, Martin FC, Michel JP, et al. Prevalence of and interventions for sarcopenia in ageing adults: a systematic review. Report of the international sarcopenia initiative (EWGSOP and IWGS). Age Ageing. 2014;43(6):748–59.
36. Nowson CA, Service C, Appleton J, Grieger JA. The impact of dietary factors on indices of chronic disease in older people: a systematic review. J Nutr Health Aging. 2018;22(2):282–96.
37. Mithal A, Bonjour JP, Boonen S, Burckhardt P, Degens H, El Hajj Fuleihan G, Josse R, Lips P, Morales Torres J, Rizzoli R, et al. Impact of nutrition on muscle mass, strength, and performance in older adults. Osteoporos Int. 2013;24(5):1555–66.

38. Beaudart C, Buckinx F, Rabenda V, Gillain S, Cavalier E, Slomian J, Petermans J, Reginster JY, Bruyere O. The effects of vitamin D on skeletal muscle strength, muscle mass, and muscle power: a systematic review and meta-analysis of randomized controlled trials. J Clin Endocrinol Metab. 2014;99(11):4336–45.
39. Muir SW, Montero-Odasso M. Effect of vitamin D supplementation on muscle strength, gait and balance in older adults: a systematic review and meta-analysis. J Am Geriatr Soc. 2011;59(12):2291–300.
40. Dewansingh P, Melse-Boonstra A, Krijnen WP, van der Schans CP, Jager-Wittenaar H, van den Heuvel E. Supplemental protein from dairy products increases body weight and vitamin D improves physical performance in older adults: a systematic review and meta-analysis. Nutr Res. 2018;49:1–22.
41. Vauzour D, Camprubi-Robles M, Miquel-Kergoat S, Andres-Lacueva C, Banati D, Barberger-Gateau P, Bowman GL, Caberlotto L, Clarke R, Hogervorst E, et al. Nutrition for the ageing brain: towards evidence for an optimal diet. Ageing Res Rev. 2017;35:222–40.
42. Moore K, Hughes CF, Ward M, Hoey L, McNulty H. Diet, nutrition and the ageing brain: current evidence and new directions. Proc Nutr Soc. 2018;77(2):1–12.
43. Hardman RJ, Kennedy G, Macpherson H, Scholey AB, Pipingas A. Adherence to a Mediterranean-style diet and effects on cognition in adults: a qualitative evaluation and systematic review of longitudinal and prospective trials. Front Nutr. 2016;3:22.
44. van de Rest O, van der Zwaluw NL, de Groot LC. Literature review on the role of dietary protein and amino acids in cognitive functioning and cognitive decline. Amino Acids. 2013;45(5):1035–45.
45. Forbes SC, Holroyd-Leduc JM, Poulin MJ, Hogan DB. Effect of nutrients, dietary supplements and vitamins on cognition: a systematic review and meta-analysis of randomized controlled trials. Can Geriatr J. 2015;18(4):231–45.
46. D'Cunha NM, Georgousopoulou EN, Dadigamuwage L, Kellett J, Panagiotakos DB, Thomas J, McKune AJ, Mellor DD, Naumovski N. Effect of long-term nutraceutical and dietary supplement use on cognition in the elderly: a 10-year systematic review of randomised controlled trials. Br J Nutr. 2018;119(3):280–98.
47. Barha CK, Galea LA, Nagamatsu LS, Erickson KI, Liu-Ambrose T. Personalising exercise recommendations for brain health: considerations and future directions. Br J Sports Med. 2017;51(8):636–9.
48. Gomez-Pinilla F. Brain foods: the effects of nutrients on brain function. Nat Rev Neurosci. 2008;9(7):568–78.
49. Beaudart C, Dawson A, Shaw SC, Harvey NC, Kanis JA, Binkley N, Reginster JY, Chapurlat R, Chan DC, Bruyere O, et al. Nutrition and physical activity in the prevention and treatment of sarcopenia: systematic review. Osteoporos Int. 2017;28(6):1817–33.
50. Daly RM. Dietary protein, exercise and skeletal muscle: is there a synergistic effect in older adults and the elderly? In: Weaver CM, Daly RM, Bischoff Ferrari HA, editors. Nutritional influences on bone health: 9th international symposium. Basel: Springer; 2016. p. 63–78.
51. Tieland M, Dirks ML, van der Zwaluw N, Verdijk LB, van de Rest O, de Groot LC, van Loon LJ. Protein supplementation increases muscle mass gain during prolonged resistance-type exercise training in frail elderly people: a randomized, double-blind, placebo-controlled trial. J Am Med Dir Assoc. 2012;13(8):713–9.
52. van de Rest O, van der Zwaluw NL, Tieland M, Adam JJ, Hiddink GJ, van Loon LJ, de Groot LC. Effect of resistance-type exercise training with or without protein supplementation on cognitive functioning in frail and pre-frail elderly: secondary analysis of a randomized, double-blind, placebo-controlled trial. Mech Ageing Dev. 2014;136-137:85–93.
53. Antoniak AE, Greig CA. The effect of combined resistance exercise training and vitamin D3 supplementation on musculoskeletal health and function in older adults: a systematic review and meta-analysis. BMJ Open. 2017;7(7):e014619.
54. Uusi-Rasi K, Patil R, Karinkanta S, Kannus P, Tokola K, Lamberg-Allardt C, Sievanen H. Exercise and vitamin D in fall prevention among older women: a randomized clinical trial. JAMA Intern Med. 2015;175(5):703–11.

55. Da Boit M, Sibson R, Sivasubramaniam S, Meakin JR, Greig CA, Aspden RM, Thies F, Jeromson S, Hamilton DL, Speakman JR, et al. Sex differences in the effect of fish-oil supplementation on the adaptive response to resistance exercise training in older people: a randomized controlled trial. Am J Clin Nutr. 2017;105(1):151–8.
56. Rodacki CL, Rodacki AL, Pereira G, Naliwaiko K, Coelho I, Pequito D, Fernandes LC. Fish-oil supplementation enhances the effects of strength training in elderly women. Am J Clin Nutr. 2012;95(2):428–36.
57. Loef M, Walach H. The omega-6/omega-3 ratio and dementia or cognitive decline: a systematic review on human studies and biological evidence. J Nutr Gerontol Geriatr. 2013;32(1):1–23.
58. Andruchow ND, Konishi K, Shatenstein B, Bohbot VD. A lower ratio of omega-6 to omega-3 fatty acids predicts better hippocampus-dependent spatial memory and cognitive status in older adults. Neuropsychology. 2017;31(7):724–34.
59. Sheppard KW, Cheatham CL. Omega-6 to omega-3 fatty acid ratio and higher-order cognitive functions in 7- to 9-y-olds: a cross-sectional study. Am J Clin Nutr. 2013;98(3):659–67.
60. Andrieu S, Guyonnet S, Coley N, Cantet C, Bonnefoy M, Bordes S, Bories L, Cufi MN, Dantoine T, Dartigues JF, et al. Effect of long-term omega 3 polyunsaturated fatty acid supplementation with or without multidomain intervention on cognitive function in elderly adults with memory complaints (MAPT): a randomised, placebo-controlled trial. Lancet Neurol. 2017;16(5):377–89.
61. Gualano B, Rawson ES, Candow DG, Chilibeck PD. Creatine supplementation in the aging population: effects on skeletal muscle, bone and brain. Amino Acids. 2016;48(8):1793–805.
62. Alves CR, Merege Filho CA, Benatti FB, Brucki S, Pereira RM, de Sa Pinto AL, Lima FR, Roschel H, Gualano B. Creatine supplementation associated or not with strength training upon emotional and cognitive measures in older women: a randomized double-blind study. PLoS One. 2013;8(10):e76301.
63. Bobeuf F, Labonte M, Dionne IJ, Khalil A. Combined effect of antioxidant supplementation and resistance training on oxidative stress markers, muscle and body composition in an elderly population. J Nutr Health Aging. 2011;15(10):883–9.
64. Nalbant O, Toktas N, Toraman NF, Ogus C, Aydin H, Kacar C, Ozkaya YG. Vitamin E and aerobic exercise: effects on physical performance in older adults. Aging Clin Exp Res. 2009;21(2):111–21.
65. Bjornsen T, Salvesen S, Berntsen S, Hetlelid KJ, Stea TH, Lohne-Seiler H, Rohde G, Haraldstad K, Raastad T, Kopp U, et al. Vitamin C and E supplementation blunts increases in total lean body mass in elderly men after strength training. Scand J Med Sci Sports. 2016;26(7):755–63.
66. Mock JT, Chaudhari K, Sidhu A, Sumien N. The influence of vitamins E and C and exercise on brain aging. Exp Gerontol. 2017;94:69–72.
67. Ng TP, Feng L, Nyunt MS, Feng L, Niti M, Tan BY, Chan G, Khoo SA, Chan SM, Yap P, et al. Nutritional, physical, cognitive, and combination interventions and frailty reversal among older adults: a randomized controlled trial. Am J Med. 2015;128(11):1225–36. e1221
68. Fielding RA, Travison TG, Kirn DR, Koochek A, Reid KF, von Berens A, Zhu H, Folta SC, Sacheck JM, Nelson ME, et al. Effect of structured physical activity and nutritional supplementation on physical function in mobility-limited older adults: results from the VIVE2 randomized trial. J Nutr Health Aging. 2017;21(9):936–42.
69. Bell KE, Snijders T, Zulyniak M, Kumbhare D, Parise G, Chabowski A, Phillips SM. A whey protein-based multi-ingredient nutritional supplement stimulates gains in lean body mass and strength in healthy older men: a randomized controlled trial. PLoS One. 2017;12(7):e0181387.
70. Rondanelli M, Klersy C, Terracol G, Talluri J, Maugeri R, Guido D, Faliva MA, Solerte BS, Fioravanti M, Lukaski H, et al. Whey protein, amino acids, and vitamin D supplementation with physical activity increases fat-free mass and strength, functionality, and quality of life and decreases inflammation in sarcopenic elderly. Am J Clin Nutr. 2016;103(3):830–40.
71. Englund DA, Kirn DR, Koochek A, Zhu H, Travison TG, Reid KF, von Berens A, Melin M, Cederholm T, Gustafsson T, et al. Nutritional supplementation with physical activity improves muscle composition in mobility-limited older adults, the VIVE2 study: a randomized, double-blind, placebo-controlled trial. J Gerontol A Biol Sci Med Sci. 2017;73(1):95–101.

72. Addison O, Marcus RL, Lastayo PC, Ryan AS. Intermuscular fat: a review of the consequences and causes. Int J Endocrinol. 2014;2014:309570.
73. Romera-Liebana L, Orfila F, Segura JM, Real J, Fabra ML, Moller M, Lancho S, Ramirez A, Marti N, Cullell M et al. Effects of a primary-care based multifactorial intervention on physical and cognitive function in frail, elderly individuals: a randomized controlled trial. J Gerontol A Biol Sci Med Sci. 2018. doi:https://doi.org/10.1093/gerona/glx259.
74. Ngandu T, Lehtisalo J, Solomon A, Levalahti E, Ahtiluoto S, Antikainen R, Backman L, Hanninen T, Jula A, Laatikainen T, et al. A 2 year multidomain intervention of diet, exercise, cognitive training, and vascular risk monitoring versus control to prevent cognitive decline in at-risk elderly people (FINGER): a randomised controlled trial. Lancet. 2015;385(9984):2255–63.

9 Sedentary Behaviors in Children and Adolescents: What Is the Influence on Bone Strength?

Simon Higgins, Staci L. Belcher, and Richard D. Lewis

Introduction

Children and adolescents are spending a considerable amount of their waking day in sitting or reclining postures [1, 2], including sedentary behaviors such as television viewing, using handheld electronic devices, sitting in school, completing homework, eating, and traveling [3–5]. This lifestyle is disconcerting because during the period of rapid adolescent growth, when being physically active is essential for optimal bone mineral accrual, a sedentary lifestyle is becoming the norm [1]. The acute and chronic implications of excessive sedentary behavior in children and adolescents have been addressed in several systematic reviews [6–9]. High amounts of sedentary behavior are associated with an increased risk of clustered cardiometabolic disease risk factors including adiposity [10], low cardiorespiratory fitness [6], and insulin resistance [6, 8], as well as greater likelihood of behavioral issues and psychosocial well-being detriments [6]. However, the evidence remains conflicting with regard to whether all types of sedentary behaviors (i.e., TV viewing time vs. total objectively measured sedentary behavior) are equally detrimental [6, 8].

One area that has received more attention in the recent years is the link between sedentary behaviors and bone health in children and adolescents [3, 11–13]. The physiological implications of excessive sedentary behaviors have been compared to periods of extended bed rest [14] and weightlessness experienced in space flight [15]; both conditions are associated with significant bone loss. Whether excess accumulation of sedentary behaviors as part of daily routines is analogous to these conditions is not known. It is hypothesized that sedentary lifestyles may attenuate the rapid skeletal growth and mineralization during adolescence [16] and potentially

S. Higgins (✉)
Department of Exercise Science, Elon University, Elon, NC, USA
e-mail: shiggins8@elon.edu

S. L. Belcher · R. D. Lewis
Department of Foods and Nutrition, University of Georgia, Athens, GA, USA

© Springer Nature Switzerland AG 2019
C. M. Weaver et al. (eds.), *Nutritional Influences on Bone Health*,
https://doi.org/10.1007/978-3-319-98464-3_9

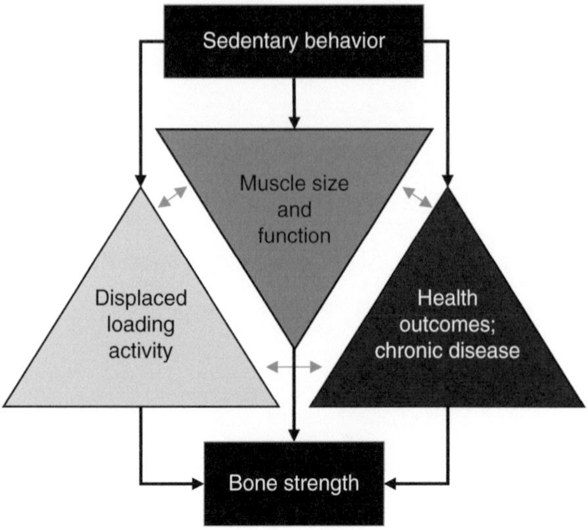

Fig. 9.1 A conceptual model for the potential detrimental effects of excess sedentary behavior on bone strength

limit peak bone mass development. Figure 9.1 presents a conceptual model describing potential pathways through which excess sedentary behavior could alter bone strength during growth.

In this chapter, sedentary behaviors will be defined and their prevalence described. We will address methodologies used in the assessment of sedentary behaviors and the links between sedentary time and health outcomes. The primary aim of the chapter will be to address the impact of total objectively measured and self-reported sedentary behavior on bone strength. This will be accompanied by an examination of the influences of patterns of sedentary time accumulation, including the analysis of shorter vs. longer duration bouts. Moreover, the effects of the displacement of physical activity (Fig. 9.1) will be addressed. The chapter will conclude by identifying directions for future research.

Defining and Measuring Sedentary Behavior

There is a clear distinction between the terms "sedentary behavior" and "physical inactivity" as well as the independent behaviors that each encompasses. It has been recommended that use of the term "sedentary behavior" should be limited to define behaviors that are seated or reclined in posture and those in which energy expenditure is $\leq$1.5 metabolic equivalents in intensity [17]. In contrast, "physical inactivity" is used to refer to someone who is not meeting physical activity guidelines of their respective country [17]. Sedentary behaviors include, but are not limited to, TV watching, non-TV screen-based activities, reading, homework, or playing video games. However, the most frequently reported sedentary behavior among children is TV watching, which consumes

Table 9.1 Commonly used cut points for the assessment of sedentary behavior and physical activity intensity in children aged 5–8 years [60]

Commonly used activity cut points in children (counts per minute, cpm)	
Sedentary	0–99 cpm
Light-intensity physical activity	101–2295 cpm
Moderate-intensity physical activity	2296–4011 cpm
Vigorous-intensity physical activity	≥4012 cpm
Moderate-to-vigorous intensity physical activity	≥2296 cpm

about 20% of their time [18]. This distinction allows researchers to capture a more accurate depiction of behaviors among populations. For example, a child may meet the physical activity recommendations for his or her age group while simultaneously acquiring many hours of sedentary behaviors during and after school. Labeling this child as only "sedentary" does not capture the positive effects of their physical activity, while labeling them exclusively as "physically active" discounts any possible negative effects of sedentary behavior on health. The distinct risks and/or benefits inherent to each behavioral pattern elicit a methodological need to distinguish between the two [8]; thus, the inclusion of formal definitions allows researchers to accurately characterize the behavioral patterns of children and adolescents.

Key methodological considerations that can influence outcomes during the objective measurement (i.e., accelerometers) of physical activity and sedentary behaviors in children and adolescents include epoch duration used during data collection and count per minute (cpm) cut points chosen to differentiate among activity intensities during analysis [19, 20]. Current recommendations suggest that epoch duration be minimized, with 5-second epochs suggested as optimal to reduce misclassification error associated with the brief bursts of activity typically observed in childhood populations [21]. With regard to cut points, Evenson et al. recommend that researchers adopt standard cpm thresholds (Table 9.1) to ensure comparability and consistency across studies [22], as differing classification methodologies can make comparison among studies more complex [18, 23].

An example of this from a sedentary behavior perspective is a study by Atkin et al., which tested different cpm cut points for sedentary behaviors in a cohort of 2327 participants (n = 1031 aged 9 and n = 1296 aged 15) with at least 1 day of valid wear time. Sedentary behaviors were defined according to the following cpm cut points: ≤100, ≤500, ≤800, or ≤ 1100, and the authors reported that the magnitude of the positive association between metabolic risk and sedentary behavior was generally greater when a larger cpm cut point was chosen [19]. Thus, caution is recommended when comparing studies that utilize differing cut points. It is essential that researchers consider these methodological differences as well as others, such as the use of uniaxial (vertical axis) vs. triaxial (vector magnitude) methods of data collection and analysis or differences in wear time and number of valid wear days when designing and comparing studies. Furthermore, measuring sedentary behavior with accelerometers has important inherent limitations. For example, a quiet standing posture can be misclassified as sedentary behavior, as accelerometers do not distinguish between sitting and standing with high accuracy [24]. Devices such as the activPAL are used to measure these more subtle postural changes such as sitting, lying down, or standing, but are not widely used due to a poor validity in the concurrent assessment of moderate-to-vigorous intensity physical activity (MVPA) [25]. Despite its limitations, accelerometry is more commonly used than postural measurement devices in the objective assessment of sedentary behaviors and is preferred to self-report data, which is susceptible to more severe misclassification, inaccuracies, and errors in reporting [26].

The Sedentary Behavior Epidemic

The US 2018 Physical Activity Guidelines Advisory Committee Scientific Report [27], in concurrence with the 2008 Physical Activity Guidelines for Americans [28], recommends that children and adolescents engage in 60 min of MVPA daily. These recommendations are consistent with recommendations from Canada [29], Australia [30], and Europe [31]. The US 2008 guidelines [28] and 2018 report [27] advised that these activities should be aerobic and muscle- and bone-strengthening, specifically including activities that apply high-impact forces to bones. However, US guidelines for the reduction of sedentary behavior in children and adolescents are yet to be proposed beyond the simple avoidance of an inactive lifestyle [27, 28]. In contrast, Canadian officials recommend that children and adolescents from the ages of 5–17 should limit recreational screen time to no more than 2 h/day and also limit motorized transport [29]. Australian guidelines are in agreement, recommending the limitation of electronic media usage to no more than 2 h/day and that children and adolescents break up long period of sitting as often as possible [30]. It is unlikely that the United States will follow suit in their 2018 Physical Activity Guidelines for Americans, as the recent Scientific Advisory Committee Report concluded that evidence supporting negative or null effects of excess sedentary behavior, on cardiometabolic or bone health, respectively, in children and adolescents was limited [27]. Nevertheless, the adoption of consistent sedentary behavior guidelines, as seen with physical activity, would mark a positive milestone in global musculoskeletal and cardiometabolic risk reduction.

Epidemiological data have revealed a striking trend of increasing sedentary behaviors across consecutive ages of children and adolescents worldwide (Fig. 9.2a, b). Utilizing data from the National Health and Nutrition Examination Survey, Matthews et al. reported that US adolescents, 16–19 years of age, had about 2 h/day more sedentary behavior than children between the ages of 6 and 11 years (Fig. 9.2b) [1]. Tanaka et al. reviewed longitudinal studies in children and adolescents and quantified that adolescents acquired an extra 30 min/day in sedentary time for every passing year [10]. Similar high volumes of sedentary behaviors that increase through adolescent growth are observed worldwide with data reported from Canada [32], Vietnam [33], Australia [34], and Britain [35]. A systematic review reported that children and

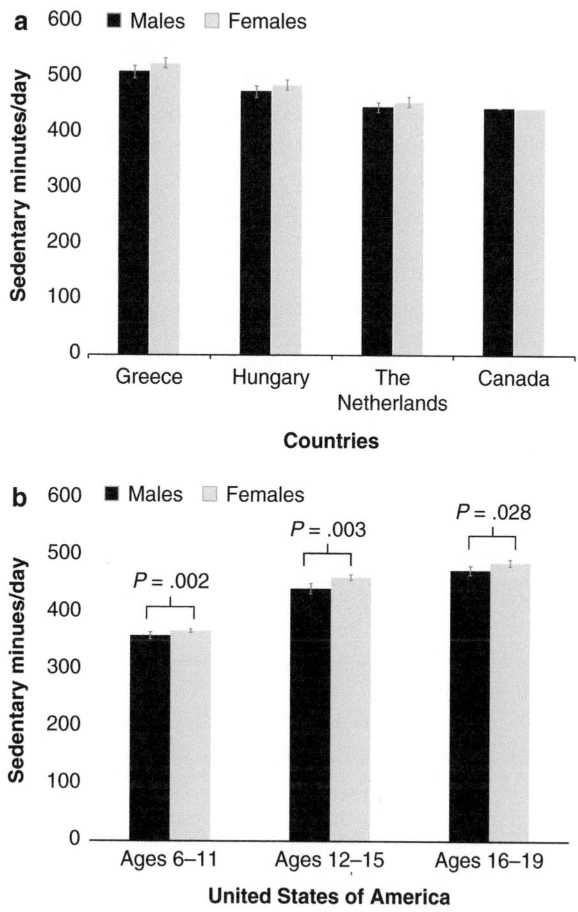

Fig. 9.2 (**a**) Sedentary behavior is common in countries around the world. Children from Greece, Hungary, and the Netherlands were 10–12 years old, and when data from all countries were combined, females were more sedentary than males ($p < 0.001$) [2]. Canadian children were 6–10 years old [31]. (**b**) In the United States, sedentary time is 2 h higher in children aged 16–19 than those aged 6–11 (linear trend by age; $p < 0.001$), and females were more sedentary than males across all age groups (all $p < 0.05$) [1]

adolescents spend an average of 49.5% and 56.6% of their after school time, respectively, engaged in sedentary behaviors [18]. Moreover, females are consistently more sedentary than males (Fig. 9.2a) [36], and sedentary time has been reported to be higher on weekend days compared to weekdays and/or school days [37].

Concern for the metabolic implications of excess sedentary behaviors in children and adolescents stems from the inclination to presume that the detrimental health effects observed in adults, independent of MVPA [27, 38, 39], also occur in youth. Specifically, strong evidence in adults supports the existence of dose-response relationships between sedentary behavior and (1) mortality from cardiovascular disease, (2) all-cause mortality, and (3) type 2 diabetes risk [27]. Data in children and adolescents are conflicting with some reporting a strong relationship between obesity and time spent in sedentary behaviors [40, 41], but others are reporting no relationships between sedentary behaviors and metabolic syndrome risk factors [40]. Froberg and Raustorp noted that most cross-sectional studies conclude there is little evidence to support the link between patterns or total volume of sedentary time and individual cardiometabolic risk after controlling for MVPA [42]. However, others have reported strong evidence from prospective studies in support of an inverse relationship between TV viewing, a common surrogate measure for sedentary behavior, and HDL cholesterol, a risk-reducing cardiometabolic factor [40]. Furthermore, trends reveal that as hours of TV viewing increase, risk for obesity (13% increase for each 1-hour per day increase of TV watching, $p < 0.001$) [43] and metabolic syndrome (odds ratio increased from 1.21 to 3.07 across screen time categories from 2 to 5 h/day, $p_{trend} < 0.01$) [44] also increase. There is moderate evidence to support a positive relationship between sedentary time and total cholesterol [41], and in adolescent females, a negative relationship between sedentary behaviors and healthy dietary behaviors has been reported [45].

Drawing conclusions across this body of work is complicated. A recent review graded the evidence of 109 prospective studies and classified only 19 studies as high quality [40]. The choice of sedentary behavior measurement methodology (subjective vs. objective), as well as differences in statistical techniques, including controlling for confounding variables such as physical activity [5, 46], will also influence the strength of evidence and conclusions. This is highlighted by the 2018 Physical Activity Guidelines Advisory Committee Scientific Report which concluded that subjectively measured sedentary behaviors (such as TV viewing time or screen time) provided stronger evidence for a detrimental effect on cardiometabolic health, including weight or adiposity, than the limited evidence provided by objective measures of total sedentary behavior [27]. Furthermore, self- and/or parent-reported sedentary behavior is common, of which reliability testing is not the norm, so accuracy within and between studies needs to be considered when drawing conclusions [47]. Finally, null effects may not be truly representative of the risk, as it has been proposed that children may not have been exposed to sedentary behavior long enough to see ill-health effects [48] as observed in adults [49].

Sedentary Behavior and Bone

The effects of sedentary behaviors on bone outcomes in children and adolescents were addressed in a 2017 systematic review [3]. Major findings were that the total time school-aged children spent in objectively measured sedentary behavior negatively predicted lower extremity bone outcomes, independent of time spent in MVPA. Conversely, subjective measures of sedentary behavior were not predictive of lower extremity, lumbar spine, or total body bone outcomes. MVPA was a strong and consistent positive predictor of bone outcomes; however, the concurrent independent effect of sedentary behavior on bone suggests that each behavior may influence bone through different mechanisms [3].

Of the 19 studies Koedijk et al. reviewed [3], only three were of a high quality [50–52], and two of the three reported data from the same cohort [50, 52]. The high-quality studies utilized objective measures of sedentary behavior and dual-energy X-ray absorptiometry (DXA)-derived bone outcomes. Among the moderate- and low-quality reports, there was significant heterogeneity with regard to the study design and measurement methodologies. Heterogeneity is presented in various ways: wide age and maturation ranges, from pre- to postpubertal children and adolescents, varying methodologies used to assess bone outcomes (DXA, peripheral quantitative computed tomography, high-resolution peripheral quantitative computed tomography [HRpQCT], and ultrasound) and sedentary behaviors (self-report, parent report, and accelerometry). Moreover, many reports lack adjustment for known confounding variables, such as height when reporting DXA-derived bone mineral content (BMC) in children. Though high-quality longitudinal data provide the greatest insight into the relationships among activity intensities and bone mineral accrual throughout youth, the majority of evidence regarding the sedentary behavior and bone relationship is currently derived from cross-sectional reports. Key cross-sectional studies assessed objectively measured total sedentary behavior and sedentary behavior distribution in tandem with self-reported screen time using questionnaires [11, 12]. The following paragraphs begin by outlining these cross-sectional papers, prior to examining the current longitudinal evidence to provide further insight.

Gabel et al. reported on a cohort of 154 males and 174 females aged 9–20 years [11]. Bone outcomes were acquired via HRpQCT and were assessed relative to time spent in objectively and subjectively measured sedentary behavior (total time and TV viewing time, respectively), as well as breaks in sedentary behavior [11]. After controlling for time spent in MVPA and other known confounders, there was no association between any iteration of sedentary behavior, or breaks in sedentary behavior, and bone architecture, volumetric bone mineral density (vBMD), or bone strength at the distal tibia [11]. In this sample, variance in bone outcomes was accounted for by maturity, muscle cross-sectional area, tibia length, dietary calcium intake, ethnicity, and, importantly, time spent in MVPA. Though this study observed no significant relationships between sedentary behavior and bone after controlling for MVPA, it is not alone in doing so [53–56] and does add to the strong confirmatory evidence of the beneficial effect of MVPA on the growing bone.

A second key cross-sectional study utilized the National Health and Nutrition Examination Survey data from the 2005 to 2006 cycle. Bone outcomes were assessed via DXA and sedentary behaviors using subjective and objective measures, TV viewing time, and accelerometry, respectively, in 677 females and 671 males aged 8–22 years [12]. In this representative sample, both objectively measured sedentary behavior and self-reported total non-screen-based sedentary behaviors were positively associated with femoral BMC, independent of MVPA, age, body mass index, ethnicity, and serum vitamin D, in males and females [12]. These counterintuitive findings agree with positive relationships seen in a key prospective report discussed later in the chapter [13]. Furthermore, the positive associations are contradictory to other data in the same manuscript that suggest that self-reported screen time was negatively associated with femoral BMC in males and females, and spinal BMC in females, independent of time in MVPA. The findings highlight the importance of recognizing the use of different measures of sedentary time, for example, subjectively measured TV viewing time or objectively measured sedentary behavior, on study outcomes. This could suggest that these notations of sedentary behavior are not capturing the same behaviors and may in fact include other detrimental behaviors such as unhealthy eating patterns as suggested in cardiometabolic data [45]. Furthermore, the authors of the above-described manuscript aimed to quantify the effects of the distribution of objectively measured sedentary behaviors throughout the day, relative to bouts of MVPA, on bone outcomes. A pattern of accrual where MVPA was less clustered and interspersed with shorter periods of sedentary behavior was negatively associated with femoral and spinal BMC in men and women. These findings suggest that long periods of sedentary behavior with clustered physical activity breaks might be a beneficial patterning of sedentary behavior intermittence. Without confirmation from clinical trials, this finding is hard to interpret from a public health perspective, especially when considering that the opposite can be said to be true in terms of the effects of sedentary behavior distribution on cardiometabolic health [6].

Since publication of the previously discussed review that included six longitudinal prospective or retrospective reports [50–52, 56–59], a noteworthy prospective study was published examining the relationships among objectively measured sedentary behavior, MVPA, and bone outcomes measured by HRpQCT [13]. Gabel et al. reported on a cohort of 136 males and 173 females from the University of British Columbia's Pediatric Bone and Physical Activity Database who were aged 9–20 years old at baseline and were followed for 4 years [13]. Time spent in MVPA, especially during the early- and mid-pubertal stages, was a positive independent predictor of bone strength (coefficient [CI], 297.3 [157.9–436.6]; 100.2 [43.1–157.3]) and bone volume fraction (coefficient [CI], 0.005 [0.001–0.09]; 0.006 [0.001–0.011]) at the distal tibia and radius, respectively [13]. Unexpectedly, total time spent in sedentary behaviors positively predicted cortical thickness (coefficient [CI], 0.10 [0.04–0.17]), trabecular thickness (coefficient [CI], 0.006 [0.003–0.009]), and cortical vBMD (coefficient [CI], 24.7 [9.9–39.5]) at the distal tibia, independent of time in MVPA [13]. Conversely, total time spent in sedentary behavior was negatively associated with total area (coefficient [CI], −58.9 [−88.0 to −29.7]) at the tibia. All analyses are controlled for known covariates of maturity, ethnicity, sex, dietary calcium, limb length, lean body mass, and muscle power. These unexpected contrasting results, together with previous cross-sectional findings, suggest that certain types and/or accrual patterns of sedentary behavior may have a beneficial effect on the status of specific bone characteristics during youth. Moreover, the effects of sedentary behaviors on bone, independent of MVPA, suggest that there may be differing mechanisms through which MVPA and sedentary behaviors affect bone, aside from the simple displacement of one another.

A second key longitudinal report utilized a nonconventional analysis technique to characterize the relationship between sedentary behavior and DXA-derived bone outcomes, relative to changes in other activity variables [51]. The study, which addresses the hypothesized pathway of sedentary behaviors displacing physical activity depicted in Fig. 9.1, included data collected over 2 years in 299 males and

303 females aged 7.2–12 years from Denmark [51]. The effects of altering time spent in sedentary behavior, with relative opposing changes in light-intensity physical activities (LPA) or MVPA, were modeled. This type of analysis is important as it helps to examine sedentary behavior in the context of total daily activity, as we cannot alter sedentary behavior without influencing the time spent in other intensities of physical activity within a human population. The models of Heidemann et al. found two major themes: (1) while holding time spent in MVPA at the mean, replacing time spent in LPA with sedentary behavior led to an increase in total body BMC but not areal bone mineral density or bone area, and (2) while maintaining LPA at the mean, an increased time spent in MVPA relative to sedentary behavior led to a proportional increase in all bone outcomes [51]. These findings suggest a potentially beneficial relationship between sedentary behavior and bone, relative to LPA, which was more pronounced in females. Furthermore, results such as these emphasize that the intensity, or more specifically the osteogenic nature (moderate-to-high impact) of activity, need be considered when discussing bone recommendations. In this way, the importance of MVPA throughout childhood is reinforced, specifically when osteogenic MVPA displaces time spent in sedentary behaviors, as this would flip the traditional displacement hypothesis. The paucity of longitudinal data suggests that to definitively characterize the sedentary behavior and bone relationship, more high-quality longitudinal studies are needed utilizing standardized measures of bone and sedentary behavior outcomes [3].

Conclusion

Children and adolescents worldwide are becoming more sedentary, and the health outcomes resulting from this lifestyle are not entirely clear. The majority of research on sedentary behaviors and health is directed to the effects on cardiometabolic health. Sedentary behaviors, independent of osteogenic MVPA, are now emerging as potentially influential factors on bone strength, with the direction of this influence being somewhat debatable. Specifically, positive relationships between sedentary behaviors and bone outcomes that persist after controlling for factors such as muscle power, lean mass, and total MVPA may support the need for rest periods between bouts of osteogenic activity to optimize the bone anabolic response, whereas data in support of the displacement hypothesis suggest that reversing the paradigm and replacing sedentary behaviors with more MVPA may help to optimize bone mineral accrual. Further high-quality longitudinal data are needed to confirm these conflicting findings. Future research opportunities exist to help better define the effects of sedentary behaviors on different types on bone. These include the effects of (1) mode (i.e., TV viewing, total non-screen-based sitting, and total objectively measured sedentary behaviors); (2) distribution pattern relative to other activity variables, for example, shorter vs. longer duration sedentary bouts (Fig. 9.3); and (3) displacement of different intensities of physical activity by sedentary behavior. Furthermore, assessment of the relationship between sedentary behavior and major effectors of

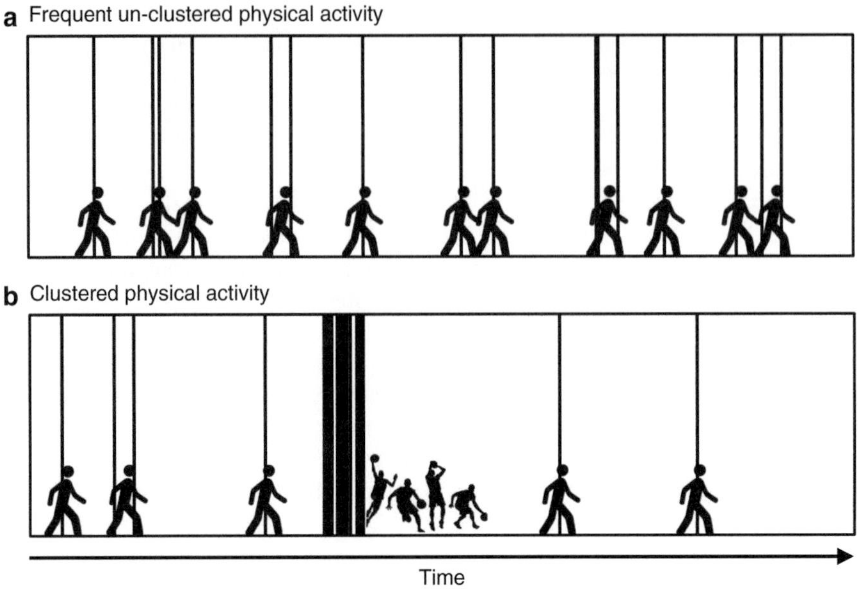

Fig. 9.3 Emerging data suggests that sedentary time accrued in long uninterrupted bouts (**b**), rather than frequent short periods (**a**), may appear beneficial due to physical activity clustering in a more osteogenic fashion [12]

bone such as fat-free soft tissue and/or neuromuscular function is also promising and may highlight potential mechanisms of the independent effects of sedentary behavior and MVPA on bone. While it is premature to generate public health recommendations with respect to sedentary behaviors and bone, it is clear that MVPA remains the most influential activity-related behavior for optimal bone accrual. Future guidelines should continue to promote activity while examining its interaction with sedentary behaviors.

References

1. Matthews CE, Chen KY, Freedson PS, Buchowski MS, Beech BM, Pate RR, Troiano RP. Amount of Time Spent in Sedentary Behaviors in the United States, 2003–2004. Am J Epidemiol. 2008;167(7):875–81. https://doi.org/10.1093/aje/kwm390.
2. Verloigne M, Van Lippevelde W, Maes L, Yıldırım M, Chinapaw M, Manios Y, Androutsos O, Kovács É, Bringolf-Isler B, Brug J, De Bourdeaudhuij I. Levels of physical activity and sedentary time among 10- to 12-year-old boys and girls across 5 European countries using accelerometers: an observational study within the ENERGY-project. Int J Behav Nutr Phys Act. 2012;9(1):34. https://doi.org/10.1186/1479-5868-9-34.
3. Koedijk JB, van Rijswijk J, Oranje WA, van den Bergh JP, Bours SP, Savelberg HH, Schaper NC. Sedentary behaviour and bone health in children, adolescents and young adults: a systematic review. Osteoporos Int. 2017;28:2507–19. https://doi.org/10.1007/s00198-017-4076-2.
4. Saunders TJ, Gray CE, Poitras VJ, Chaput JP, Janssen I, Katzmarzyk PT, Olds T, Connor Gorber S, Kho ME, Sampson M, Tremblay MS, Carson V. Combinations of physical activity,

sedentary behaviour and sleep: relationships with health indicators in school-aged children and youth. Appl Physiol Nutr Metab. 2016;41(6 Suppl 3):S283–93. https://doi.org/10.1139/apnm-2015-0626.

5. Cliff DP, Hesketh KD, Vella SA, Hinkley T, Tsiros MD, Ridgers ND, Carver A, Veitch J, Parrish AM, Hardy LL, Plotnikoff RC, Okely AD, Salmon J, Lubans DR. Objectively measured sedentary behaviour and health and development in children and adolescents: systematic review and meta-analysis. Obes Rev. 2016;17(4):330–44. https://doi.org/10.1111/obr.12371.
6. Carson V, Hunter S, Kuzik N, Gray CE, Poitras VJ, Chaput JP, Saunders TJ, Katzmarzyk PT, Okely AD, Connor Gorber S, Kho ME, Sampson M, Lee H, Tremblay MS. Systematic review of sedentary behaviour and health indicators in school-aged children and youth: an update. Appl Physiol Nutr Metab. 2016;41(6 Suppl 3):S240–65. https://doi.org/10.1139/apnm-2015-0630.
7. Tremblay MS, LeBlanc AG, Kho ME, Saunders TJ, Larouche R, Colley RC, Goldfield G, Connor Gorber S. Systematic review of sedentary behaviour and health indicators in school-aged children and youth. Int J Behav Nutr Phys Act. 2011;8:98. https://doi.org/10.1186/1479-5868-8-98.
8. Saunders TJ, Chaput JP, Tremblay MS. Sedentary behaviour as an emerging risk factor for cardiometabolic diseases in children and youth. Can J Diabetes. 2014;38(1):53–61. https://doi.org/10.1016/j.jcjd.2013.08.266.
9. Mitchell JA, Byun W. Sedentary behavior and health outcomes in children and adolescents. Am J Lifestyle Med. 2014;8(3):173–99. https://doi.org/10.1177/1559827613498700.
10. Tanaka C, Reilly JJ, Huang WY. Longitudinal changes in objectively measured sedentary behaviour and their relationship with adiposity in children and adolescents: systematic review and evidence appraisal. Obes Rev. 2014;15(10):791–803. https://doi.org/10.1111/obr.12195.
11. Gabel L, McKay HA, Nettlefold L, Race D, Macdonald HM. Bone architecture and strength in the growing skeleton: the role of sedentary time. Med Sci Sports Exerc. 2015;47(2):363–72. https://doi.org/10.1249/mss.0000000000000418.
12. Chastin SF, Mandrichenko O, Skelton DA. The frequency of osteogenic activities and the pattern of intermittence between periods of physical activity and sedentary behaviour affects bone mineral content: the cross-sectional NHANES study. BMC Public Health. 2014;14:4. https://doi.org/10.1186/1471-2458-14-4.
13. Gabel L, Macdonald HM, Nettlefold L, McKay HA. Physical activity, sedentary time, and bone strength from childhood to early adulthood: a mixed longitudinal HR-pQCT study. J Bone Miner Res. 2017;32(7):1525–36. https://doi.org/10.1002/jbmr.3115.
14. Thyfault JP, Du M, Kraus WE, Levine JA, Booth FW. Physiology of sedentary behavior and its relationship to health outcomes. Med Sci Sports Exerc. 2015;47(6):1301–5. https://doi.org/10.1249/MSS.0000000000000518.
15. Caillot-Augusseau A, Lafage-Proust MH, Soler C, Pernod J, Dubois F, Alexandre C. Bone formation and resorption biological markers in cosmonauts during and after a 180-day space flight (Euromir 95). Clin Chem. 1998;44(3):578–85.
16. Bailey DA, McKay HA, Mirwald RL, Crocker PRE, Faulkner RA. A six-year longitudinal study of the relationship of physical activity to bone mineral accrual in growing children: the University of Saskatchewan Bone Mineral Accrual Study. J Bone Miner Res. 1999;14(10):1672–9. https://doi.org/10.1359/jbmr.1999.14.10.1672.
17. Sedentary Behaviour Research Network. Letter to the Editor: Standardized use of the terms 'sedentary' and 'sedentary behaviours'. Appl Physiol Nutr Metab. 2012;37(3):540–2. https://doi.org/10.1139/h2012-024.
18. Arundell L, Fletcher E, Salmon J, Veitch J, Hinkley T. A systematic review of the prevalence of sedentary behavior during the after-school period among children aged 5-18 years. Int J Behav Nutr Phys Act. 2016;13(1):93. https://doi.org/10.1186/s12966-016-0419-1.
19. Atkin AJ, Ekelund U, Moller NC, Froberg K, Sardinha LB, Andersen LB, Brage S. Sedentary time in children: influence of accelerometer processing on health relations. Med Sci Sports Exerc. 2013;45(6):1097–104. https://doi.org/10.1249/MSS.0b013e318282190e.

20. Ojiambo R, Cuthill R, Budd H, Konstabel K, Casajus JA, Gonzalez-Aguero A, Anjila E, Reilly JJ, Easton C, Pitsiladis YP. Impact of methodological decisions on accelerometer outcome variables in young children. Int J Obes. 2011;35(Suppl 1):S98–103. https://doi.org/10.1038/ijo.2011.40.
21. McClain JJ, Abraham TL, Brusseau TA Jr, Tudor-Locke C. Epoch length and accelerometer outputs in children: comparison to direct observation. Med Sci Sports Exerc. 2008;40(12):2080–7. https://doi.org/10.1249/MSS.0b013e3181824d98.
22. Evenson KR, Wen F, Hales D, Herring AH. National youth sedentary behavior and physical activity daily patterns using latent class analysis applied to accelerometry. Int J Behav Nutr Phys Act. 2016;13:55. https://doi.org/10.1186/s12966-016-0382-x.
23. Reilly JJ, Penpraze V, Hislop J, Davies G, Grant S, Paton JY. Objective measurement of physical activity and sedentary behaviour: review with new data. Arch Dis Child. 2008;93(7):614–9. https://doi.org/10.1136/adc.2007.133272.
24. Hart TL, Ainsworth BE, Tudor-Locke C. Objective and subjective measures of sedentary behavior and physical activity. Med Sci Sports Exerc. 2011;43(3):449–56. https://doi.org/10.1249/MSS.0b013e3181ef5a93.
25. Aminian S, Hinckson EA. Examining the validity of the ActivPAL monitor in measuring posture and ambulatory movement in children. Int J Behav Nutr Phys Act. 2012;9:119. https://doi.org/10.1186/1479-5868-9-119.
26. Chinapaw MJ, Proper KI, Brug J, van Mechelen W, Singh AS. Relationship between young peoples' sedentary behaviour and biomedical health indicators: a systematic review of prospective studies. Obes Rev. 2011;12(7):e621–32. https://doi.org/10.1111/j.1467-789X.2011.00865.x.
27. U.S. Department of Health and Human Services. 2018 Physical activity guidelines advisory committee scientific report. Office of Disease Prevention and Health Promotion. 2018. https://health.gov/paguidelines/second-edition/report/pdf/PAG_Advisory_Committee_Report.pdf. Accessed 12 Mar 2018.
28. U.S. Department of Health and Human Services. Physical activity guidelines for Americans. Office of Disease Prevention and Health Promotion. 2008. https://health.gov/paguidelines/guidelines/. Accessed 22 Feb 2018.
29. Tremblay MS, Carson V, Chaput J-P, Connor Gorber S, Dinh T, Duggan M, Faulkner G, Gray CE, Gruber R, Janson K, Janssen I, Katzmarzyk PT, Kho ME, Latimer-Cheung AE, Le Blanc C, Okely AD, Olds T, Pate RR, Phillips A, Poitras VJ, Rodenburg S, Sampson M, Saunders TJ, Stone JA, Stratton G, Weiss SK, Zehr L. Canadian 24-hour movement guidelines for children and youth: an integration of physical activity, sedentary behaviour, and sleep. Appl Physiol Nutr Metab. 2016;41(6 (Suppl. 3)):S311–27. https://doi.org/10.1139/apnm-2016-0151.
30. Australian Government Department of Health. Australia's physical activity and sedentary behaviour guidelines. The Department of Health. 2017. http://www.health.gov.au/internet/main/publishing.nsf/content/health-pubhlth-strateg-phys-act-guidelines#apaadult. Accessed 22 Feb 2018.
31. E.U. Working Group "Sport & Health". EU physical activity guidelines: recommended policy actions in support of health-enhancing physical activity. 2008. http://ec.europa.eu/assets/eac/sport/library/policy_documents/eu-physical-activity-guidelines-2008_en.pdf. Accessed 22 Feb 2018.
32. Colley RC, Garriguet D, Janssen I, Craig CL, Clarke J, Tremblay MS. Physical activity of Canadian children and youth: accelerometer results from the 2007 to 2009 Canadian Health Measures Survey. Health Rep. 2011;22(1):15–23.
33. Trang NH, Hong TK, van der Ploeg HP, Hardy LL, Kelly PJ, Dibley MJ. Longitudinal sedentary behavior changes in adolescents in Ho Chi Minh City. Am J Prev Med. 2013;44(3):223–30. https://doi.org/10.1016/j.amepre.2012.10.021.
34. Hardy LL, Dobbins T, Booth ML, Denney-Wilson E, Okely AD. Sedentary behaviours among Australian adolescents. Aust N Z J Public Health. 2006;30(6):534–40. https://doi.org/10.1111/j.1467-842X.2006.tb00782.x.
35. Brodersen NH, Steptoe A, Boniface DR, Wardle J. Trends in physical activity and sedentary behaviour in adolescence: ethnic and socioeconomic differences. Br J Sports Med. 2007;41(3):140–4. https://doi.org/10.1136/bjsm.2006.031138.

36. Stierlin AS, De Lepeleere S, Cardon G, Dargent-Molina P, Hoffmann B, Murphy MH, Kennedy A, O'Donoghue G, Chastin SF, De Craemer M. A systematic review of determinants of sedentary behaviour in youth: a DEDIPAC-study. Int J Behav Nutr Phys Act. 2015;12(1):133. https://doi.org/10.1186/s12966-015-0291-4.
37. Bucksch J, Sigmundova D, Hamrik Z, Troped PJ, Melkevik O, Ahluwalia N, Borraccino A, Tynjala J, Kalman M, Inchley J. International trends in adolescent screen-time behaviors from 2002 to 2010. J Adolesc Health. 2016;58(4):417–25. https://doi.org/10.1016/j.jadohealth.2015.11.014.
38. Biswas A, Oh PI, Faulkner GE, Bajaj RR, Silver MA, Mitchell MS, Alter DA. Sedentary time and its association with risk for disease incidence, mortality, and hospitalization in adults: a systematic review and meta-analysis. Ann Intern Med. 2015;162(2):123–32. https://doi.org/10.7326/m14-1651.
39. Tremblay MS, Colley RC, Saunders TJ, Healy GN, Owen N. Physiological and health implications of a sedentary lifestyle. Appl Physiol Nutr Metab. 2010;35(6):725–40. https://doi.org/10.1139/h10-079.
40. van Ekris E, Altenburg TM, Singh AS, Proper KI, Heymans MW, Chinapaw MJ. An evidence-update on the prospective relationship between childhood sedentary behaviour and biomedical health indicators: a systematic review and meta-analysis. Obes Rev. 2016;17(9):833–49. https://doi.org/10.1111/obr.12426.
41. de Rezende LF, Rodrigues Lopes M, Rey-Lopez JP, Matsudo VK, Luiz Odo C. Sedentary behavior and health outcomes: an overview of systematic reviews. PLoS One. 2014;9(8):e105620. https://doi.org/10.1371/journal.pone.0105620.
42. Froberg A, Raustorp A. Objectively measured sedentary behaviour and cardio-metabolic risk in youth: a review of evidence. Eur J Pediatr. 2014;173(7):845–60. https://doi.org/10.1007/s00431-014-2333-3.
43. Zhang G, Wu L, Zhou L, Lu W, Mao C. Television watching and risk of childhood obesity: a meta-analysis. Eur J Pub Health. 2016;26(1):13–8. https://doi.org/10.1093/eurpub/ckv213.
44. Mark AE, Janssen I. Relationship between screen time and metabolic syndrome in adolescents. J Public Health (Oxf). 2008;30(2):153–60. https://doi.org/10.1093/pubmed/fdn022.
45. Costigan SA, Barnett L, Plotnikoff RC, Lubans DR. The health indicators associated with screen-based sedentary behavior among adolescent girls: a systematic review. J Adolesc Health. 2013;52(4):382–92. https://doi.org/10.1016/j.jadohealth.2012.07.018.
46. Katzmarzyk PT, Barreira TV, Broyles ST, Champagne CM, Chaput JP, Fogelholm M, Hu G, Johnson WD, Kuriyan R, Kurpad A, Lambert EV, Maher C, Maia J, Matsudo V, Olds T, Onywera V, Sarmiento OL, Standage M, Tremblay MS, Tudor-Locke C, Zhao P, Church TS. Physical Activity, Sedentary Time, and Obesity in an International Sample of Children. Med Sci Sports Exerc. 2015;47(10):2062–9. https://doi.org/10.1249/mss.0000000000000649.
47. Lubans DR, Hesketh K, Cliff DP, Barnett LM, Salmon J, Dollman J, Morgan PJ, Hills AP, Hardy LL. A systematic review of the validity and reliability of sedentary behaviour measures used with children and adolescents. Obes Rev. 2011;12(10):781–99. https://doi.org/10.1111/j.1467-789X.2011.00896.x.
48. Chinapaw M, Altenburg T, Brug J. Sedentary behaviour and health in children – evaluating the evidence. Prev Med. 2015;70:1–2. https://doi.org/10.1016/j.ypmed.2014.10.029.
49. Same RV, Feldman DI, Shah N, Martin SS, Al Rifai M, Blaha MJ, Graham G, Ahmed HM. Relationship between sedentary behavior and cardiovascular risk. Curr Cardiol Rep. 2016;18(1):6. https://doi.org/10.1007/s11886-015-0678-5.
50. Ivuskans A, Maestu J, Jurimae T, Latt E, Purge P, Saar M, Maasalu K, Jurimae J. Sedentary time has a negative influence on bone mineral parameters in peripubertal boys: a 1-year prospective study. J Bone Miner Metab. 2015;33(1):85–92. https://doi.org/10.1007/s00774-013-0556-4.
51. Heidemann M, Molgaard C, Husby S, Schou AJ, Klakk H, Moller NC, Holst R, Wedderkopp N. The intensity of physical activity influences bone mineral accrual in childhood: the childhood health, activity and motor performance school (the CHAMPS) study, Denmark. BMC Pediatr. 2013;13:32. https://doi.org/10.1186/1471-2431-13-32.

52. Vaitkeviciute D, Latt E, Maestu J, Jurimae T, Saar M, Purge P, Maasalu K, Jurimae J. Physical activity and bone mineral accrual in boys with different body mass parameters during puberty: a longitudinal study. PLoS One. 2014;9(10):e107759. https://doi.org/10.1371/journal.pone.0107759.
53. Sioen I, Michels N, Polfliet C, De Smet S, D'Haese S, Roggen I, Deschepper J, Goemaere S, Valtuena J, De Henauw S. The influence of dairy consumption, sedentary behaviour and physical activity on bone mass in Flemish children: a cross-sectional study. BMC Public Health. 2015;15:717. https://doi.org/10.1186/s12889-015-2077-7.
54. Herrmann D, Pohlabeln H, Gianfagna F, Konstabel K, Lissner L, Marild S, Molnar D, Moreno LA, Siani A, Sioen I, Veidebaum T, Ahrens W. Association between bone stiffness and nutritional biomarkers combined with weight-bearing exercise, physical activity, and sedentary time in preadolescent children. A case-control study. Bone. 2015;78:142–9. https://doi.org/10.1016/j.bone.2015.04.043.
55. Vicente-Rodriguez G, Ortega FB, Rey-Lopez JP, Espana-Romero V, Blay VA, Blay G, Martin-Matillas M, Moreno LA. Extracurricular physical activity participation modifies the association between high TV watching and low bone mass. Bone. 2009;45(5):925–30. https://doi.org/10.1016/j.bone.2009.07.084.
56. Bounds W, Skinner J, Carruth BR, Ziegler P. The relationship of dietary and lifestyle factors to bone mineral indexes in children. J Am Diet Assoc. 2005;105(5):735–41. https://doi.org/10.1016/j.jada.2005.02.046.
57. Wang MC, Crawford PB, Hudes M, Van Loan M, Siemering K, Bachrach LK. Diet in midpuberty and sedentary activity in prepuberty predict peak bone mass. Am J Clin Nutr. 2003;77(2):495–503. https://doi.org/10.1093/ajcn/77.2.495.
58. McVeigh JA, Zhu K, Mountain J, Pennell CE, Lye SJ, Walsh JP, Straker LM. Longitudinal trajectories of television watching across childhood and adolescence predict bone mass at age 20 years in the Raine study. J Bone Miner Res. 2016;31(11):2032–40. https://doi.org/10.1002/jbmr.2890.
59. Wosje KS, Khoury PR, Claytor RP, Copeland KA, Kalkwarf HJ, Daniels SR. Adiposity and TV viewing are related to less bone accrual in young children. J Pediatr. 2009;154(1):79–85.e72. https://doi.org/10.1016/j.jpeds.2008.06.031.
60. Evenson KR, Catellier DJ, Gill K, Ondrak KS, McMurray RG. Calibration of two objective measures of physical activity for children. J Sports Sci. 2008;26(14):1557–65. https://doi.org/10.1080/02640410802334196.

Effects of Low Energy Availability on Bone Health in Exercising Premenopausal Women

10

Nancy I. Williams and Mary Jane De Souza

Introduction

Bone health in premenopausal women is an important concern due to the clinical consequences of osteoporosis later in life. Osteoporosis is characterized by low bone mass, increasing bone fragility, and a deterioration of bone microarchitecture. An estimated 53.6 million US adults over age 50 suffer from either osteoporosis or low bone mass at the femoral neck or lumbar spine [1]. Associated reductions in bone strength increase the risk of debilitating fractures which represent a major healthcare cost burden estimated to grow to over 25 billion by 2025 [2]. Approximately one out of two Caucasian women and one out of five men will experience an osteoporosis-related fracture in her or his lifetime [3]. Although osteoporosis is less frequent in African Americans, those with osteoporosis have the same elevated fracture risk as Caucasians. The development of optimal peak bone mass during the adolescent years and the associated rate of decline in bone mass with aging are the key determinants of bone health. Because both can be influenced by lifestyle behaviors such as exercise and dietary intake, an understanding of the effects of energy deficiency and exercise on bone health in premenopausal women is paramount [4].

Effects of Exercise on Bone

The skeleton naturally adapts to optimize its structure in response to mechanical loading. There is substantial evidence that regular physical activity can improve bone mineral density (BMD) [5] and in particular peak bone mass [4]. The beneficial effects of exercise on bone mass and structure are maximized during the child

N. I. Williams (✉) · M. J. De Souza
Women's Health and Exercise Laboratories, Department of Kinesiology, The Pennsylvania State University, University Park, PA, USA
e-mail: niw1@psu.edu; mjd34@psu.edu

© Springer Nature Switzerland AG 2019
C. M. Weaver et al. (eds.), *Nutritional Influences on Bone Health*,
https://doi.org/10.1007/978-3-319-98464-3_10

and adolescent years when bone mass is accruing [5]. A recent meta-analysis, which limited only to randomized controlled exercise intervention trials lasting 24–104 weeks, frequency of 2–7 days per week, and including exercises eliciting both ground and/or joint reaction forces in premenopausal women, documented small but significant increases in both the femoral neck and lumbar spine BMD [6]. The minimum number of women needed to see an effect of exercise was estimated to be ten; however, whether or not the gains in BMD are sufficient to reduce fracture risk in the spine and/or hip are unknown.

Exercise is most effective when it evokes high-magnitude strains or high strain rates. The forces on bone (i.e., compression, bending, shearing, and twisting) vary depending on the type of exercise and dimensions such as speed, strength, power, endurance, and motor coordination [7]. Accordingly, cross-sectional studies in young female athletes document differences in BMD ranging from 5 to 18.5% among sports depending on skeletal loading characteristics [8]. Weight-bearing activities that evoke high and/or irregular strain rates such as squash and weightlifting exhibit a threefold higher weight-adjusted BMD at weight-bearing sites than low or non-weight-bearing sports such as speed skating, cycling, or swimming [8]. Notably, BMD in the low and non-weight-bearing sports does not differ significantly from that in regularly physically active or sedentary women.

Exercise influences bone through direct and indirect actions. Although the mechanisms are not fully elucidated, there are numerous ways that mechanical strains are sensed and transduced into biological signals that affect the balance of bone formation and resorption. Forces imparted on bone directly activate mechanoreceptors located on osteocytes which transduce mechanical stimuli into biological signals primarily through the Wnt-β-catenin canonical signaling pathway to trigger bone remodeling by directing osteoblast activity and osteoclastic resorption [7]. While exercise is known to be osteogenic, particularly during adolescence, the effects depend on the type of mechanical stimuli created by a particular activity. Bone responds optimally when mechanical forces are dynamic rather than static such that bone formation increases with the degree of bone deformation, although at a certain level this effect plateaus [9]. Similarly, extending the duration of skeletal loading is not associated with proportional increases in bone mass. Rather, adaptive bone responses are most responsive to brief, intermittent exercise. Lastly, responsiveness is improved when forces imparted on bone depart from the usual loading pattern, i.e., are relatively "abnormal," exhibiting variations in both orientation and magnitude [9]. Indirect pathways whereby exercise exerts osteogenic effects include muscle contraction and hormonal influences. Muscle contraction forces represent over 70% of the forces indirectly imparted on bone [10]. Accordingly, lean body mass is a key determinant of BMD in adults, and indices of bone strength and peak rates of bone mineral acquisition are preceded by gains in muscle [7]. In contrast, sarcopenia with aging is accompanied by bone loss [11]. Muscle contraction, acting through tendon attachments, can activate bone mechanoreceptors [7].

Exercise impacts bone metabolism indirectly through its acute and chronic effects on numerous hormones, adipokines, and enterokines. Acute exercise produces transient alterations in anabolic hormones such as growth hormone [12], insulin-like growth factor-1 [13], and estradiol [14]. Cortisol, parathyroid hormone, ghrelin, leptin, and other bone acting factors can also indirectly influence bone formation and resorption [7]. The effects of chronic training on many hormones depend on energy availability status such that increases in hormones such as ghrelin and cortisol are greater during conditions of low energy availability and/or weight loss [15]. It is important to note that optimizing the effects of exercise on bone not only requires adequate calcium and vitamin D, but estradiol also plays an important role. Mechanotransduction via the Wnt signaling pathway is heavily dependent on estrogen receptor activation, which is especially relevant in models of low energy availability-induced hypoestrogenism [16].

Early Observations of Bone Loss in Premenopausal Women

In light of the positive impact of exercise on bone and the overall health benefits of regular physical activity [17], it is not surprising that early reports of osteoporosis and low bone mass in female endurance runners in the 1980s drew widespread concern [18]. Drinkwater et al. in the 1980s and early 1990s showed that female endurance runners who were amenorrheic had alarmingly low BMDs at the spine. This paradoxical finding was documented in a series of studies that identified the close association between the menstrual status of athletes and BMD [18–21]. Changes in BMD were documented in amenorrheic runners followed for 15.5 months who regained menses or who remained amenorrheic and compared to athletes with regular menstrual cycles. Vertebral (L1–L4) bone mineral density increased 6.3% in those who resumed menses through a combination of weight gain and reduced training and decreased 3.4% in those who remained amenorrheic. However, the improvement in BMD in those who resumed menses did not fully restore BMD when compared to the athletes with regular menstrual cycles and remained 12% lower than the menstruating control group. This result was concerning and led to speculation that bone loss in premenopausal exercising women with suppressed menstrual function was irreversible. Contemporaneous studies showed that exercise in young women severely disrupted the menstrual cycle [22] and that a surprising proportion of female ballet dancers suffered from clinical eating disorders and amenorrhea [23]. These studies were foundational to three decades of subsequent research in female athletes, women with anorexia nervosa, and female military recruits on the medical condition known as the female athlete triad [24].

The Female Athlete Triad

The first position stand on the female athlete triad was published in 1997 and described a syndrome of three interrelated conditions: disordered eating, amenorrhea, and osteoporosis [25]. Cross-sectional studies subsequently documented the clinically relevant endpoints for each of the three triad components to include eating disorders, amenorrhea, and osteoporosis. The components of the triad are physiologically and behaviorally interrelated because low energy availability, i.e., energy available for vital bodily processes, is associated with disordered eating and plays a causal role in the development of menstrual disturbances [26–28]. Moreover, both low energy availability (EA) and the hypoestrogenic environment associated with amenorrhea play a causal role in bone loss [29–31]. In 2007, the triad was redefined as a syndrome of low energy availability with or without disordered eating, functional hypothalamic amenorrhea, and osteoporosis [24]. The new triad model represented each component as the pathological endpoint of one of the three interrelated spectrums ranging from a healthy endpoint to subclinical and clinical conditions (Fig. 10.1) [24]. At the "healthy" end of the continuum, each triad component is considered to be optimized, i.e., energy intake matches energy expenditure, ovulatory menstrual cycles are maintained, and bone mass is normal [24]. At the "unhealthy" end of the continuum, each triad component presents the clinical endpoints of the syndrome, including low EA with or without disordered eating, functional hypothalamic amenorrhea, and osteoporosis [24]. Although recent reports have focused on the general physiological effects of chronic low energy availability [32], the most clinically relevant sequelae are its effects on the menstrual cycle and reproductive hormones and on the skeleton. Equally concerning is the fact that the pathway to low energy availability can include severe clinical eating disorders. Other documented physiological consequences include dyslipidemia, impaired endothelial function [33–35], fatigue, and decrements in competitive performance [36], but the prevalence of these effects and their clinical relevance has not been established. Much progress has been made in our understanding of the underlying behaviors and physiology of these conditions [37–39] as well as the

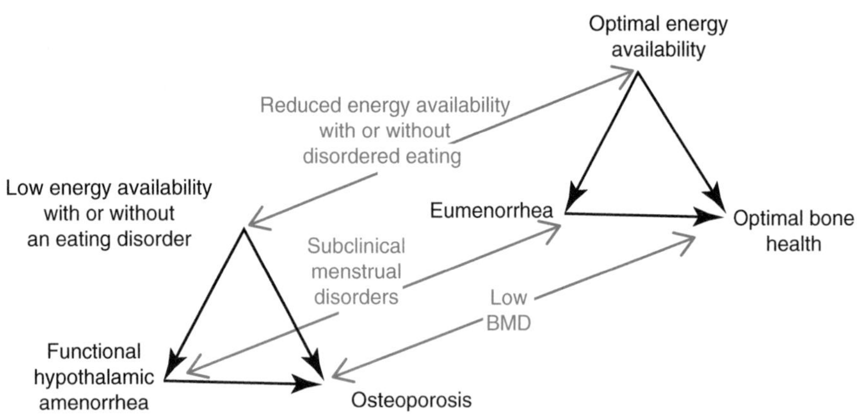

Fig. 10.1 Current model of the female athlete triad. Adapted from Nattiv et al. [24]. The spectrums of energy availability, menstrual function, and bone mineral density along which female athletes are distributed (narrow arrows). An athlete's condition moves along each spectrum at a different rate, in one direction or the other, according to her diet and exercise habits. Energy availability, defined as dietary energy intake minus exercise energy expenditure, affects bone mineral density both directly via metabolic hormones and indirectly via effects on menstrual function and thereby estrogen (thick arrows)

creation and use of practical recommendations for prevention, screening, treatment, and return to play [24, 40–42]. The prevalence of triad components is greatest in sports emphasizing leanness, aesthetics, and high energy expenditure, but it can range up to 60% for menstrual disturbances, 20% for eating disorders/disordered eating, and 5% for osteoporosis [24]. Subclinical manifestations, i.e., disordered eating practices, anovulation and luteal phase defects, and low bone mass, occur at even higher prevalence rates [24]. A high proportion, i.e., approximately 11%, of women experience bone stress injuries in association with the triad [43]. A key concern is whether young women who are amenorrheic and who lose bone or fail to achieve peak bone mass can recover bone with subsequent weight gain and/or resumption of menses [24]. The interrelatedness of the triad components underscores the key roles that energy availability and estrogen exposure play in the bone health of young exercising women.

Low Energy Availability and Menstrual Disturbances

The primary mechanism that leads to the induction of menstrual disturbances with exercise is energy deficiency and/or low energy availability. In a variety of mammalian species, the availability of oxidizable metabolic fuels modulates the hypothalamic control of the reproductive axis such that reproduction succeeds when food availability is optimal and is suppressed during times of famine or during periods of high energy expenditure associated with thermoregulation or foraging behaviors [44]. In contrast to animals in the wild where food availability depends on environmental factors, the underlying causes of low energy availability in exercising women include the conscious restriction of food intake (dietary cognitive restraint) in response to high demands for a slim physique and low body weight, high body dissatisfaction, and according to some reports, inadvertent undereating [45–47]. Numerous cross-sectional studies comparing measures of eating attitudes and metabolic endpoints between exercising women with eumenorrheic and ovulatory cycles versus their counterparts with menstrual disturbances have found evidence of adaptive changes indicative of energy conversation to accommodate the imbalance created by restrictive eating and high exercise energy expenditure. These include reductions in resting metabolic rate; decreased concentrations of leptin, triiodothyronine, and insulin-like growth factor-1; and increased ghrelin and cortisol [26, 48–50].

The seminal prospective exercise and feeding study by Bullen et al. shed light on the susceptibility of the menstrual cycle to weight loss induced by an abrupt increase in exercise training combined with caloric restriction [22]. Women were studied over two menstrual cycles and randomized either to a weight maintenance or a weight loss group, while both groups increased daily running up to 10 miles per day. While the weight maintenance group exhibited menstrual disturbances, modest decreases of 4 ± 0.3 kg in the weight loss group were associated with a significantly higher prevalence of delayed menses (75% vs. 8%) and loss of the LH surge (81% vs. 42%). The causal role of energy deficiency reported in studies using a monkey model of exercise-related amenorrhea was reported by Williams et al. [51] in another prospective study that capitalized on the advantages of an animal model. Using a monkey model of amenorrhea, food intake and exercise were controlled, and the development of full-scale amenorrhea (at least 3 months with no menstrual bleeding) could be observed. Monkeys developed amenorrhea ($n = 8$) while running up to 12.3 ± 0.9 km/day for 7–24 months with no change in food intake when compared to a control group who sat on the treadmill [27]. The transition to amenorrhea was abrupt, immediately preceded in most cases by only one abnormal menstrual cycle. Amenorrhea was then reversed in all monkeys ($n = 4$) who were provided increased food intake (138–181% of calorie intake during amenorrhea) even though daily training persisted [51]. Circulating triiodothyronine concentrations declined significantly with the onset of menses and increased significantly with the reversal of menses, presumably indicating that alterations in cellular metabolism closely parallel the modulation of the reproductive axis. In a subsequent randomized controlled trial, Williams et al. [49] showed that an energy deficit of −470 to 810 kcal/day leads to significant menstrual disruptions (luteal phase defects and anovulation) in accordance with the magnitude of the daily energy deficit during three menstrual cycles of 5× per week moderate to vigorous exercise training (Fig. 10.2). The average percent energy deficit of −22% to −42% of baseline energy needs was the main predictor of the frequency of menstrual disturbances, not the modest weight loss of −0.9 to −3.8 kg. This study confirmed the prior monkey studies and extended earlier findings by quantifying the actual magnitude of energy deficit and the time frame over which menstrual disturbances are induced with moderate exercise training combined with caloric restriction.

The previous studies document the causal role of low energy availability on the induction of menstrual disturbances and the associated effects on circulating estradiol, an important factor in bone formation and resorption. Even modest reductions in energy availability that are not associated with dramatic weight loss can reduce the exposure to circulating estrogen [52]. Further advances in the role energy availability plays in the disruption of bone metabolism come from the elegant short-term (4–5 days) prospective studies of Loucks et al. [28, 53–57]. In a series of laboratory experiments in sedentary women where levels of energy availability were clamped while subjects performed daily treadmill walking, Loucks et al. showed that LH pulsatility patterns were not significantly disrupted until energy availability was below a certain threshold [28]. These experiments employed the assessment of LH pulsatility as a proxy indicator of GnRH neuronal activity. When energy availability was reduced below a threshold of 30 kcals/kg/LBM/day, altered release characteristics of LH from the pituitary gland resulted, most notably, in a decrease in LH pulse frequency. At an energy availability of 10 kcals/kg/LBM/day, urinary N-telopeptide (NTX) concentrations and indices of bone resorption/formation uncoupling were increased. Osteocalcin (OC) and serum type I procollagen carboxy-terminal propeptide (PICP) were suppressed at all levels of reduced energy availability. The increase in NTX was in association with a significant decrease in circulating estradiol, and the changes in the markers of bone formation, i.e., OC and PICP, were associated with declines in triiodothyronine, IGF-1, and insulin, respectively. These

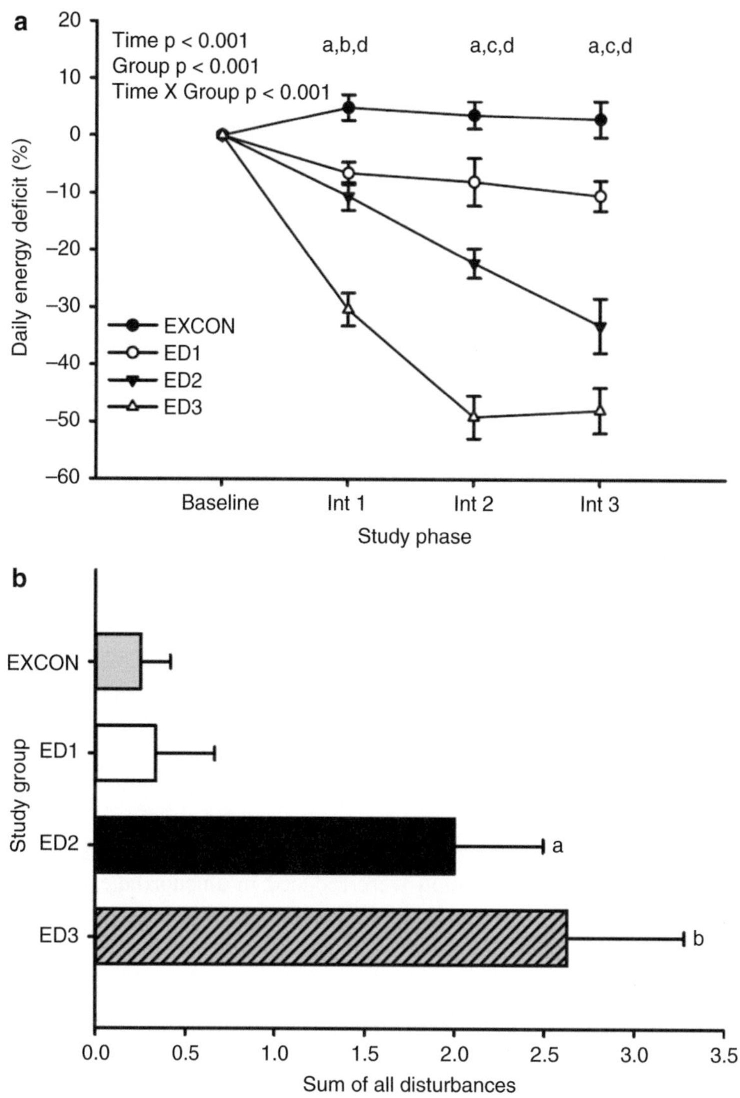

Fig. 10.2 Effects of low, moderate, and high energy deficiency on the induction of menstrual disturbances. Adapted from Williams et al. [51]. The causal role of low energy availability is illustrated in this randomized clinical trial where the magnitude of the daily energy deficit is significantly associated with the induction of menstrual disturbances, i.e., luteal phase defects, oligomenorrhea, and anovulation in ovulatory untrained women in response to laboratory-based exercise training with controlled feeding. Average daily energy deficit (%) experienced across study phases (**a**) and sum of all menstrual disturbances across the intervention for each group (**b**). Data are reported as means_SE. (**a**) [a]ED1 (low energy deficit) significantly different from EXCON (exercising controls; energy balance); [b]ED2 (moderate energy deficit) significantly different from EXCON; [c]ED2 significantly different from EXCON and ED1; [d]ED3 (high energy deficit) significantly different from EXCON, ED1, and ED2. (**b**) [a]Significantly different from EXCON; [b]significantly different from EXCON and ED1. Data are reported as means_SE

results and others [58–60] indicate the close correspondence between short-term changes in energy availability and bone metabolism which precede changes in bone mass or structure.

Low Energy Availability and Amenorrhea Effects on Bone

Bone strength is dependent on a variety of factors including the quality of the bone tissue, the structural integrity of the trabecular and cortical compartments, and finally, the quantity of bone present [61]. Although the measurement of areal BMD (aBMD) is the primary surrogate of bone strength used for the clinical diagnosis of osteoporosis, other measures of bone microarchitecture using HR-pQCT and techniques to estimate bone strength in humans provide valuable insights into the underlying mechanisms for determining increased fracture risk. Because changes in BMD and bone microarchitecture happen slowly, studies examining mechanisms underlying the effects of low energy availability and/or hypoestrogenism have been limited to cross-sectional association studies and observational or randomized trials to *reverse* bone loss in patients with existing bone health issues. Much of what is believed to be true or is being tested in exercising women with the female athlete triad has first been observed in women with anorexia nervosa where the prevalence of osteopenia and osteoporosis is 92% and 38%, respectively [62]. Clinical observations in amenorrheic athletes and in adolescents with anorexia who display long-term energy deficiency document low aBMD at several bone sites [37, 63, 64], compromised bone microarchitecture [65–67], and lower estimates of bone strength [67, 68]. Christo et al. [63] found lower BMD Z-scores at the spine and total body in amenorrheic athletes compared to eumenorrheic athletes and age-matched controls 12–18 years who ran >30 miles per week or exercise >4 h/week. Markers of bone formation and bone resorption were reduced in amenorrheic athletes compared to controls, and BMI, lean mass, insulin-like growth factor I, and menstrual status were predictors of BMD Z-scores. In young, amenorrheic athletes, lumbar BMD Z-scores were lower compared to eumenorrheic athletes and nonathletes, and hip and femoral neck scores were highest in eumenorrheic athletes. Athletes had greater total area, trabecular area, and cortical perimeter than nonathletes, whereas cortical area and thickness were lower in amenorrheic athletes. Trabecular number was lower and trabecular separation was higher in amenorrheic versus eumenorrheic and nonathletes, and menstrual status accounted for 18–24% of the variability in the tibial trabecular number and separation [66]. Estimations of bone strength using finite element analysis from high-resolution peripheral computed tomography (HR-pQCT) images were compromised in amenorrheic athletes in endurance sports at the distal radius and tibia compared to eumenorrheic athletes and nonathletes. These studies demonstrate the importance of menstrual status on key variables that impact fracture risk [69].

Prolonged low energy availability and estrogen deficiency, though causally related, can have independent and combined effects on BMD, bone geometry, and estimated bone strength [29, 70]. In a cross-sectional study of young physically active women that isolated the effects of energy and estrogen deficiency, energy deficiency was associated with lower total volumetric BMD (vBMD), trabecular volumetric BMD, cortical area, and bone strength index (BSI) at the distal tibia and lower total vBMD, smaller cortical area and cortical thickness, and larger endosteal circumference at the proximal tibia compared to the energy replete participants [70]. Estrogen deficiency (as noted in amenorrheic exercising women) was associated with lower total and cortical vBMD, lower BSI, and larger total and trabecular area at the distal radius than non-estrogen-deficient (eumenorrheic) exercising women. When energy deficiency and estrogen deficiency were both present, total and trabecular area at the distal tibia were higher, perhaps due to greater periosteal expansion and/or less endosteal expansion. The independent effects of energy status on tibial vBMD, geometry, and estimated bone strength reported in the latter study extend earlier findings of independent effects of energy and estrogen status on bone markers [29]. These findings underscore the idea that treatment strategies to prevent or treat bone loss in active women need to account for both “pathways” to compromised bone health. Since energy deficiency precedes the suppression of the menstrual cycle, a focus on preventing low energy availability by ensuring that food intake matches energy demands is the recommended strategy for maintaining healthy bone in exercising women [40].

The underlying mechanisms that mediate bone loss due to low energy availability and associated hypoestrogenism include associated changes in body composition, i.e., reductions in lean body mass and fat mass, the direct effects of inadequate estrogen exposure, and negative alterations in metabolic hormones that impact bone such as decreased leptin, insulin, IGF-1, and increased growth hormone and cortisol [29, 30, 71–73]. Lean body mass is a strong independent predictor of bone mass in a variety of populations, likely due to the effects of mechanical forces imparted on bone through muscle [7, 11]. Studies of bone health in exercising women need to take this important variable into account in addition to metabolic and reproductive factors, and preservation of lean mass during times of low energy availability should be prioritized. Insulin receptors are located on osteoblasts and osteoclasts, and insulin has been shown to increase bone formation and decrease bone resorption. Leptin receptors are also present on osteoblasts and chondrocytes, but leptin plays a key role in modulating other hormones such as cortisol, IGF-1, and PTH, all of which can influence bone metabolism [74].

Another factor to consider when examining mechanisms of bone loss in exercising amenorrheic women is the duration of amenorrhea and past and current menstrual status [19, 75]. Although most studies document associations between current menstrual status and bone parameters, the cumulative effects of menstrual cessation are important to consider because bone accrual in girls occurs primarily during adolescence between the ages of 11 and 14 years. Delayed menarche and/or amenorrhea during the first and second decades of life may attenuate peak bone mass and plays a major role in bone health later in life. Recently, Mallinson et al. demonstrated that the cumulative effect of current and past menstrual irregularity predicted low femoral neck cross-sectional moment of inertia and cross-sectional area and diameter at the femoral neck [76].

Reversal of Bone Loss in Exercising Women

A key question is whether reductions in BMD and associated decrements in bone microarchitecture and bone strength in exercising women can be reversed with increased energy availability and the restoration of normal menstrual cycles. This is an important question because there are no pharmacological therapies that have proven to outpace the 2–3% loss of BMD/year in amenorrheic women for bone loss in premenopausal women [77]. Menstrual recovery is an important contributor to the improvement of bone health. The reversal of amenorrhea in exercising women has been addressed in retrospective [78] and prospective studies [79–81], but none of these studies are randomized controlled trials. Overall, the results support that modest increases (approximately 300 kcal/day) in energy availability by increasing caloric intake and/or decreasing exercise training, and by increasing body weight, can lead to the resumption of ovulatory cycles in amenorrheic women. With respect to bone, early observational work from Drinkwater [21] indicates that the resumption of menses is possible, but the recovery of bone mass is incomplete. In the latter study [21], the restoration of menses due to reduced training, increased caloric intake, and/or injury was associated with an increase in lumbar spine BMD over 15.5 month follow-up period in 6/7 participants. However, lumbar BMD in those who regained menses was 12% lower than their regularly menstruating counterparts [21], leaving open the possibility that complete recovery of bone takes longer than 15 months, requires a greater energy surplus, or is not possible. In a case study of an amenorrheic distance runner with osteoporosis studied over 8 years, changes in BMD of the lumbar spine, hip, and total body were examined in response to pharmacological and nutritional interventions [82]. At age 22.9 years, the patient had primary amenorrhea, a BMI of 15.8 kg m^{-2}, and low T scores of −2.50 at the spine and −1.54 at the hip. Two years of oral contraceptive therapy were ineffective at increasing BMD, while BMI remained low. The patient remained on oral contraceptive therapy and started gaining weight at age 25 years. From the ages of 25.4 to 30.8 years, the patient attained a BMI of 21.3 kg m^{-2}, experiencing gains in BMD of 25.5% at the spine and 19.5% at the hip which represented a normalization of BMD to 94% of normal, spine, and 96% of normal, hip. She ceased taking oral contraceptives at age 27.6 and her menstrual cycles resumed. These results are promising because they demonstrate that "catch-up" increases in BMD are possible after a period of suspended bone accrual due to 12 years of food restriction and amenorrhea. However, this was a case study, so the increase in bone mass cannot be compared to any reference group to determine if the recovery of bone was on par with exercising, eumenorrheic peers. Whether the idea of "catch-up" increases in bone are generalizable to the majority of exercising women with triad-related bone loss is not known. Having a history of anorexia increases the risk of fracture over one's lifetime, and bone density and quality remain low. Up to 25 years after the diagnosis of anorexia or triad conditions, cross-sectional studies show varied results as BMD is normal, reduced, or indicative of osteopenia or osteoporosis [40].

Prospective studies examining the reversal of bone loss in anorexia demonstrate that the resumption of menstrual function is important for spine BMD recovery, whereas weight gain is necessary for the recovery of hip BMD [77]. In the absence of weight gain and menstrual resumption, young women with anorexia experience a 2.6% decline in BMD at the spine and 2.4% at the hip. If both were improved, a 3.1% increase in the spine and 1.8% increase at the hip were observed. Independent of weight gain, menstrual recovery was associated with an increase in the spine but not hip BMD. Weight gain, independent of menstrual recovery, was associated with increases in the hip, but not spine BMD. The most important determinant of BMD increases associated with weight gain fat-free mass, not total body weight or fat mass [77]. These results and others [83] suggest that hormonal and nutritional factors may operate independently to differentially influence bone recovery in patients with anorexia (Fig. 10.3).

Regarding women who are experiencing triad conditions but not considered to be anorexic, the only randomized controlled trial to date to examine the impact of increased energy availability on menstrual cyclicity and bone health in exercising women with menstrual disturbances has been conducted by Williams and De Souza at Penn State University and the University of Toronto (unpublished). Preliminary findings from this 12-month trial indicate that gradual increases in energy availability (20–30%) are associated with the resumption of menses in amenorrheic women. The resumption of menstrual bleeding occurred in a significantly greater proportion of women who were assigned to the refeeding group (58% or 11/19) vs. those in the control group who maintained their normal intake (8% or 1/12) ($p < 0.05$). Interestingly, most women who recovered did so within 3 months of beginning the intervention and weight gain were modest. Future publication of the results of this study will address whether menstrual recovery was associated with improvements in bone metabolism and bone density over the 12 months of the study. The latter study has the potential to contribute significantly to the field because the randomization of subjects to treatment or control conditions allows for the control of factors associated with the spontaneous resumption of menses and/or other factors that cause changes in bone health.

Practical Recommendations for Prevention and Treatment of Bone Loss in Exercising Women

Although more research is necessary to determine optimal strategies for preventing and reversing bone loss in exercising women, there is an immediate need for specific guidelines for managing cases of triad-related bone loss based on what is currently known. A recent consensus statement provides the most up-to-date and evidence-based guidelines for addressing triad-related bone loss in exercising women with respect to treatment and return to play [40]. The statement includes practical recommendations for increasing energy availability for menstrual and bone recovery but also includes an algorithm that uses a point system where six different risk factors for low bone mass and stress fracture/bone stress injury are assigned a value of 0, low risk; 1, moderate risk; and 2, high risk. A cumulative risk score is calculated that provides guidance for clinicians to make decisions on full or

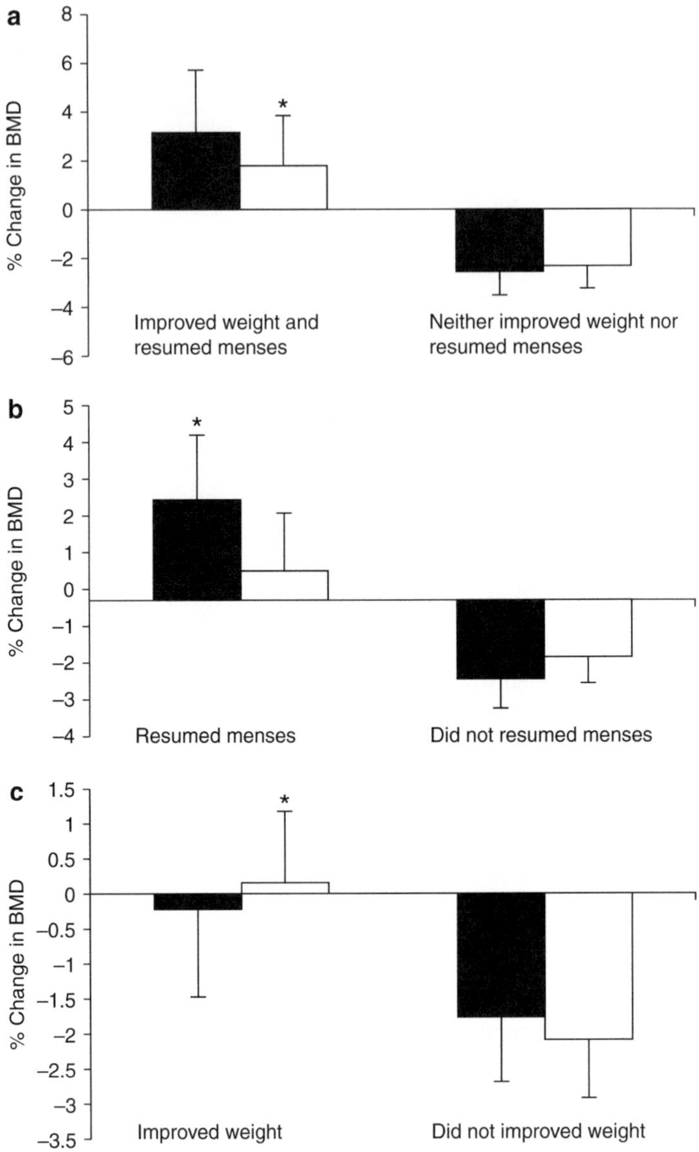

Fig. 10.3 Determinants of skeletal recovery in anorexia. Adapted from Miller et al. [77]. Annualized percent change in BMD at the lumbar spine and hip in women not receiving oral contraceptives. (**a**) Women who both improved weight and resumed menses increased BMD at the spine and hip, compared with those who neither improved weight nor resumed menses (spine, 3.1 ± 2.7 vs. −2.6 ± 1.0%, $p = 0.064$; hip, 1.8 ± 2.1 vs. −2.4 ± 0.9%, $p = 0.045$). (**b**) Women who resumed menses increased lumbar spine BMD, compared with those who did not improve menstrual function (2.7 ± 1.7 vs. −2.2 ± 0.8%, $p = 0.018$). However, there was no increase in hip BMD. (**c**) Women who improved weight increased hip BMD, compared with those who did not improve weight (0.15 ± 1.0 vs. −2.1 ± 0.8%, $p = 0.038$). However, there was no increase in lumbar spine BMD. *Black bars* lumbar spine BMD, *white bars*, hip BMD. Improved weight, at subsequent visit, increased body weight by at least 10% or to more than 85% of ideal body weight. * $p < 0.05$

provisional clearance to play and includes recommendations for monitoring and follow-up. The risk factors that are scored include low energy availability with or without disordered eating/eating disorders, low BMI, delayed menarche, oligomenorrhea/amenorrhea, low BMD, and history of stress fracture/bone stress injury. Follow-up studies will likely lead to refinement of this approach as more evidence is gathered regarding the validity of the scoring system and the relative weight of each risk factor.

Summary and Conclusions

Over three decades of research has documented the physiological, behavioral, and clinical interrelatedness of energy availability, menstrual function, and bone health in exercising women. While the osteogenic benefits of exercise are well established, these gains are dependent on optimal energy availability and adequate estrogen exposure. Energy availability is causally related to the induction and reversal of menstrual disturbances, and 20–30% reductions in energy availability are associated with early indications of reproductive hormone suppression and negative alterations in bone metabolism. Low energy availability and hypoestrogenism can have both independent and combined effects on bone mass and site-specific bone microarchitecture, and these effects are most concerning if they occur during adolescence when bone accrual is maximal. Key determinants for the recovery bone loss associated with menstrual disturbances are weight gain and the restoration of menses, but more research is necessary to determine if complete recovery of bone mass and bone quality is possible. Future research should focus on optimizing evidence-based modifications in diet and exercise regimens that are acceptable to women's lifestyles and promote lifelong reproductive and bone health.

References

1. Wright NC, Looker AC, Saag KG, Curtis JR, Delzell ES, Randall S, et al. The recent prevalence of osteoporosis and low bone mass in the United States based on bone mineral density at the femoral neck or lumbar spine. J Bone Miner Res. 2014;29(11):2520–6.
2. van den Bergh JP, van Geel TA, Geusens PP. Osteoporosis, frailty and fracture: implications for case finding and therapy. Nat Rev Rheumatol. 2012;8(3):163–72.
3. Cosman F, de Beur SJ, LeBoff MS, Lewiecki EM, Tanner B, Randall S, et al. Clinician's guide to prevention and treatment of osteoporosis. Osteoporos Int. 2014;25(10):2359–81.
4. Weaver CM, Gordon CM, Janz KF, Kalkwarf HJ, Lappe JM, Lewis R, et al. The National Osteoporosis Foundation's position statement on peak bone mass development and lifestyle factors: a systematic review and implementation recommendations. Osteoporos Int. 2016;27(4):1281–386.
5. Bailey CA, Brooke-Wavell K. Exercise for optimising peak bone mass in women. Proc Nutr Soc. 2008;67(1):9–18.
6. Kelley GA, Kelley KS, Kohrt WM. Exercise and bone mineral density in premenopausal women: a meta-analysis of randomized controlled trials. Int J Endocrinol. 2013;2013:741639.
7. Bonnet N, Ferrari SL. Exercise and the skeleton: how it works and what it really does. IBMS BoneKEy. 2010;7(7):235–48.

8. Heinonen A, Oja P, Kannus P, Sievanen H, Haapasalo H, Manttari A, et al. Bone mineral density in female athletes representing sports with different loading characteristics of the skeleton. Bone. 1995;17(3):197–203.
9. Lanyon LE. The success and failure of the adaptive response to functional load-bearing in averting bone fracture. Bone. 1992;13(Suppl 2):S17–21.
10. Kohrt WM, Bloomfield SA, Little KD, Nelson ME, Yingling VR, American College of Sports M. American College of Sports Medicine Position Stand: physical activity and bone health. Med Sci Sports Exerc. 2004;36(11):1985–96.
11. Robling AG. Is bone's response to mechanical signals dominated by muscle forces? Med Sci Sports Exerc. 2009;41(11):2044–9.
12. Nindl BC, Hymer WC, Deaver DR, Kraemer WJ. Growth hormone pulsatility profile characteristics following acute heavy resistance exercise. J Appl Physiol (1985). 2001;91(1):163–72.
13. Wideman L, Weltman JY, Hartman ML, Veldhuis JD, Weltman A. Growth hormone release during acute and chronic aerobic and resistance exercise: recent findings. Sports Med. 2002;32(15):987–1004.
14. Jurkowski JE, Jones NL, Walker C, Younglai EV, Sutton JR. Ovarian hormonal responses to exercise. J Appl Physiol Respir Environ Exerc Physiol. 1978;44(1):109–14.
15. Leidy HJ, Dougherty KA, Frye BR, Duke KM, Williams NI. Twenty-four-hour ghrelin is elevated after calorie restriction and exercise training in non-obese women. Obesity (Silver Spring). 2007;15(2):446–55.
16. Armstrong VJ, Muzylak M, Sunters A, Zaman G, Saxon LK, Price JS, et al. Wnt/beta-catenin signaling is a component of osteoblastic bone cell early responses to load-bearing and requires estrogen receptor alpha. J Biol Chem. 2007;282(28):20715–27.
17. Garber CE, Blissmer B, Deschenes MR, Franklin BA, Lamonte MJ, Lee IM, et al. American College of Sports Medicine position stand. Quantity and quality of exercise for developing and maintaining cardiorespiratory, musculoskeletal, and neuromotor fitness in apparently healthy adults: guidance for prescribing exercise. Med Sci Sports Exerc. 2011;43(7):1334–59.
18. Drinkwater BL, Nilson K, Chesnut CH 3rd, Bremner WJ, Shainholtz S, Southworth MB. Bone mineral content of amenorrheic and eumenorrheic athletes. N Engl J Med. 1984;311(5):277–81.
19. Drinkwater BL, Bruemmer B, Chesnut C 3rd, Chait A. Menstrual history as a determinant of current bone density in young athletes. J Clin Endocrinol Metab. 1993;77(6):1605–9.
20. Drinkwater BL, Nilson K, Ott S, Chesnut CH 3rd. Bone mineral content of amenorrheic and eumenorrheic athletes. JAMA. 1986;256(3):380–2.
21. Drinkwater BL, Nilson K, Ott S, Chesnut CH 3rd. Bone mineral density after resumption of menses in amenorrheic athletes. JAMA. 1986;256(3):380–2.
22. Bullen BA, Skrinar GS, Beitins IZ, von Mering G, Turnbull BA, McArthur JW. Induction of menstrual disorders by strenuous exercise in untrained women. N Engl J Med. 1985;312(21):1349–53.
23. Brooks-Gunn J, Warren MP, Hamilton LH. The relation of eating problems and amenorrhea in ballet dancers. Med Sci Sports Exerc. 1987;19(1):41–4.
24. Nattiv A, Loucks AB, Manore MM, Sanborn CF, Sundgot-Borgen J, Warren MP. American College of Sports Medicine position stand. The female athlete triad. Med Sci Sports Exerc. 2007;39(10):1867–82.
25. Otis CL, Drinkwater B, Johnson M, Loucks A, Wilmore J. American College of Sports Medicine position stand. The female athlete triad. Med Sci Sports Exerc. 1997;29(5):i–ix.
26. De Souza MJ, Lee DK, VanHeest JL, Scheid JL, West SL, Williams NI. Severity of energy-related menstrual disturbances increases in proportion to indices of energy conservation in exercising women. Fertil Steril. 2007;88(4):971–5.
27. Williams NI, Caston-Balderrama AL, Helmreich DL, Parfitt DB, Nosbisch C, Cameron JL. Longitudinal changes in reproductive hormones and menstrual cyclicity in cynomolgus monkeys during strenuous exercise training: abrupt transition to exercise-induced amenorrhea. Endocrinology. 2001;142(6):2381–9.
28. Loucks AB, Thuma JR. Luteinizing hormone pulsatility is disrupted at a threshold of energy availability in regularly menstruating women. J Clin Endocrinol Metab. 2003;88(1):297–311.

29. De Souza MJ, West SL, Jamal SA, Hawker GA, Gundberg CM, Williams NI. The presence of both an energy deficiency and estrogen deficiency exacerbate alterations of bone metabolism in exercising women. Bone. 2008;43(1):140–8.
30. De Souza MJ, Williams NI. Beyond hypoestrogenism in amenorrheic athletes: energy deficiency as a contributing factor for bone loss. Curr Sports Med Rep. 2005;4(1):38–44.
31. Ihle R, Loucks AB. Dose-response relationships between energy availability and bone turnover in young exercising women. J Bone Miner Res. 2004;19(8):1231–40.
32. Mountjoy M, Sundgot-Borgen J, Burke L, Carter S, Constantini N, Lebrun C, et al. The IOC consensus statement: beyond the female athlete triad – Relative Energy Deficiency in Sport (RED-S). Br J Sports Med. 2014;48(7):491–7.
33. Hoch AZ, Jurva JW, Staton MA, Thielke R, Hoffmann RG, Pajewski N, et al. Athletic amenorrhea and endothelial dysfunction. WMJ. 2007;106(6):301–6.
34. Friday KE, Drinkwater BL, Bruemmer B, Chesnut C 3rd, Chait A. Elevated plasma low-density lipoprotein and high-density lipoprotein cholesterol levels in amenorrheic athletes: effects of endogenous hormone status and nutrient intake. J Clin Endocrinol Metab. 1993;77(6):1605–9.
35. O'Donnell E, De Souza MJ. The cardiovascular effects of chronic hypoestrogenism in amenorrhoeic athletes – a critical review. Sports Med. 2004;34(9):601–27.
36. Vanheest JL, Rodgers CD, Mahoney CE, De Souza MJ. Ovarian suppression impairs sport performance in junior elite female swimmers. Med Sci Sports Exerc. 2014;46(1):156–66.
37. Gibbs JC, Williams NI, De Souza MJ. Prevalence of individual and combined components of the female athlete triad. Med Sci Sports Exerc. 2013;45(5):985–96.
38. Sundgot-Borgen J, Torstveit MK. Prevalence of eating disorders in elite athletes is higher than in the general population. Clin J Sport Med. 2004;14(1):25–32.
39. Nichols JF, Rauh MJ, Lawson MJ, Ji M, Barkai HS. Prevalence of the female athlete triad syndrome among high school athletes. Arch Pediatr Adolesc Med. 2006;160(2):137–42.
40. De Souza MJ, Nattiv A, Joy E, Misra M, Williams NI, Mallinson RJ, et al. 2014 Female Athlete Triad Coalition consensus statement on treatment and return to play of the female athlete triad: 1st International Conference held in San Francisco, CA, May 2012, and 2nd International Conference held in Indianapolis, IN, May 2013. Clin J Sport Med. 2014;24(2):96–119.
41. De Souza MJ, Williams NI, Nattiv A, Joy E, Misra M, Loucks AB, et al. Misunderstanding the female athlete triad: refuting the IOC consensus statement on Relative Energy Deficiency in Sport (RED-S). Br J Sports Med. 2014;48(20):1461–5.
42. Tenforde AS, Carlson JL, Chang A, Sainani KL, Shultz R, Kim JH, et al. Association of the female athlete triad risk assessment stratification to the development of bone stress injuries in collegiate athletes. Am J Sports Med. 2017;45(2):302–10.
43. Barrack MT, Gibbs JC, De Souza MJ, Williams NI, Nichols JF, Rauh MJ, et al. Higher incidence of bone stress injuries with increasing female athlete triad-related risk factors: a prospective multisite study of exercising girls and women. Am J Sports Med. 2014;42(4):949–58.
44. Wade GN, Schneider JE, Li HY. Control of fertility by metabolic cues. Am J Physiol. 1996;270(1 Pt 1):E1–19.
45. Reed JL, De Souza MJ, Kindler JM, Williams NI. Nutritional practices associated with low energy availability in division I female soccer players. J Sports Sci. 2014;32(16):1499–509.
46. Gibbs JC, Williams NI, Mallinson RJ, Reed JL, Rickard AD, De Souza MJ. Effect of high dietary restraint on energy availability and menstrual status. Med Sci Sports Exerc. 2013;45(9):1790–7.
47. Sundgot-Borgen J. Eating disorders among male and female elite athletes. Br J Sports Med. 1999;33(6):434.
48. Loucks AB, Laughlin GA, Mortola JF, Girton L, Nelson JC, Yen SS. Hypothalamic-pituitary-thyroidal function in eumenorrheic and amenorrheic athletes. J Clin Endocrinol Metab. 1992;75(2):514–8.
49. Williams NI, Leidy HJ, Hill BR, Lieberman JL, Legro RS, De Souza MJ. Magnitude of daily energy deficit predicts frequency but not severity of menstrual disturbances associated with exercise and caloric restriction. Am J Physiol Endocrinol Metab. 2015;308(1):E29–39.

50. Loucks AB, Mortola JF, Girton L, Yen SS. Alterations in the hypothalamic-pituitary-ovarian and the hypothalamic-pituitary-adrenal axes in athletic women. J Clin Endocrinol Metab. 1989;68(2):402–11.
51. Williams NI, Helmreich DL, Parfitt DB, Caston-Balderrama A, Cameron JL. Evidence for a causal role of low energy availability in the induction of menstrual cycle disturbances during strenuous exercise training. J Clin Endocrinol Metab. 2001;86(11):5184–93.
52. Williams NI, Reed JL, Leidy HJ, Legro RS, De Souza MJ. Estrogen and progesterone exposure is reduced in response to energy deficiency in women aged 25–40 years. Hum Reprod. 2010;25(9):2328–39.
53. Loucks AB, Callister R. Induction and prevention of low-T3 syndrome in exercising women. Am J Physiol. 1993;264(5 Pt 2):R924–30.
54. Loucks AB, Heath EM. Dietary restriction reduces luteinizing hormone (LH) pulse frequency during waking hours and increases LH pulse amplitude during sleep in young menstruating women. J Clin Endocrinol Metab. 1994;78(4):910–5.
55. Loucks AB, Heath EM. Induction of low-T3 syndrome in exercising women occurs at a threshold of energy availability. Am J Physiol. 1994;266(3 Pt 2):R817–23.
56. Loucks AB, Verdun M. Slow restoration of LH pulsatility by refeeding in energetically disrupted women. Am J Physiol. 1998;275(4 Pt 2):R1218–26.
57. Loucks AB. The response of luteinizing hormone pulsatility to 5 days of low energy availability disappears by 14 years of gynecological age. J Clin Endocrinol Metab. 2006;91(8):3158–64.
58. Zanker CL, Swaine IL. Responses of bone turnover markers to repeated endurance running in humans under conditions of energy balance or energy restriction. Eur J Appl Physiol. 2000;83(4–5):434–40.
59. Talbott SM, Shapses SA. Fasting and energy intake influence bone turnover in lightweight male rowers. Int J Sport Nutr. 1998;8(4):377–87.
60. Talbott SM, Rothkopf MM, Shapses SA. Dietary restriction of energy and calcium alters bone turnover and density in younger and older female rats. J Nutr. 1998;128(3):640–5.
61. de Bakker CMJ, Tseng WJ, Li Y, Zhao H, Liu XS. Clinical evaluation of bone strength and fracture risk. Curr Osteoporos Rep. 2017;15(1):32–42.
62. Miller KK, Grinspoon SK, Ciampa J, Hier J, Herzog D, Klibanski A. Medical findings in outpatients with anorexia nervosa. Arch Intern Med. 2005;165(5):561–6.
63. Christo K, Prabhakaran R, Lamparello B, Cord J, Miller KK, Goldstein MA, et al. Bone metabolism in adolescent athletes with amenorrhea, athletes with eumenorrhea, and control subjects. Pediatrics. 2008;121(6):1127–36.
64. Grinspoon S, Thomas E, Pitts S, Gross E, Mickley D, Miller K, et al. Prevalence and predictive factors for regional osteopenia in women with anorexia nervosa. Ann Intern Med. 2000;133(10):790–4.
65. Mitchell DM, Tuck P, Ackerman KE, Cano Sokoloff N, Woolley R, Slattery M, et al. Altered trabecular bone morphology in adolescent and young adult athletes with menstrual dysfunction. Bone. 2015;81:24–30.
66. Ackerman KE, Nazem T, Chapko D, Russell M, Mendes N, Taylor AP, et al. Bone microarchitecture is impaired in adolescent amenorrheic athletes compared with eumenorrheic athletes and nonathletic controls. J Clin Endocrinol Metab. 2011;96(10):3123–33.
67. Faje AT, Karim L, Taylor A, Lee H, Miller KK, Mendes N, et al. Adolescent girls with anorexia nervosa have impaired cortical and trabecular microarchitecture and lower estimated bone strength at the distal radius. J Clin Endocrinol Metab. 2013;98(5):1923–9.
68. Singhal V, Tulsiani S, Campoverde KJ, Mitchell DM, Slattery M, Schorr M, et al. Impaired bone strength estimates at the distal tibia and its determinants in adolescents with anorexia nervosa. Bone. 2018;106:61–8.
69. Solmi M, Veronese N, Correll CU, Favaro A, Santonastaso P, Caregaro L, et al. Bone mineral density, osteoporosis, and fractures among people with eating disorders: a systematic review and meta-analysis. Acta Psychiatr Scand. 2016;133(5):341–51.

70. Southmayd EA, Mallinson RJ, Williams NI, Mallinson DJ, De Souza MJ. Unique effects of energy versus estrogen deficiency on multiple components of bone strength in exercising women. Osteoporos Int. 2017;28(4):1365–76.
71. De Souza MJ, Williams NI. Physiological aspects and clinical sequelae of energy deficiency and hypoestrogenism in exercising women. Hum Reprod Update. 2004;10(5):433–48.
72. Lawson EA, Donoho D, Miller KK, Misra M, Meenaghan E, Lydecker J, et al. Hypercortisolemia is associated with severity of bone loss and depression in hypothalamic amenorrhea and anorexia nervosa. J Clin Endocrinol Metab. 2009;94(12):4710–6.
73. Misra M, Miller KK, Cord J, Prabhakaran R, Herzog DB, Goldstein M, et al. Relationships between serum adipokines, insulin levels, and bone density in girls with anorexia nervosa. J Clin Endocrinol Metabol. 2007;92(6):2046–52.
74. Upadhyay J, Farr OM, Mantzoros CS. The role of leptin in regulating bone metabolism. Metabolism. 2015;64(1):105–13.
75. Keen AD, Drinkwater BL. Irreversible bone loss in former amenorrheic athletes. Osteoporos Int. 1997;7(4):311–5.
76. Mallinson RJ, Williams NI, Gibbs JC, Koehler K, Allaway HCM, Southmayd E, et al. Current and past menstrual status is an important determinant of femoral neck geometry in exercising women. Bone. 2016;88:101–12.
77. Miller KK, Lee EE, Lawson EA, Misra M, Minihan J, Grinspoon SK, et al. Determinants of skeletal loss and recovery in anorexia nervosa. J Clin Endocrinol Metab. 2006;91(8):2931–7.
78. Arends JC, Cheung MY, Barrack MT, Nattiv A. Restoration of menses with nonpharmacologic therapy in college athletes with menstrual disturbances: a 5-year retrospective study. Int J Sport Nutr Exerc Metab. 2012;22(2):98–108.
79. Dueck CA, Manore MM, Matt KS. Role of energy balance in athletic menstrual dysfunction. Int J Sport Nutr. 1996;6(2):165–90.
80. Kopp-Woodroffe SA, Manore MM, Dueck CA, Skinner JS, Matt KS. Energy and nutrient status of amenorrheic athletes participating in a diet and exercise training intervention program. Int J Sport Nutr. 1999;9(1):70–88.
81. Lagowska K, Kapczuk K, Jeszka J. Nine-month nutritional intervention improves restoration of menses in young female athletes and ballet dancers. J Int Soc Sports Nutr. 2014;11(1):52.
82. Fredericson M, Kent K. Normalization of bone density in a previously amenorrheic runner with osteoporosis. Med Sci Sports Exerc. 2005;37(9):1481–6.
83. Misra M, Prabhakaran R, Miller KK, Goldstein MA, Mickley D, Clauss L, et al. Weight gain and restoration of menses as predictors of bone mineral density change in adolescent girls with anorexia nervosa-1. J Clin Endocrinol Metab. 2008;93(4):1231–7.

11 Lifestyle Intervention to Improve Mobility in Apparently Healthy Chinese Elders: A Hypothesis Generating Study

Marie-Noelle Horcajada and Elizabeth A. Offord

Introduction

As the aging population increases worldwide, there is an increasing awareness of the importance of "quality of life." Physical functionality or mobility is a core indicator of healthy aging in the elderly population [1].

Thus it is important to find means to prevent or attenuate decline of key physiological functions required to live an active, independent life [2].

Nutrition plays an important role in maintenance of musculoskeletal health during aging. Nutrients, such as Ca, vit D, and proteins, are commonly deficient in the aging population and are important for maintenance of bone mass and strength [3–5]. Certain nutrient deficiencies in elderly have been linked to loss of muscle strength, lower performance in functional tests, and increased risk of falls [1, 6]. Iron and zinc are recognized deficiencies in China [7]. A cross-sectional study in postmenopausal women in Korea found a relationship between bone mineral density and dietary intake of b-carotene, vitamin C, zinc, and vegetables [8]. Vitamin C is also a cofactor for collagen synthesis, important for soft tissues such as cartilage, and may enhance the anticatabolic effect of hyaluronic acid in human chondrocyte cells [9]. While micronutrient deficiency can be addressed by eating regular foods rich in those nutrients [7], many consumers do not readily follow a balanced diet. Thus nutritional food supplements are one way to contribute to meeting unmet dietary needs.

Muscle weakness, bone fragility, joint pain, and discomfort are frequently experienced symptoms of musculoskeletal aging leading to reduced mobility and quality of life. In particular, symptomatic knee pain (often linked to later diagnosis of osteoarthritis) is likely to increase due to increasing life expectancy and the obesity

M.-N. Horcajada (✉) · E. A. Offord
Nestlé Institute of Health Sciences, Nestlé Research Center, Lausanne, Switzerland
e-mail: marienoelle.horcajada@rdls.nestle.com; elizabeth.offord-cavin@rdls.nestle.com

© Springer Nature Switzerland AG 2019

C. M. Weaver et al. (eds.), *Nutritional Influences on Bone Health*,
https://doi.org/10.1007/978-3-319-98464-3_11

epidemic, affecting not only the older adults but also the adult (obese) population of <65 years [10].

While no pharmacological agents are available for managing joint discomfort and pain today, many dietary supplements exist with varying degrees of effectiveness. The most widely studied ones are glucosamine and chondroitin. Specifically a recent Cochrane review concluded that chondroitin alone or combined with glucosamine led to significant improvement in joint pain [11]. Today, there is still a lack of consensus, due to several factors including differences in formulation (e.g., glucosamine sulfate vs glucosamine chloride) and study design [12, 13].

Several international guidelines [14, 15] recommend non-pharmacological interventions such as exercise and weight management at early stages of joint discomfort or osteoarthritis. Exercise may include a mixture of strength training, motion, and aerobic exercise [16]. Indeed, resistance exercise has been shown to be effective on pain relief, alleviation of pain and stiffness, and improvement of physical function [17]. Interestingly, a first, recent systematic review/meta-analysis on the effects of traditional Chinese exercise (TCE) which combines low-level aerobic exercise, strength, balance, and coordination showed beneficial effects on reducing pain, improving physical function, and alleviating stiffness in diagnosed OA patients after TCE interventions for an average 12 weeks' duration [18]. These conclusions are consistent with previous reviews on the benefits of Tai Chi on knee OA [19–22]. Furthermore, the combination of resistance exercise and Tai Chi on knee OA was also beneficial on symptoms [18].

Overall, there is good evidence that exercise is effective in improving physical function and mobility in older adults. However, there is general poor adherence to intensive exercise programs. Rather incorporating lifestyle programs with physical activity such as walking or Tai Chi as balance of aerobics, resistance and balance may be more appropriate and when combined with nutrition may be effective ways for maintaining musculoskeletal health in elderly.

Due to the multifactorial nature of OA, there is an increasing interest in the implementation of a more holistic lifestyle approach. In a first trial (IDEA), the combination of an intensive diet-induced weight loss of 10% combined with exercise was significantly more effective at reducing pain in men and women with symptomatic knee OA than either intervention alone [23].

Very few studies have been conducted on individuals at risk but not yet diagnosed with OA. In the first OA prevention trial of its kind, the PROOF study showed that oral glucosamine sulfate (GS), with or without a personalized diet and exercise program, led to a decrease in the incidence of knee OA as defined by joint structural damage progression over 2.5 years [24]. This was observed in a group of overweight and obese women with no diagnosis of knee OA and without treatment for knee symptoms at baseline [25].

The aim of the current study was to test the feasibility of combined nutrition and exercise approach in healthy, older adults experiencing joint pain and discomfort but not yet formally diagnosed as OA, to test if such an intervention would alleviate symptoms and improve physical functionality and quality of life. This trial was conducted in a Chinese population using a mix of Tai Chi and resistance exercise and a nutritional, dairy supplement containing Ca, vit D, vit C, zinc corresponding to frequently missing nutrients, and glucosamine sulfate for alleviation of joint discomfort [26].

Methods

Subjects

In total, 54 apparently healthy subjects (mean age 55.8 ± 2.26 years, mean BMI 23.8 ± 1.59 kg/m^2) were included in the present study (Table 11.1, mean ± SEM). Forty-two subjects completed the study (23% dropout rate).

All participating subjects were non-diagnosed for osteoarthritis. All subjects must have presented with knee pain (mild or medium discontinuity), dull pain being improved after rest, or becoming serious after knee moves, or going upstairs, and knee pain scored between 2 and 6 out of 10 by use of a visual analog scale (VAS) of pain assessment at baseline. The study protocol was approved by the Medical Ethics Committee of the Peking University Third Hospital (medical ethics trial 2015-004). All participants in the trial provided their written and signed informed consent.

Design

This study was a single-center, single-arm, open-design format where each subject acted as their own control. The intervention in the present study consisted of a progressive physical activity program combined with nutritional supplementation for a total duration of 24 consecutive weeks. For the first 8 weeks, all subjects consumed the nutritional supplement in the absence of the physical activity program while monitoring total daily step count. At the third month, the physical activity program was introduced while maintaining the ingestion of the nutritional supplement.

Table 11.1 Subject (n = 54) characteristics at baseline and 6 months

	Mean ± SEM (baseline)	Mean ± SEM (6 months)
Age (years)	55.8 ± 2.26	N/A
Sex	Men: 7	N/A
	Women: 47	
Weight (kg)	62.5 ± 3.05	62.2 ± 3.19
Height (cm)	161.8 ± 2.60	N/A
BMI (kg/m^2)	23.8 ± 1.59	23.9 ± 1.71
Calcium intake (mg/day)	672 ± 15.7	520 ± 13.7
Proteins intake (g/day)	76.7 ± 5.2	74.1 ± 4.8

Experimental Product

For the duration of the intervention, all subjects consumed an oral supplement reconstituted in 180 mL of warm water twice per day for the duration of the study. Total daily intake of the supplement contained 50 g milk powder, 850 mg calcium, 8 μg vitamin D3, 35 mg vitamin C, 6.5 mg zinc, and 1400 mg glucosamine sulfate.

Exercise Program

The exercise intervention program was a progressive incremental exercise program that included muscle strength training, balance training, daily aerobic exercises, and Tai Chi. Specifically, muscle strength training was performed 2 days per week for 30 min per day; Tai Chi was performed once per week for 20 min. Balance training was performed at home, twice per week for 10 min per session. A 10 min warm-up and cooldown was performed before and following each exercise session. As the exercise program was progressive overtime, the amount of exercise increased by 10–15% per month based on the previous month's physical activity level. For muscle strength training, this meant an increase in the load and for aerobic exercise an increase in the target number of steps. A pedometer (Garmin SA) was provided to each subject, which was used to monitor daily step count throughout the duration of the study. The data from the pedometer were automatically uploaded to the cloud (Medidata, US) twice a week upon attendance at the research center training site.

Assessment and Measurement

Primary Outcomes

Six-Minute Walking Test (6MWT) This test was used to objectively assess submaximal functional exercise capacity. The test was performed indoors, on a 30 m long walking course defined by two cones. Each participant was instructed to walk as fast as they could around the 30 m course for a total duration of 6 min. Upon completion of the 6 min trial, the distance in meters each subject walked (accurate to 0.1 m) was recorded.

Isokinetic Strength The maximal torque and total work of the quadriceps extensor and flexor muscles was assessed using the isokinetic biomechanics test and trainer (CON-TREX, Physiomed Elektromedizin, Germany) at an angular velocity of 60°/s and repeated five times. Each set was separated by 90 s rest intervals.

Secondary Outcomes

Balance Test The subjects were asked to stand with one leg on a flat even platform area (0.5 × 0.5 m) until they no longer were able to keep their balance and the suspended foot touched the ground. Each subject was allowed six attempts (three attempts each foot) and the longest in duration attempt was recorded.

Serum Biomarkers: Bone, Joint, and Inflammation Total serum P1NP (procollagen type 1 amino terminal propeptide kit, Roche Diagnostics GmbH), CTX-1 (C-terminal telopeptides of type I collagen, β-CrossLaps/serum kit, Roche Diagnostics GmbH), CTX-2 (C-terminal telopeptides of type II collagen kit, IDS Ltd.), and IL-6 (interleukin-6, Immulite 2006 kit, Siemens) levels were measured by electrochemiluminescence immunoassay, at baseline, 1, 2, and 6 months of intervention.

Vitamin D Fasting serum 25-OH-D3 was measured at baseline, 2- and 6-month intervention by electrochemiluminescence immunoassay (25-hydroxyvitamin D3 test kit, Roche Diagnostics, GmbH).

Knee Pain Intensity Subjective assessment was performed at baseline and each month of intervention, using a visual analog scale (VAS). The scale was anchored by "no pain" (score of 0) and "pain as bad as it could be" (score of 10). Subjects were asked to place a line perpendicular to the VAS line at the point that represents their pain intensity.

Knee Injury and Osteoarthritis Outcome Score (KOOS) The KOOS subscales are divided into pain, symptoms, activity of daily life (ADL), sport, and quality of life (QoL). At baseline, 2, 4, and 6 months of intervention, subjects completed the KOOS survey to record their perceived levels of each KOOS subscale item (0–100) [27].

Food Frequency Questionnaire (FFQ) To determine the daily dietary protein and calcium intake at baseline and 6 months, a FFQ based on Chinese food and dietary habits was used.

Statistical Analysis

Sample size calculations were based on the data presented in Ng et al. [28] where it is assumed that 6 min walk test is similar to self-paced test. KOOS was also expected to produce similar results to WOMAC score. Sample size calculations were done via a one-sided *t*-test, at a significance level of 2.5% (since there are two primary outcomes) and with a statistical power of 80%. All the calculations were done in NCSS 2007 software (PASS 2005 feature). Taking into account projected 35% dropout rate, 55 subjects were planned to be recruited. Primary analysis focused on the change from baseline to 6 months for combined nutrition and exercise. For this purpose, ANCOVA model correcting for baseline was used introducing compliance to the physical program as a factor (number of daily steps). For the co-primary factors, type I error rate was set to 2.5%. The rest of analyses were done without adjustment for multiplicity. In addition, longitudinal analysis using a mixed model with repeated measures was conducted on all endpoints to valorize the data, and estimates at each visit compared to baseline have been produced. Intent-to-treat (ITT) analysis and per-protocol analysis were performed on co-primary factors; the rest of parameters were only evaluated on ITT.

Results

Throughout the study, the subjects were supposed to take two sachets of products daily. This was tracked via diaries and by counting the difference between the number of dispensed and returned sachets. Compliance for product intake was 98% for subjects who completed the study.

Functional Outcomes

There was a significant difference in the distance walked during the 6 min walking distance test. Specifically there was an increase of 27 and 38 m at months 5 and 6, respectively ($P < 0.05$) compared to baseline (Fig. 11.1). The isokinetic peak torque assessment showed a statistically significant increase in peak knee flexor torque at 6 months compared to baseline ($P < 0.05$), as well as the total work flexor (data not shown). However, no significant difference was observed for peak knee extension torque at any time point. A statistically significant improvement ($P < 0.05$) in single-leg balance outcomes was observed at month 4 (17.52 ± 1.28), 5 (19.21 ± 1.4), and 6 (19.67 ± 1.33) of intervention relative to baseline (13.94 ± 1.08). Values are expressed as mean ± SEM, in s.

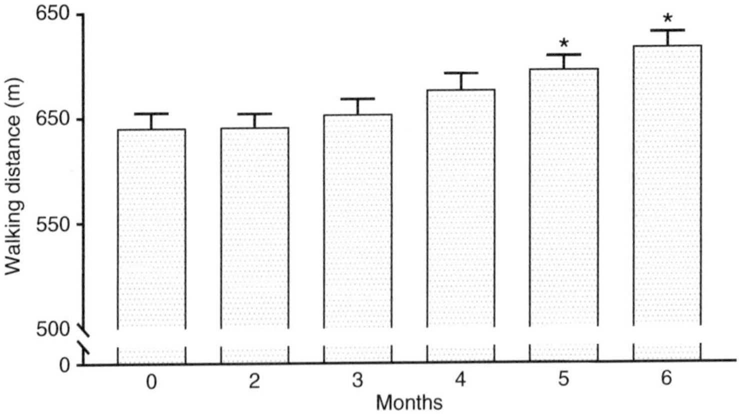

Fig. 11.1 Data showing the distance covered during the 6 min walking distance (6MWD) test throughout the duration of the trial. $^*P < 0.05$ relative to baseline (0 months). Values are expressed as mean ± SEM

Volunteer-Reported Outcome Measures

VAS Score

There was a significant decrease in reported knee pain at 6-month intervention relative to baseline (VAS score baseline 3.37 ± 0.11 vs 1.95 ± 0.17; $p < 0.0001$). A statistically significant decrease was already observed from 2-month intervention ($p < 0.001$) (Table 11.2).

KOOS Score

KOOS pain, activity, and sport scores were significantly improved at 6-month intervention. KOOS QoL score (change from baseline) was significantly improved at 4- and 6-month (51%) intervention time points. No significant modification to the KOOS symptoms was achieved. See Table 11.2 for a summary of all KOOS subcategory scores.

Food Frequency Questionnaire

At baseline, daily calcium and proteins intake were (mean ± SEM in g/day) 672.0 ± 15.7 and 76.7 ± 5.2, respectively, and were not significantly different from that at 6 months: 520 ± 13.7 and 74.1 ± 4.8, respectively (Table 11.1).

Table 11.2 Five-KOOS scores (i.e., pain, symptoms, function in daily leaving (adl), function in sport and recreation (sport), knee-related quality of life (qol)) and VAS scores throughout the duration of the trial

	Months	Mean ± SEM
KOOS pain	0	57.46 ± 2.95
	2	59.72 ± 2.99
	6	60.67 ± 2.15*
KOOS symptoms	0	59.85 ± 3.62
	2	63.01 ± 3.37
	6	63.16 ± 3.48
KOOS ADL	0	64.03 ± 2.69
	2	65.81 ± 2.77
	6	66.56 ± 3.01*
KOOS sport	0	49.44 ± 3.92
	2	50.54 ± 4.21
	6	54.21 ± 4.27*
KOOS QoL	0	35.53 ± 4.17
	2	37.28 ± 3.93
	6	53.95 ± 4.19**
VAS score	0	3.37 ± 0.11
	1	2.76 ± 0.12
	2	2.69 ± 0.13*
	3	2.20 ± 0.16**
	4	2.57 ± 0.17
	5	2.15 ± 0.14**
	6	1.95 ± 0.17**

*$p < 0.05$; **$p < 0.001$ relative to baseline (0 months)

Biomarkers

No statistical significant variations in fasting serum 25-OH-D3 at 2 months (52.00 ± 4.35) or 6-month intervention (47.02 ± 7.25) compared to baseline (49.81 ± 3.78) were observed. Values are expressed as mean ± SEM, in ng mL^{-1}.

The change from baseline (0.91 ± 0.03) in serum CTX-2 levels at 6-month intervention (0.71 ± 0.02) was statistically significant ($p < 0.0001$) but remained unchanged at 1- and 2-month intervention. Values are expressed as mean ± SEM, in μg L^{-1}.

Compared to baseline, a significant decrease in blood CTX-1 was measured already at 1-month intervention and also at each following visit, i.e., 2- and 6-month intervention ($p < 0.001$) (Fig. 11.2a). A parallel decrease in P1NP was observed but only at 2- and 6-month intervention compared to baseline ($p < 0.05$) (Fig. 11.2b). Finally, IL-6 serum levels did not show any significant changes throughout the study (data not shown).

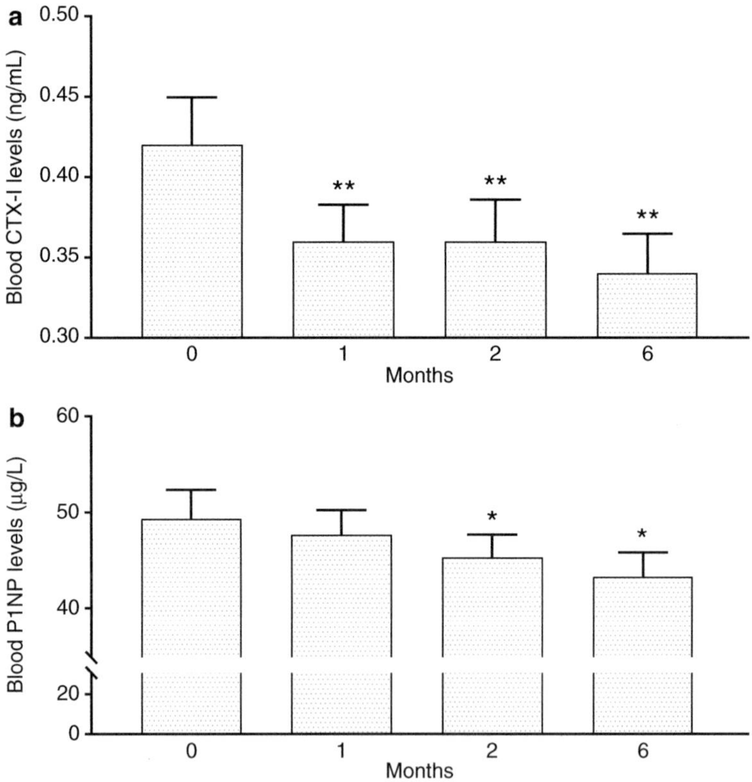

Fig. 11.2 Data showing serum levels of biomarkers, (**a**) bone resorption (CTX-1, ng/mL) and (**b**) bone formation (P1NP, μg/L) throughout the duration of the trial. *$P < 0.05$; **$P < 0.001$ relative to baseline (0 months)

Discussion

Design and Target Population

This study explored the combination of providing key nutrients for musculoskeletal health combined with low-intensity exercise to alleviate self-reported, age-related symptoms of mild knee pain (baseline VAS score: 3.37 ± 0.835) and to improve parameters of physical function over 6-month intervention. The subjects were recruited as otherwise healthy aging, Chinese seniors with normal BMI (23.8 ± 1.59 kg/m^2) with no reports of previously diagnosed joint disease (no further radiography was performed).

The milk-based nutritional supplement provided several of the frequently missing nutrients from diets of the aging population (Ca, vitamin D, Zn), important for preservation of bone and muscle. Indeed dietary calcium at the beginning and end of the study was around 600 mg/day. The supplement provided additional 800 mg/day ensuring volunteers to meet daily calcium recommendations. Moreover, the experimental product provided vitamin C for collagen synthesis and glucosamine sulfate for relief of joint pain. The form (sulfate) and dose (1500 mg) of glucosamine were in accordance with reports of meta-analysis of the effects of glucosamine formulations on knee pain in osteoarthritic populations concluding that glucosamine sulfate but not glucosamine hydrochloride is effective on pain reduction [29].

The progressive exercise program consisted of a mixture of aerobic, balance, and strength routines, commonly practiced by Chinese seniors, e.g., Tai Chi. As the participants in the study were neither overweight nor obese, the low-intensity physical activity component was chosen to improve functional outcomes through increases in leg strength and balance and not weight loss per se which has also previously been shown to improve function in OA patients [23]. Furthermore, the weight of the subjects did not change during the study (Table 11.1); thus any change in pain symptoms or physical function was not due to reduced mechanical strain on the joints.

The aim of this study was to test the effect of the combined nutrition and exercise program as a feasible lifestyle program for Chinese seniors to manage age-related concerns related to mobility. The study design did not allow us to distinguish the effects of nutrition and physical activity on final outcomes of physical functionality or pain, rather each subject was monitored for evolution with respect to their own baseline values, followed by 2 months of nutrition alone and 4 months of nutrition and exercise. Similar to a previous study of this kind in diagnosed hip or knee osteoarthritis subjects [28], our study was designed as an exploratory, single-arm, baseline-controlled, open-label trial but in a normal aging population experiencing mild joint discomfort.

Effect of First 2 Months of Nutrition Alone

During the first 2 months, the subjects were given the nutritional supplement alone while controlling their normal step counts. Our aim was to normalize the nutritional status of the subjects for important micronutrients such as Ca and vit D and to monitor their regular activity before starting the exercise program. We were surprised to observe several early responses in bone and cartilage turnover already within this 2-month period. As shown in Fig. 11.2a and b, the bone resorption marker CTX1 was reduced by an average of 15% ($p < 0.01$). This may be a response to the milk-based supplement containing Ca as has previously been reported for bone resorption markers [30] or to the restoration of missing nutrients, e.g., calcium. More surprising was the finding that CTX-2 (a marker of cartilage breakdown) decreased by 5%, although this effect size did not reach significance at 2 months. Whether this response is due to any single component of the nutritional supplement or to the mix remains to be verified. Interestingly glucosamine sulfate has been shown to reduce cartilage breakdown, but not bone metabolism biomarkers in healthy subjects with normal cartilage metabolism [31].

Concerning self-reported knee pain and joint discomfort, a 20% decrease in knee pain (VAS score, table, $p < 0.001$) was shown to be significant after 2-month intervention (reaching 42% at 6-month intervention, $p < 0.001$), whereas no effect was seen with the KOOS questionnaire for quality of life at 2 months.

Effect of Combined Nutrition + Exercise

The progressive exercise program consisted of a mixture of aerobic, balance, and strength routines, commonly practiced by Chinese seniors, e.g. Tai Chi. We observed a significant increase in the time the participants were able to stand on one leg from the fourth to the sixth month inclusive. In addition we also observed an increase in the distance covered in the 6MWD as well as significant increases in knee flexion strength after 6 months of intervention (Fig. 11.1), a finding in line with previous reports [32].

Beyond physical functionality outcomes, our program (nutritional blend combined with physical activity) resulted in improvement in self-reported joint discomfort and mild knee pain of subjects at 6 months relative to baseline. Indeed, pain VAS score was decreased by 42% ($P < 0.001$) at 6-month intervention. Furthermore, KOOS pain (5.5%, $p < 0.05$), activity (4%, $p < 0.05$), and sport (5.5%, $p < 0.05$) scores were significantly improved at the end of the intervention. This might partly explain the reported KOOS QoL score that was significantly improved at 4 (28.5%, $p < 0.05$) and 6 months (51%, $p < 0.01$) (Table 11.2). Ng et al. [28] also showed that combining a progressive walking program and daily oral supplement with glucosamine sulfate (1500 mg) helped to alleviate OA symptoms of the hip and knee in their OA diagnosed subjects, by 6–12 weeks of intervention, using the WOMAC questionnaire.

Further to the initial effect of nutrition alone at 2 months on biomarkers of bone and cartilage turnover, we further observed a significant decrease (20%, $p < 0.001$) in bone turnover markers of resorption (CTX1) after 1 month and subsequently coupled decrease in bone formation (PINP) after 2 months (Fig. 11.2a and b, respectively). A decrease in cartilage breakdown biomarker (CTX2) was observed (22%,

$p < 0.001$) at the end of the combined nutrition and exercise phase. Two months of nutritional intervention alone did not seem to impact cartilage turnover but mainly bone turnover. Interestingly, the biomarkers measured in this study have been shown to increase in progressive knee OA early stages compared to nonprogressive OA and controls [33].

Conclusion

In conclusion, this study provided initial data to support the hypothesis that a combined nutrition and exercise program improves mobility and quality of life in healthy aging individuals experiencing mild knee pain and joint discomfort. Despite the limitations of a single-arm trial, which does not allow us to distinguish the relative contribution of nutrition or physical activity, we can nevertheless speculate that the nutritional supplement did contribute to the overall effects as shown by initial observations with nutrition alone in the first 2 months of the study (biomarkers of bone turnover, pain score). The significant improvement in functional tests was observed after the combined period of nutrition and exercise at 6 months, underlining the importance of the physical activity component of the program without excluding a complimentary indirect effect of nutrition over time.

Larger, more rigorous confirmatory trials are warranted to investigate the influence of nutrition +/_ exercise to improve nutritional status and physical functionality in the senior population experiencing symptoms of musculoskeletal aging such as joint pain and discomfort.

References

1. Milaneschi Y, Tanaka T, Ferrucci L. Nutritional determinants of mobility. Curr Opin Clin Nutr Metab Care. 2010;13(6):625–9.
2. Collino S, Martin FP, Karagounis LG, Horcajada MN, Moco S, Franceschi C, et al. Reprint of: Musculoskeletal system in the old age and the demand for healthy ageing biomarkers. Mech Ageing Dev. 2014;136-137:94–100.
3. Dawson-Hughes B. Calcium and protein in bone health. Proc Nutr Soc. 2003;62(2):505–9.
4. de Souza Genaro P, Martini LA. Effect of protein intake on bone and muscle mass in the elderly. Nutr Rev. 2010;68(10):616–23.
5. Liao RX, Yu M, Jiang Y, Xia W. Management of osteoporosis with calcitriol in elderly Chinese patients: a systematic review. Clin Interv Aging. 2014;9:515–26.
6. Annweiler C, Montero-Odasso M, Schott AM, Berrut G, Fantino B, Beauchet O. Fall prevention and vitamin D in the elderly: an overview of the key role of the non-bone effects. J Neuroeng Rehabil. 2010;7:50.
7. Koyama T, Yoshita K, Sakurai M, Miura K, Naruse Y, Okuda N, et al. Relationship of consumption of meals including grain, fish and meat, and vegetable dishes to the prevention of nutrient deficiency: the INTERMAP Toyama study. J Nutr Sci Vitaminol (Tokyo). 2016;62(2): 101–7.
8. Kim DE, Cho SH, Park HM, Chang YK. Relationship between bone mineral density and dietary intake of beta-carotene, vitamin C, zinc and vegetables in postmenopausal Korean women: a cross-sectional study. J Int Med Res. 2016;44(5):1103–14.

9. Huang TL, Yang CH, Yanai G, Liao JY, Sumi S, Yang KC. Synergistic effect of l-ascorbic acid and hyaluronic acid on the expressions of matrix metalloproteinase-3 and -9 in human chondrocytes. J Biomed Mater Res B Appl Biomater. 2018;106(5):1809–17.
10. Deshpande BR, Katz JN, Solomon DH, Yelin EH, Hunter DJ, Messier SP, et al. Number of persons with symptomatic knee osteoarthritis in the US: impact of race and ethnicity, age, sex, and obesity. Arthritis Care Res (Hoboken). 2016;68(12):1743–50.
11. Singh JA, Noorbaloochi S, MacDonald R, Maxwell LJ. Chondroitin for osteoarthritis. Cochrane Database Syst Rev. 2015;1:Cd005614.
12. Kucharz EJ, Kovalenko V, Szanto S, Bruyere O, Cooper C, Reginster JY. A review of glucosamine for knee osteoarthritis: why patented crystalline glucosamine sulfate should be differentiated from other glucosamines to maximize clinical outcomes. Curr Med Res Opin. 2016;32(6):997–1004.
13. Henrotin Y. Non-pharmacological therapies for the management of osteoarthritis in guidelines: discrepancies and translating evidence in practices, Nonpharmacological therapies in the management of osteoarthritis. Emirate of Sharjah: Bentham Science Publishers; 2012. p. 21–34.
14. McAlindon TE, Bannuru RR, Sullivan MC, Arden NK, Berenbaum F, Bierma-Zeinstra SM, et al. OARSI guidelines for the non-surgical management of knee osteoarthritis. Osteoarthr Cartil. 2014;22(3):363–88.
15. Combe B, Landewe R, Daien CI, Hua C, Aletaha D, Alvaro-Gracia JM, et al. 2016 update of the EULAR recommendations for the management of early arthritis. Ann Rheum Dis. 2017;76(6):948–59.
16. Fransen M, McConnell S, Harmer AR, Van der Esch M, Simic M, Bennell KL. Exercise for osteoarthritis of the knee: a Cochrane systematic review. Br J Sports Med. 2015;49(24):1554–7.
17. Li Y, Su Y, Chen S, Zhang Y, Zhang Z, Liu C, et al. The effects of resistance exercise in patients with knee osteoarthritis: a systematic review and meta-analysis. Clin Rehabil. 2016;30(10):947–59.
18. Zhang Y, Huang L, Su Y, Zhan Z, Li Y, Lai X. The effects of traditional chinese exercise in treating knee osteoarthritis: a systematic review and meta-analysis. PLoS One. 2017;12(1):e0170237.
19. Ye J, Cai S, Zhong W, Cai S, Zheng Q. Effects of tai chi for patients with knee osteoarthritis: a systematic review. J Phys Ther Sci. 2014;26(7):1133–7.
20. Yan JH, Gu WJ, Sun J, Zhang WX, Li BW, Pan L. Efficacy of Tai Chi on pain, stiffness and function in patients with osteoarthritis: a meta-analysis. PLoS One. 2013;8(4):e61672.
21. Lauche R, Langhorst J, Dobos G, Cramer H. A systematic review and meta-analysis of Tai Chi for osteoarthritis of the knee. Complement Ther Med. 2013;21(4):396–406.
22. Wang C, Schmid CH, Iversen MD, Harvey WF, Fielding RA, Driban JB, et al. Comparative effectiveness of tai chi versus physical therapy for knee osteoarthritis: a randomized trial. Ann Intern Med. 2016;165(2):77–86.
23. Messier SP, Mihalko SL, Legault C, Miller GD, Nicklas BJ, DeVita P, et al. Effects of intensive diet and exercise on knee joint loads, inflammation, and clinical outcomes among overweight and obese adults with knee osteoarthritis: the IDEA randomized clinical trial. JAMA. 2013;310(12):1263–73.
24. Runhaar J, van Middelkoop M, Reijman M, Willemsen S, Oei EH, Vroegindeweij D, et al. Prevention of knee osteoarthritis in overweight females: the first preventive randomized controlled trial in osteoarthritis. Am J Med. 2015;128(8):888–95.e4.
25. Runhaar J, Deroisy R, van Middelkoop M, Barretta F, Barbetta B, Oei EH, et al. The role of diet and exercise and of glucosamine sulfate in the prevention of knee osteoarthritis: further results from the PRevention of knee Osteoarthritis in Overweight Females (PROOF) study. Semin Arthritis Rheum. 2016;45(4 Suppl):S42–8.
26. Chang C, Karagounis LG, Yu Y, Yin J, Donato-Capel L, Shevlyakova M, et al. Combining nutritional supplementation and progressive physical activity program improves functionality and quality of life in healthy 50y+ volunteers with knee joint discomfort: a baseline-control trial. Osteoarthr Cartil. 2017;25:S293–S4.

27. Roos EM, Roos HP, Lohmander LS, Ekdahl C, Beynnon BD. Knee injury and osteoarthritis outcome score (KOOS) – development of a self-administered outcome measure. J Orthop Sports Phys Ther. 1998;28(2):88–96.
28. Ng NT, Heesch KC, Brown WJ. Efficacy of a progressive walking program and glucosamine sulphate supplementation on osteoarthritic symptoms of the hip and knee: a feasibility trial. Arthritis Res Ther. 2010;12(1):R25.
29. Wu D, Huang Y, Gu Y, Fan W. Efficacies of different preparations of glucosamine for the treatment of osteoarthritis: a meta-analysis of randomised, double-blind, placebo-controlled trials. Int J Clin Pract. 2013;67(6):585–94.
30. Katsuyama H, Sunami S, Fukunaga M. Influence of nutrients intake on bone turnover markers. Clin Calcium. 2005;15(9):1529–34.
31. Momomura R, Naito K, Igarashi M, Watari T, Terakado A, Oike S, et al. Evaluation of the effect of glucosamine administration on biomarkers of cartilage and bone metabolism in bicycle racers. Mol Med Rep. 2013;7(3):742–6.
32. Messier SP. Physical activity and weight loss interventions in older adults with knee osteoarthritis. N C Med J. 2007;68(6):436–8.
33. Nguyen LT, Sharma AR, Chakraborty C, Saibaba B, Ahn ME, Lee SS. Review of prospects of biological fluid biomarkers in osteoarthritis. Int J Mol Sci. 2017;18(3):E601.

Part IV

Prebiotics

12 Diet, Microbiota, and Bone Health

René Rizzoli

Introduction

The largest number of cells (10e14) within the human body is located in the intestinal tract. This number is much higher than the number of cells in any human body organ. The estimated number of different species varies between 1000 and 5000 comprising gram-positive (*Firmicutes*, *Bifidobacteria*) and gram-negative (*Bacteroidetes*, *Proteobacteria*) bacteria, archaea, eukarya, as well as fungi and viruses [1]. These organisms are collectively called the gut microbiota (GM). They mostly refer to the large intestine content, but all parts of the GI tract are colonized with an increasing density from the duodenum to the distal colon. GM is now considered as an organ modulating the expression of genes involved in mucosal barrier function, immune system, food digestion, and energy metabolism as it is capable of fermenting undigested nutrients into short-chain fatty acids with local and systemic effects [1–3]. Conversely, colonocyte metabolic products change the lumen environment and the types of bacteria that can grow [4]. The microbiome refers to the aggregate collection of genomes and genes present in gut microbiota. *Dysbiosis* is a state of microbial imbalance in the gut. It refers to a change in microbiota structure and/or function [2]. *Gnotobiotic* animals are animals raised under germ-free conditions and then colonized with well-defined microbes.

Microbiota is acquired during natural delivery, perhaps even during fetal life since meconium appears to be non-sterile [5], feeding, with a marked change when solid foods are introduced [6]. There is also a vertical transmission through suckling, bathing, and cutaneous contact (for review see [7]). Children born by cesarean section have less bifido- and lactobacteria than those by natural delivery [8]. Though relatively stable during adult life [9], microbiota modifications can be observed

R. Rizzoli
Service of Bone Diseases, Geneva University Hospitals and Faculty of Medicine, Geneva, Switzerland
e-mail: rene.rizzoli@unige.ch

© Springer Nature Switzerland AG 2019

C. M. Weaver et al. (eds.), *Nutritional Influences on Bone Health*,
https://doi.org/10.1007/978-3-319-98464-3_12

according to age [10, 11], sex [12], diet [13, 14], living conditions, geography [11, 15], and diseases requiring antibiotic treatment and various drugs [16, 17]. For instance, the variability of the microbiota increases with aging, with greater proportion of *Bacteroides* species and enterobacteriaceae populations and less bifidobacteriaceae [10, 11].

Over the last 12 years, GM has gathered increasing interest with associations or causal relationships suggested or demonstrated for a large variety of disorders including bowel inflammatory diseases, irritable bowel syndrome, colorectal cancer, obesity, metabolic syndrome, type 2 diabetes, atherosclerosis, nonalcoholic fatty liver, malnutrition, asthma, autoimmune diseases, psoriasis, multiple sclerosis, infections, anxiety, depression, and autism [18]. A link of microbiota has been recognized with periodontitis, rheumatoid arthritis, spondyloarthropathy, and frailty [19]. The present review summarizes the associations between diet, bone health, and GM.

Potential Mechanisms How Microbiota Can Influence Bone

Various mechanisms have been proposed to link microbiota composition and/or products to bone metabolism.

Intestinal Wall Permeability

Sex hormone deprivation increases intestinal permeability [19], allowing the translocation of bacteria and increasing antigens entering the epithelial mucosa. Higher levels of inflammation markers can then be detected. A possible mechanism is the reduction in gap junction protein transcripts caused by sex hormone deficiency [20]. This increase in gut permeability can be prevented by the administration of probiotics [19], leading to a lower generation of osteoclastogenic cytokines. Intestinal wall thickness and surface increases have been reported in relation with changes in microbiota [21], accounting for increases in solutes absorption. Products of GM metabolism regulate metabolism and reduce autophagy in mammalian colon [22, 23]. High protein diet-mediated changes in luminal environment are associated with the maintenance of colonic homeostasis [24].

Immune System Modulation

Germ-free (GF) animals, hence lacking microbiota, have immature mucosal immune system [25]. CD4 T-cells are decreased as are TNFalpha and IL6 productions [26]. GF mice have less CD4+ T-cells and germinal centers in the spleen, suggesting that microbiota can modulate immune system development [25]. Presence of bioactive TNFalpha is necessary for the progression of ovariectomy-induced bone loss [27]. An association between inflammation and bone loss is well recognized [28]. T-cell depletion by anti-CD4 and anti-CD8 antibody administration prevents ovariectomy-induced bone loss in mice [29].

Microbial Metabolites

Products from fatty acid metabolism, like short-chain fatty acids (SCFAs: acetate, propionate, butyrate), can directly modify local intestinal metabolism [22] and support intestinal barrier function. In addition, these SCFAs can directly influence bone metabolism and mass. SCFA (acetate, propionate, or butyrate) given in the drinking water increased trabecular volume and reduced osteoclast number and biochemical markers of bone resorption in mice [3]. Furthermore, propionate or butyrate administration prevented ovariectomy-induced as well as inflammation-dependent bone loss. SCFAs were able to inhibit osteoclast differentiation and bone resorption [3]. Butyrate is also an inhibitor of histone deacetylase and stimulates osteoblast differentiation [30]. Butyrate increases bone formation with increased bone sialoprotein and osteoprotegerin production [31].

Nutrients Digestion

GM is involved in the digestion and release of dietary nutrients, which are then excreted in the urine [32, 33]. Changes in microbiota metabolism or composition can modify bowel content pH, by producing short-chain fatty acids, influencing thereby calcium availability and increasing its absorption [34, 35]. Since an increase in net intestinal calcium absorption could be achieved by just ingesting more calcium, a change in intestinal absorption is unlikely to markedly account for the effects of GM on bone metabolism.

Endocrine Pathway Modifications

An increase in calcium absorption leads to a reduction in PTH production and thus a decrease in bone resorption [36]. The gut endocrine system could be affected too, as GF animals have a lower serotonin secretion, in relation to reduced tryptophan hydroxylase-1 expression in the large intestine [26]. Serotonin has been shown to lower bone formation [37]. GF mice are protected against sex hormone deficiency-induced increase in bone turnover and accelerated bone loss [19]. In these mice, there is no increased production of osteoclastic cytokines in response to sex hormone deprivation. GM is required for sex hormone deprivation-mediated bone loss [19]. Another hormone system influenced by GM is IGF-I [38]. Indeed, while, in the short term, colonization of adult mice reduced bone mass, it increased bone formation in the long term, resulting in the correction of bone mass and increased longitudinal and radial bone growth. Serum IGF-I levels were increased in response to microbial colonization. Antibiotic treatment of conventional mice, in contrast, decreased serum IGF-I and decreased bone formation [38]. Supplementation of antibiotic-treated mice with SCFAs restored IGF-I and bone mass to levels seen in nonantibiotic-treated mice. Along the same line, lower serum IGF-I levels have been reported in GF mice [39].

Direct Evidence for an Important Role of Microbiota in Bone Metabolism

To appraise the role of GM in bone metabolism, the first step was to investigate bone properties under an extreme situation, i.e., the total lack of microbiota such as in germ-free animals. Osteoclast number was reduced, while bone formation rate was maintained, suggesting that higher bone mass and microstructure in GF mice were related to a decrease in bone resorption [26]. This study shows that GM is a major regulator of bone mass, since relative bone volume, trabecular number, and cortical area were markedly higher in germ-free mice [26]. Some animals were recolonized with a normal gut microbiota by 3 weeks of age. They displayed a reduction in trabecular bone mineral density and cortical area as compared to GF mice, together with higher levels of osteoclast precursors, supporting a microbiota influence on bone, which is mediated by inflammation-related bone resorption. GF animals had decreased frequency of CD4+ T-cells and CD11b+/GR 1 osteoclast precursor as well as lower bone IL6 and TNFalpha mRNA expression. These mice also displayed lower serotonin levels, but the latter were not changed upon recolonization despite normalization of bone mass, suggesting that low serotonin level is not the primary cause of high bone mass in GF animals [26].

The negative effects of normal GM on the bone are observed in mice with a C57BL/6 background. In contrast, normal GM support growth and bone development in Balb/c and CB6F1 mice [38, 39], indicating that the GM influence on bone physiology is controlled by mouse genetic background. It appears that GM has pro-osteoclastic immunoregulation in CH57BL/6 strain, while it exerts a pro-anabolic effect through IGF-I in Balb/b and CB6F1 mice.

Modulation of Microbiota Composition and/or Metabolism and Effects on Bone

Antibiotics

Low-dose antibiotics have been used as growth promoter in poultry and cattle industry [40]. Subtherapeutic doses of antibiotics such as penicillin, vancomycin, and chlortetracycline in early life led to changes in fecal microbiome, particularly in genes involved in carbohydrate metabolism, with increased short-chain fatty acid production and changes in hepatic lipid metabolism gene expression [41]. By 3 weeks but not by 7 weeks, this treatment was associated with an increase in bone mineral density. There was no change in circulating IGF-I, insulin, leptin, ghrelin, nor peptide YY, but only a higher level of gastric inhibitory polypeptide (GIP). An increase in fat mass was present at both time points. Extending this observation, it was then shown that altering the intestinal microbiota during a critical development window had lasting metabolic consequences [42]. Low-dose penicillin from birth on or from weaning led to fat mass increase in males and higher bone mineral density in female mice but not in males. This study suggests that antibiotics during growth can exert some sex-specific influence on bone [42]. Though a link with microbiota was not suggested at that time, tetracycline administration was shown to prevent ovariectomy-induced bone loss [43]. The same treatment was associated with higher bone strength [44].

Sex Hormones

Sex hormone deprivation (ovariectomy, OVX) caused much less cortical and trabecular bone loss in GF animals than in controls [19], through lower bone resorption. OVX was associated with higher number of TNFalpha+CD4+ and TNFalpha+CD8+ cells in the bone marrow in controls but not in GF animals. GM may thus be necessary to provide the antigens for T-cell production of TNFalpha. Therefore GM composition may modulate postmenopausal bone loss. Ovariectomy increased microbiota diversity and number of *Bacteroidetes* phylum and reduced short-chain fatty acid levels [45]. In a RCT in healthy postmenopausal women, 2 months of isoflavone supplementation increased several microorganisms, including *Bifidobacterium* genus [46].

Diet

Food is a major factor to determine the types and proportion of the microorganisms present in gut microbiota. Conversely, microbiota contributes to influence food nutritional value. The microbiota of older people displays a greater interindividual variation than that of younger adults. Microbiota composition correlates with residence location, frailty, comorbidities, markers of inflammation, and nutritional status [10, 11]. Diet-driven alterations of microbiota may influence the rate of health decline with aging. The fiber content of the diet markedly influences microbiota composition, by its prebiotic properties [35] as does the ingestion of foods containing probiotics [47]. Diet rapidly alters the human gut microbiome. An animal-based diet increased fat and protein intakes and led to higher beta diversity, without affecting alpha diversity [13].

Microbiota collected from malnourished children impaired the growth of gnotobiotic mice [48]. When these malnourished subjects received a supplementation containing peanuts, sugar, milk, vitamins, and minerals, their microbiota transplanted into the mice corrected the impaired growth. Several taxa in recipient animals correlated with lean mass gain; liver, muscle, and brain metabolism; and bone morphology [49]. When mice having received microbiota from controls or from malnourished children were cohoused, taxa from the former invaded the latter and prevented growth alteration of the recipient animals [49]. When two invading species, *Ruminococcus gnavus* and *Clostridium symbosum*, were added to the microbiota of undernourished donors, growth and metabolic abnormalities of the recipient mice were improved. These observations highlight that normal growth depends on normal postnatal microbiota development.

A series of diet modulations can alter GM composition. A high fat diet reduces GM diversity in mice [50]. Artificial sweeteners induce glucose intolerance together with changes in GM [51].

Adherence to a Mediterranean diet, which provides fibers, fermented dairy products, and polyphenols, is associated with various health benefits. Changes in GM have been reported [52–54]. Regarding bone, higher adherence to such a diet is associated with lower hip fracture risk [55, 56].

Prebiotics

Prebiotics are nondigestible fiber compounds that pass undigested in the upper part of the gastrointestinal tract and stimulate the growth and/or activity of bacteria that colonize the large bowel by acting as a substrate for them [57]. Prebiotics refer to galacto-oligosaccharides (GOS), inulin, resistant starch, polydextrose, fructooligosaccharides (FOS), xylooligosaccharides, and lactulose. Oligosaccharides are composed of 3–10 sugars. Their length influences the site of fermentation [58]. Foods particularly rich in fibers are shown in Table 12.1. They resemble oligosaccharides occurring naturally in human milk. Some GOS can also be found in peas and beans.

Effects on Gut

The mode of action implies the fermentation of fibers within the large intestine leading to the production of short-chain fatty acids such as acetate, propionate, valerate, isovalerate, or butyrate and isobutyrate [35, 57, 59, 60]. The changes observed are an increase of calcium bioavailability through a reduction in bowel content pH [34, 60], an increase in caecum weight and microvilli surface [21, 60], histone acetylation with epigenetic modulation [61], as well as microbiota modifications, with increases in the bifidobacteria species capable of causing deconjugation of phytoestrogens [62]. Doses of GOS, FOS, fiber dextrin, inulin, and agave fructans, up to

Table 12.1 Fiber content of various vegetables

Prebiotics	Fiber/weight (%)	Daily serving needed (g) (aim: ≥6 g/day fiber)
Chicory roots	65	9
Raw Jerusalem artichokes	31	19
Raw dandelion greens	24	25
Raw garlic	17	34 (bulb >50 g)
Raw leeks	12	51
Raw onion	9	70
Cooked onion	5	120
Raw asparagus	5	120
Raw wheat bran	5	120
Baked wheat flour	5	125
Raw banana	1	600

From MyFoodData

20 g/day in human, increased the number of bifidobacteria and lactobacilli and decreased that of coliforms [57]. Soy bars increase bifidobacteria and eubacteria [63]. It is also possible that prebiotics may have direct effects, without metabolism, on the immune system [64].

A large series of evidence, both in experimental animals (Table 12.2) and in humans (Table 12.3), supports a significant role of prebiotics on intestinal absorption, calcium retention, and bone mineral mass/density [57]. In various experimental models, prebiotic ingestion leads to increased intestinal calcium absorption in male rats [65, 66] and female mice and rats [59, 67]. For review see [35, 57, 68, 69]. Growing male rats exposed to GOS displayed a decrease in cecal pH and increases in bifidobacteria, calcium and magnesium absorption, tibia strength, and BMD [60]. OVX-induced bone loss was attenuated by prebiotics [66, 70–72]. In an old study, lactitol increased the net and fractional calcium absorption in intact male rats, with a higher positive calcium balance [34]. Interestingly, cecal pH was lower in lactitol-treated animals. When cecal calcium collected from lactitol-treated rats and controls was injected into duodenal loops to assess the absorbability of calcium present in the large intestine, calcium absorption was 50% higher for cecal content from the lactitol group [34]. Rats possess a potent vitamin D-dependent calcium absorptive mechanism in the large intestine, which is usually poorly used, because of calcium complexed to various anions which is not available to the transport system [73]. By modifying bowel content pH, bioavailability of calcium is thus increased.

Effects on Bone

At the bone level, FOS administration increased cortical and trabecular bone in mice and BMC in male rats [59, 65, 74]. Diet enriched in fibers enhanced cortical thickness, cortical BMC, and trabecular BMD in rats [60]. FOS was also associated with higher bone strength [75]. Such an improvement in strength was also observed in ovariectomized rats receiving FOS [76]. Difructose anhydride III improved post-gastrectomy osteopenia in rats [77]. Regarding bone metabolism, agave fructans increased osteocalcin levels [59], GOS/FOS stimulated osteoblast proliferation [78], and FOS-inulin lowered the ratio for bone resorption/bone formation in ovariectomized rats [72]. Femur and tibia breaking strength as well as distal femur total and trabecular volumetric BMD, as well as proximal tibia volumetric BMD, increased in response to GOS supplementation [60]. It has been shown that onion and a mixture of vegetables decreased bone resorption, through a mechanism independent of their supply in base excess [79, 80]. Though microbiota changes were not evaluated in these studies, the high fiber content of these nutrients (Table 12.1) suggests that these observations might be related to a prebiotic effect. Calcium supplementation appears to modulate gut microbiota in a prebiotic manner in diet-induced obese mice [81].

Human sialylated milk oligosaccharides are less abundant in mother milk of severely stunted offsprings [82]. Using gnotobiotic mice and piglets, it has been shown that human sialylated milk oligosaccharides added to microbiota collected from undernourished children were able to increase muscle mass and modify bone morphology. This type of oligosaccharides is present in whey. They stimulate the

Table 12.2 Effects on bone metabolism of prebiotics in mammalian experimental animals

First author	Date	Model	Prebiotics	Intestine	Bone mass/density
Ammann [34]	1988	Intact rats	Lactitol, 1 week	Incr. Ca absorption, decr. cecal pH	Incr. Ca balance
Brommage [141]	1993	Intact rats	Lactulose	Incr. Ca absorption	
Bueno-Vergas [142]	2016	Pregnant rats	FOS and inulin		Incr. BV/TV and TrTh Offspring: incr. vert. trabecular and cortical bone
Bryk [78]	2015	Intact rats	GOS and FOS	Incr. Ca, decr. pH, incr. cecum weight, incr. lactobacilli	Incr. femur BMC, TrBMD and stiffness
Chaplin [81]	2015	Intact mice	Calcium	Incr. cecum weight, incr. bifidobacteria and bacteroidetes	
Charbonneau [82]	2016	Mice	Human milk oligosaccharides		Incr. femur cortical and trabecular bone No effects in germ-free mice
Chonan [66]	1995	OVX rats	GOS ≥10 days	Incr. Ca absorption	Prevention bone loss 8 ash weight
Coudray [143]	2003	Intact rats	FOS or inulin, 4 weeks	Incr. Ca and Mg absorption	Incr. Ca balance (with both FOS and inulin)
Delzenne [144]	1995	Intact rats	FOS		Incr. Ca and Mg balance
Garcia-Vieyra [59]	2014	OVX mice	Agave fructans or inulin		Prevention bone loss, incr. osteocalcin
Hirama [145]	2003	Gastrectomized rats	FOS, 4 weeks		Prevention of BV/TV and cortical bone loss
Legette [67]	2012	OVX rats	Inulin or polydextrose, 4 weeks	Incr. Ca and Mg absorption Incr. cecal SCFAs Incr. cecal wall weight	Incr. Ca retention (polydextrose)
Mathey [75]	2014	OVX rats	FOS, 90 days		Incr. Femur BMD, maximal load Decr. Dpd Improved isoflavone effects

Mitamura [70]	2006	OVX rats	Difructose anhydride, 4 and 8 weeks	Incr. Ca and Mg absorption	Incr. distal femur BMD Incr. femur strength
Ohta [146]	1998	Intact rats	FOS	Incr. Ca absorption	
Ohta [71]	2002	OVX mice	FOS ± isoflavone	Incr. equol production from isoflavone	Prevention bone loss
Roberfroid [65]	2002	Intact male rats	Inulin		Incr. WB BMC and WB BMD
Shiga [77]	2006	Gastrectomized rats	Difructose anhydride	Incr. Ca absorption Incr. cecal SCFAs	Partial prevention of bone loss Decr. Dpd
Scholz-Ahrens [147]	2002	OVX rats	FOS ± calcium		Prevention trabecular bone loss (increasing Ca → not same effect)
Takahara [74]	2000	Intact male rats	FOS	Incr. Ca and Mg absorption	Incr. femur BV/TV
Tousen [148]	2016	OVX mice	Starch and soya	Incr. equol production, incr. *Bifidobacteria*	Incr. vBMD, incr. polar moment of inertia, decr. IL-7 and CD4 expression in bone marrow
Varley [149]	2010	Pigs	Inulin	Decr. colon *Enterobacteriaceae*	No effect on bone
Weaver [60]	2011	Intact rats	GOS, 8 weeks	Incr. Ca and Mg absorption, decr cecal pH, incr. cecal wall weight, incr. *Bifidobacteria*	Incr. femur and tibia vBMD, incr. femur and tibia breaking strength
Yang [76]	2013	OVX rats	*Anoectochilus formosanus* or inulin12 weeks	Incr. Ca absorption Decr. cecal pH, incr. SCFAs, Incr. cecal wall weight	Incr. Ca retention Incr. tibia BMD, incr. BV/TV Incr. femur maximal load and stiffness
Younes [150]	2001	Intact male rats	Resistant starch or inulin	Incr. Ca and Mg absorption	Incr. Ca balance
Zafar [72]	2004	OVX rats	FOS and inulin, 3 weeks	Incr. Ca absorption	Incr. femur BMD Incr. Ca balance

GOS galacto-oligosaccharides, *OVX* ovariectomized, *FOS* fructooligosaccharides, *SCFA* short-chain fatty acids, *Dpd* deoxypyridinoline, *Ca* calcium, *Mg* magnesium

Table 12.3 Effects of prebiotics on bone metabolism in human

First author	Date	Subjects	Prebiotics	Intestine	Bone/calcium balance
Abrams [87]	2005	98 (9–13 years) boys and girls	8 g/day fructans, 8 weeks and 1 year	+28 and 19% Ca absorption	Incr. WB BMC and WB BMD
Abrams [151]	2007	13 (18–27 years) men and women	8 g/d inulin-type fructans, 8 weeks	8/13 → incr. Ca absorption >3% (35%)	
Abrams [152]	2007	98 (9–13 years) boys and girls	8 g/day fructans, 8 weeks and 1 year	32/48 = responders	Responders at 8 weeks had higher WB BMC increase
Boler [153]	2011	21 (21–28 years) men	±21 g/day polydextrose or soluble maize fibers	Lower fecal pH More bifidobacteria	
Coudray [154]	1997	9 (19–24 years) men	±40 g/day inulin, 4 weeks	+58% Ca absorption	
Dahl [155]	2005	15 (23–57 years), institutionalized, wheel chair bound	+13 g/day inulin, 3 weeks		No difference NTX nor fasting urinary calcium
Griffin [96]	2002	59 (12 years girls), 1500 mg/day calcium	±8 g/day oligofructose ± inulin, 3 weeks	Oligofructose and inulin → +18% Ca absorption	
Hicks [156]	2012	55 (2-months) infants	±GOS/polydextrose 4 g/l	No difference in Ca absorption	
Holloway [97]	2007	15 (72 years) PM women	±10 g/day inulin and oligofructose, 6 weeks	+5% Ca absorption +5% Mg absorption	
Holscher [95]	2015	21 (21–28 years) men	±21 g/day polydextrose or soluble maize fibers	Incr. *Bacteroidetes*/*Firmicutes* ratio	
Jakeman [157]	2016	14 (40–80 years) PM women	±10 ± 20 g/day soluble corn fibers, 50 days		+4.8 and +7% Ca retention +8% ALP
Slevin [99]	2014	PM women	FOS 2 years		Decr. CTX
Tahiri [158]	2001	11 (59 years) PM women	±10 g/day short-chain FOS, 5 weeks	+12% Mg absorption	
Tahiri [159]	2003	12 (59 years) PM women	±10 g/day short-chain FOS, 5 weeks	No difference in Ca absorption (may if >6 years PM)	

Teuri [160]	1999	15 (20–29 years) women	±15 g/day inulin		No difference in PTH nor urinary calcium
Van den Heuvel [161]	1998	12 (20–30 years) males	±15 g/day FOS and GOS and inulin, 3 weeks	No difference in Ca absorption	
Van den Heuvel [89]	1999	12 (14–16 years) boys	±15 g/day oligofructose, 9 days	+11% Ca absorption	
Van den Heuvel [98]	1999	12 (56–64 years) PM women	±5 ± 10 g/day lactulose, 9 days	Incr. Ca absorption (10 g)	
Van den Heuvel [93]	2000	12 (55–65 years) PM women	±20 g/day GOS, 9 days, +2 × 200 ml yogurt	+16% Ca absorption	No difference in urinary calcium
Van den Heuvel [162]	2009	14 (12–14 years) girls	± 10 g/day short-chain FOS	+18% Mg absorption No difference in Ca absorption	No difference in PTH, 1,25(OH)^{2}D nor Dpd
Walton [92]	2012	37 ≥ 50 years men and women	±8 g/day GOS, 3 weeks	More bifidobacteria, more butyrate	
Whisner [90]	2013	31 (10–13 years) girls	±5 ± 10 g/day GOS, 3 weeks (above 14 g/day of fibers)	Incr. Ca absorption More bifidobacteria	
Whisner [91]	2014	24 (12–15 years) boys and girls	±12 g/day soluble maize fibers, 3 weeks	+12% Ca absorption, ≥24 h more *Bacteroidetes*	Ca retention not affected
Whisner [100]	2016	28 (11–14 years) girls	±10 or 20 g/day soluble corn fibers, 4 weeks	+13% Ca absorption More bifidobacteria and greater variability Decr. fecal pH (20 g)	

PM postmenopausal, *GOS* galacto-oligosaccharides, *FOS* fructooligosaccharides, *Ca* calcium, *Mg* magnesium, *Dpd* deoxypyridinoline growth of *Bifidobacterium* and *Lactobacillus* species [83]. In breast-fed infants, there is an inverse relationship between IL6 in intestinal secretion and *Bacteroides fragilis* in the gut lumen [84]. In addition, human milk contains various glycans with prebiotic properties contributing to infant immune system development [85]. Fermentation products enhanced intestinal barrier function by stimulating the assembly of tight junctions [86]. Infant formulas are supplemented with GOS usually to prevent or treat constipation.

Human Studies

In a randomized controlled trial conducted in adolescents, 8 g/day of FOS and inulin for 1 year increased whole-body BMC [87]. Adolescence is a time for rapid growth that represents an opportunity to influence peak bone mass [88]. In male adolescents, the consumption of 15 g of oligofructose per day was shown to stimulate fractional calcium absorption [89]. Among healthy adolescent girls aged 10–13 years who consumed smoothie drinks twice daily with 0, 2.5, or 5 g GOS for 3-week periods, increase in the fractional calcium absorption was seen with both 5 and 10 g/day doses of GOS compared with the control (0.444, 0.419, and 0.393, respectively), although a dose-response relationship was not observed [90]. The increase in calcium absorption was the greatest after 24 h, consistent with distal gut absorption. Whether a small increase in fractional calcium absorption with GOS supplementation may result in a biologically significant increment in bone mineral accrual leading to higher peak bone mass in the long term remains to be demonstrated. This was accompanied by a higher amount of bifidobacteria in the stools [90]. Using a similar stable calcium absorption method, the same authors detected a 12% higher intestinal calcium absorption in adolescent boys and girls exposed to maize and corn fibers [91]. Fecal bifidobacteria was shown to increase with GOS treatment, which suggests that calcium absorption may be mediated by the gut microbiota, specifically bifidobacteria [90, 92]. Differences in calcium absorption were correlated with various bacteria genera at the end of the study [91]. Prebiotic agents, such as GOS, have been demonstrated to increase calcium absorption in postmenopausal women too [93].

In various populations of different ages from adolescents to postmenopausal women, and with various treatment durations, from 9 days to 1 year, higher intestinal calcium absorption was consistently detected in response to prebiotics [87, 89, 93–96, 97]. In a small study of 12 postmenopausal women, lactulose consumption (5 or 10 g/day) was shown to increase calcium absorption in a dose-response manner [98]. Bone turnover marker levels were reduced with FOS administration in postmenopausal women by 12 and 24 months, however without any change in BMD [99].

The amount of prebiotics required to produce significant bone effects is limited by the tolerance. Indeed, undigested saccharide/fiber fermentation in the large intestine may be associated with flatulence and abdominal discomfort, precluding amounts of prebiotic ingestion sufficient to reach meaningful biological effects. However, in the studies by Whisner [90, 91, 100], this issue was addressed, and the tolerance to prebiotic amounts associated with increased calcium absorption was reported as good in adolescent girls.

Probiotics

Besides modulating microbiota by changing the substrate for its metabolism, another approach to modify it is to directly provide some bacteria to the GI tract, i.e., administering probiotics. Probiotics are live microorganisms which, when administered in adequate amounts, confer a health benefit on the host [101]. By adequate, one means an amount able to trigger the targeted effect. It depends on strain specificity, process and matrix, and sought targeted effect. With concentration of around $10^{e}7$ to $10^{e}8$ probiotic bacteria per gram, serving size is around 100–200 mg. Various species are provided as probiotics, such as *Lactobacillus*, *Bifidobacteria*, *Escherichia*, *Enterococcus*, and *Bacillus subtilis*. Yeasts like *Saccharomyces* have been used too. Probiotics are available in the form of yogurt, milk-based foods, powder, capsules, or solutions like ice cream and beer.

On purpose the use of probiotics in poultry industry will not be reviewed here, but it may be mentioned that *Bacillus subtilis* given to hens increased the number of eggs and the strength of the eggshell [102] and *Bacilli licheniformis* and *Bacilli subtilis* increased tibia mass [103].

Effects on Bone

Regarding bone, *Lactobacillus reuteri* increased femoral and vertebral BMD in male but not in female intact mice [104]. It prevented OVX-induced bone loss [105] and type 1 diabetes-associated osteopenia [106] (Table 12.4). These two models differ by their bone turnover pattern. The former is associated with an increased osteoclastic bone resorption whereas the latter rather with low bone formation. This would suggest that the probiotic *Lactobacillus reuteri* is also capable of stimulating osteoblast activity by preventing TNFalpha suppression of Wnt10b production in bone [106]. *Lactobacillus paracasei* prevented OVX-dependent bone loss [107, 108], together with a decrease in TNFalpha and IL1beta expression in cortical bone. OVX-induced bone loss was also prevented by *Lactobacillus helveticus* fermented milk [109]. *Bacillus longum* together with the prebiotic yacon flour increased BMC in rats [110]. The same probiotics partially prevented OVX-induced bone loss, without significantly affecting bone strength [111]. The role of probiotics in attenuating sex hormone deficiency-exerted bone damage has been extensively studied by [19]. In this study, hypogonadal GF mice did not show a bone loss like hypogonadal mice with intact gut microflora. In GF mice, there was no increase in osteoclasts in response to hypogonadism. When microflora was reintroduced in these GF animals, there was a reversal of the osteoprotection observed in the absence of microflora. Estrogen deficiency altered the gut barrier function leading to endotoxemia. This did not occur in GF mice, which in addition did not show an increase in TNFalpha-expressing CD4+ T-cells. In this model, the probiotics *Lactobacillus rhamnosus* prevented estrogen deficiency-mediated bone loss and decreased TNFalpha and RANKL expression in the intestine and bone marrow in hypogonadal mice [19].

In a model of collagen-induced arthritis in rats, *Lactobacillus casei* decreased TNFalpha and IL6 and increased the anti-inflammatory cytokine IL10 [112]. In rodents, the administration of *Bacillus subtilis* reduced periodontitis-induced bone

Table 12.4 Effects of probiotics on bone metabolism in mammalian experimental animals

Author	Date	Model	Probiotics	Bone mass/ density	Biochemistry
Britton [105]	2014	OVX mice	*L. reuteri*, 3×/ week, 4 weeks	Prevention femur and vert. trabecular bone loss	Decr. RANKL expression and osteoclast number. Decr. CD4+ T-cells. *L. reuteri* → soluble factor depressing osteoclastogenesis
Chiang [108]	2011	OVX mice	*L. paracasei* and *L. plantarum* fermented soy skim milk, 8 weeks	Prevention femur trabecular bone loss	
Kimoto-Nira [163]	2007	Senescent intact mice	Heat killed *Lactococcus lactis*	Decr. bone loss with heat killed but not with living bacteria fermented milk	
Li [19]	2016	E2 depleted mice	*L. rhamnosus* or VLS3 (8 strains), 4 weeks	Full prevention of vert. BV/TV decr. Incr. in BV/TV in Sham	
McCabe [104]	2013	Intact male mice	*L. reuteri*, 3×/ week, 4 weeks	Incr. femur and vert. vBMD, TbN and TrTh, in males but NOT in females	Incr. BFR, decr. gut TNFα expression
Narva [109]	2007	OVX rats	*L. helveticus* fermented milk, 12 ×	Prevention bone loss	Decr. turnover
Ohlsson [107]	2014	OVX mice	*L. paracasei* or *L. paracasei* and *L. plantarum* 2 + 3 daily	Prevention cortical bone loss	Decr. cortical bone TNFα, IL-1β RANKL/OPG expression Incr. TGFβ expression in bone marrow
Parvaneh [111]	2015	OVX rats	*B. longum*, daily, 16×	Attenuation decr. BMD	Incr. osteocalcin, decr. CTX Incr. BMP2 and Sparc bone expression, incr. fecal *Bifidobacteria*
Rodriguez [110]	2012	Intact rats	*B. longum* and yacon flour (FOS)	Incr. tibia Ca and Pi content	
Zhang [106]	2016	T1D mice	*L. reuteri*, 3×/ week, 4 weeks	Incr. BMD, incr. TbN and TbTh, incr. OB surfaces (in controls too), incr. MOI	Prevention of Wnt10b suppression in bone

T1D type 1 diabetes, *MOI* cross-sectional moment of inertia, *OVX* ovariectomized, *L. Lactobacillus*, *B. Bifidobacterium*

loss [113]. *Saccharomyces cerevisiae* prevented alveolar bone loss, through decreased expression of IL1beta, TNFalpha, and IL10 [114].

Human Studies

In humans, the main source of probiotics is fermented dairy products [115], which also provide calcium, protein phosphorus, and zinc (Fig. 12.1). The problem is to provide a sufficient amount of bacteria capable of reaching the distal part of the gastrointestinal tract. However, it has been reported that yogurt consumers had lower level of *Enterobacteriaceae* and higher beta-galactosidase activity, the latter and *Bifidobacterium* population being positively correlated to the amount of fermented products ingested [116]. In a 12-year follow-up of the Framingham Offspring Study, yogurt intake was associated with hip (trochanter) BMD. Yogurt intake showed a weak positive protective trend for hip fracture, while no other dairy groups showed a significant association [117]. In both cross-sectional and longitudinal study in 65-year-old women, yogurt consumers had higher lumbar spine BMD and distal

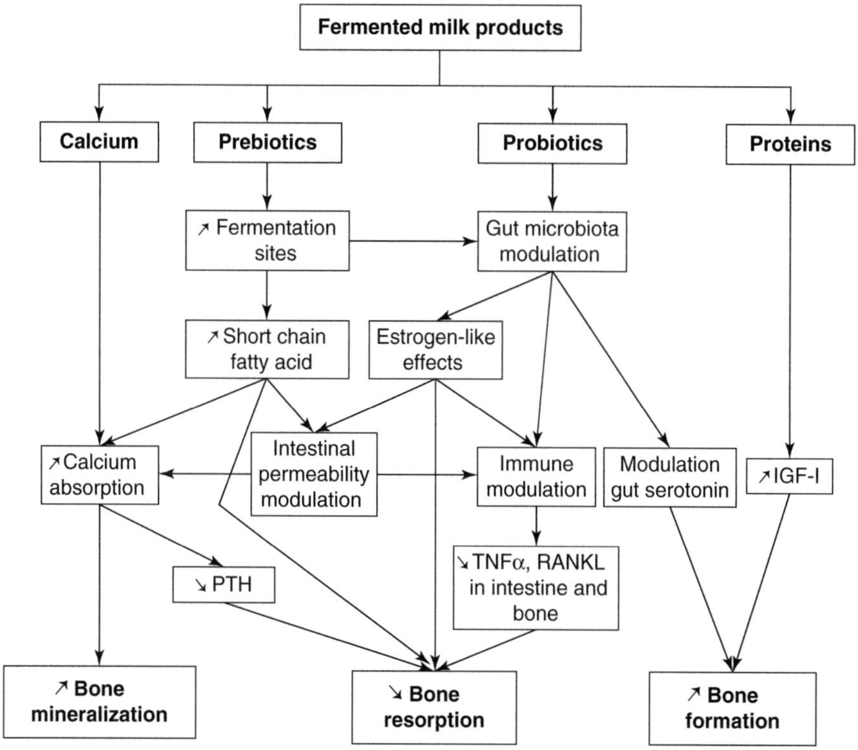

Fig. 12.1 Effects of fermented dairy products on bone. Adapted from Rizzoli and Biver [115], with permission of the publisher. In addition to nutrients like calcium, phosphorus, and protein, fermented dairy products provide pre- and probiotics which influence gut wall permeability, solute absorption, and modulate immune system and hormone production, leading to changes in bone turnover

tibia cortical area. Over a 3-year follow-up, those ingesting one or more yogurt per day had attenuated decrease of total hip BMD, distal radius cortical area, and thickness [118]. In a long-term follow-up of postmenopausal women, the combination of fruits and vegetables (fibers) with fermented milk (yogurt or soured milk, probiotics) was associated with the lowest rates of hip fracture in high consumers (HR, 0.81 (95% CI, 0.68–0.97) for ≥2 servings/day of fermented milk and ≥5 servings/day of fruits and vegetables compared with low consumption of both fruit and vegetables and fermented milk) [119]. In the same cohort, women with a high intake of cheese or fermented milk products compared with women with low intakes had lower mortality and fracture rates. For each serving the rate of mortality and hip fractures was reduced by 10–15% ($P < 0.001$) [120]. The effects of fermented dairy products on bone have been recently reviewed [115]. However, since the calcium and protein contained in fermented dairy products are able to influence bone metabolism, it is difficult to identify the specific effects of probiotics in these products. In addition, some specific effects of fermented dairy products have been reported, as compared to milk and non-fermented dairy product, or independently of calcium and protein intakes [109, 121–123].

Oral supplementation with *Lactobacillus reuteri* increased circulating 25-OH-vitamin D levels [124]. In a 6-month randomized controlled trial, healthy 1–6-year-old children received milk supplemented or not with 5 × 10^e8 *Lactobacillus reuteri*. The latter group had a greater weight and height monthly gain [125].

A major problem with probiotic administration is certainly the amount of bacteria ingested. In adult monozygotic tweens, two servings a day of fermented milk products containing five different species of bacteria did not modify large intestine bacterial species composition. In contrast when the same bacteria were given by gavage to gnotobiotic mice, there was a rapid change (in less than 24 h) in microbiome encoded enzymes involved in carbohydrate metabolism [126]. In the same study, *Bifidobacterium animalis* subspecies *lactis* upregulated a locus involved in xylooligosaccharide catabolism in both mice and human metatranscriptome.

Physical Activity

Physical activity in childhood and adolescence influences microbiota development [127]. In adults, exercise is associated with a higher GM diversity [128] and protein intakes positively correlating with GM diversity. This suggests an influence on GM of dietary adaptation to exercise. Comparing elite athletes to sedentary controls showed even greater differences at the metagenomic and metabolomic levels than at GM composition, with enhanced pathways for amino acids and carbohydrate metabolism leading to higher SCFAs production [129]. The latter have an impact on immunity, colonic epithelial function, brain, and bone. Exercise training-induced compositional and functional changes in GM were primarily observed in lean but not in obese individuals and were reversed when training was discontinued [130].

Pharmacological Agents

Vitamin D deficiency has been associated with gut barrier alterations and dysbiosis [131]. An interaction between vitamin D and microbiota is exemplified by the fact that cecal content and stools of VDR knockout animals are depleted in lactobacilli and enriched in clostridium and bacteroides [132]. In human, there were some differences in microbiota species according to vitamin D intakes or circulating levels [133]. Furthermore, *Lactobacillus rhamnosus* and *Lactobacillus plantarum* increased VDR expression in both mouse and human intestinal epithelial cells [134]. The protective effects of these probiotics on *Salmonella*-induced colitis were demonstrated in VDR+/+, but not in VDR−/−, animals. High-dose vitamin D (<70,000 IU/week) modifies microbiome in human with a response, which varies according to the region of the gastrointestinal tract [135].

In long-term proton-pump inhibitor users (≥5 years), there was a change in beta diversity, i.e., between groups, with a decrease in bacteroidetes and an increase in firmicutes, without modification of alpha diversity, i.e., the within individual microorganism diversity [136]. A meta-analysis has shown an association between PPI use and enteric infections [137]. In a large study conducted in healthy tweens, gut microbial diversity was negatively correlated with PPI use, the latter being also associated with an overrepresentation of proximal gastrointestinal tract bacteria in the distal parts of the intestine [138]. In a study involving both healthy and patients with gastrointestinal tract disease, a less healthy microbiome pattern was detected in PPI users, with the development of pathogenic bacteria [139].

Investigating the gut microbiota of type 2 diabetes patients, it was found that metformin treatment modified the dysbiosis associated with this metabolic disease [140]. Indeed, patients with type 2 diabetes treated with metformin had higher levels of *Escherichia* species and less *Intestinibacter* species. The former bacteria have the potential to produce SCFAs, such as butyrate and propionate, which can stimulate intestinal gluconeogenesis contributing thereby to lower blood glucose and to reduce bone resorption [3].

Conclusion

Gut microbiota plays a major role in protecting intestinal barrier function and developing the intestinal immune system. An implication of GM in the pathogenesis of a large series of disorders has been suggested, though a direct causal relationship remains to be established. Bone mass accrual, bone homeostasis, and prevention of sex hormone deficiency-induced bone loss seem to benefit from pre- or probiotic ingestion, which modifies microbiota composition and metabolism. GM appears to be a major player in the various determinants of musculoskeletal health. With pre- and probiotics, some issues remain to be further elucidated. Referring to the McCabe paper [104], is the response to probiotic sex-specific or more readily detectable in subjects with high bone turnover like children or adolescents? The doses in terms of both efficacy and tolerance are crucial factors. Timing and duration of the administration should be further studied, as well as the offset of the effects upon pre- or probiotic discontinuation.

Furthermore, it remains to be demonstrated in well-conducted long-term randomized controlled trials whether interventions changing GM composition and/or function are capable of preventing bone loss and/or reducing fracture risk. Genetic background, sex, immune status, age, dietary intakes, living conditions, geography, and medications are likely important confounding factors necessary to consider in evaluating the effects of GM changes on bone health.

References

1. Consortium HMP. Structure, function and diversity of the healthy human microbiome. Nature. 2012;486:207–14.
2. Gordon JI. Honor thy gut symbionts redux. Science. 2012;336:1251–3.
3. Lucas S, Omata Y, Hofmann J, et al. Short-chain fatty acids regulate systemic bone mass and protect from pathological bone loss. Nat Commun. 2018;9:55.
4. Cani PD. Gut cell metabolism shapes the microbiome. Science. 2017;357:548–9.
5. Valles Y, Artacho A, Pascual-Garcia A, Ferrus ML, Gosalbes MJ, Abellan JJ, Francino MP. Microbial succession in the gut: directional trends of taxonomic and functional change in a birth cohort of Spanish infants. PLoS Genet. 2014;10:e1004406.
6. Avershina E, Storro O, Oien T, Johnsen R, Pope P, Rudi K. Major faecal microbiota shifts in composition and diversity with age in a geographically restricted cohort of mothers and their children. FEMS Microbiol Ecol. 2014;87:280–90.
7. Cho I, Blaser MJ. The human microbiome: at the interface of health and disease. Nat Rev Genet. 2012;13:260–70.
8. Kalliomaki M, Collado MC, Salminen S, Isolauri E. Early differences in fecal microbiota composition in children may predict overweight. Am J Clin Nutr. 2008;87:534–8.
9. Lahti L, Salojarvi J, Salonen A, Scheffer M, de Vos WM. Tipping elements in the human intestinal ecosystem. Nat Commun. 2014;5:4344.
10. Claesson MJ, Cusack S, O'Sullivan O, et al. Composition, variability, and temporal stability of the intestinal microbiota of the elderly. Proc Natl Acad Sci U S A. 2011;108(Suppl 1):4586–91.
11. Claesson MJ, Jeffery IB, Conde S, et al. Gut microbiota composition correlates with diet and health in the elderly. Nature. 2012;488:178–84.
12. Biagi E, Nylund L, Candela M, et al. Through ageing, and beyond: gut microbiota and inflammatory status in seniors and centenarians. PLoS One. 2010;5:e10667.
13. David LA, Maurice CF, Carmody RN, et al. Diet rapidly and reproducibly alters the human gut microbiome. Nature. 2014;505:559–63.
14. Beaumont M, Portune KJ, Steuer N, et al. Quantity and source of dietary protein influence metabolite production by gut microbiota and rectal mucosa gene expression: a randomized, parallel, double-blind trial in overweight humans. Am J Clin Nutr. 2017;106:1005–19.
15. Faith JJ, Guruge JL, Charbonneau M, et al. The long-term stability of the human gut microbiota. Science. 2013;341:1237439.
16. Devkota S. MICROBIOME. Prescription drugs obscure microbiome analyses. Science. 2016;351:452–3.
17. Maier L, Pruteanu M, Kuhn M, et al. Extensive impact of non-antibiotic drugs on human gut bacteria. Nature. 2018;555:623–8.
18. Sekirov I, Russell SL, Antunes LC, Finlay BB. Gut microbiota in health and disease. Physiol Rev. 2010;90:859–904.
19. Li JY, Chassaing B, Tyagi AM, et al. Sex steroid deficiency-associated bone loss is microbiota dependent and prevented by probiotics. J Clin Invest. 2016;126:2049–63.
20. Collins FL, Schepper JD, Rios-Arce ND, et al. Immunology of gut-bone signaling. Adv Exp Med Biol. 2017;1033:59–94.

21. Mineo H, Amano M, Minaminida K, Chiji H, Shigematsu N, Tomita F, Hara H. Two-week feeding of difructose anhydride III enhances calcium absorptive activity with epithelial cell proliferation in isolated rat cecal mucosa. Nutrition. 2006;22:312–20.
22. Donohoe DR, Garge N, Zhang X, Sun W, O'Connell TM, Bunger MK, Bultman SJ. The microbiome and butyrate regulate energy metabolism and autophagy in the mammalian colon. Cell Metab. 2011;13:517–26.
23. Ma N, Guo P, Zhang J, He T, Kim SW, Zhang G, Ma X. Nutrients mediate intestinal Bacteria-mucosal immune crosstalk. Front Immunol. 2018;9:5.
24. Beaumont M, Andriamihaja M, Armand L, et al. Epithelial response to a high-protein diet in rat colon. BMC Genomics. 2017;18:116.
25. Macpherson AJ, Harris NL. Interactions between commensal intestinal bacteria and the immune system. Nat Rev Immunol. 2004;4:478–85.
26. Sjogren K, Engdahl C, Henning P, Lerner UH, Tremaroli V, Lagerquist MK, Backhed F, Ohlsson C. The gut microbiota regulates bone mass in mice. J Bone Miner Res. 2012;27:1357–67.
27. Ammann P, Rizzoli R, Bonjour JP, Bourrin S, Meyer JM, Vassalli P, Garcia I. Transgenic mice expressing soluble tumor necrosis factor-receptor are protected against bone loss caused by estrogen deficiency. J Clin Invest. 1997;99:1699–703.
28. Terashima A, Takayanagi H. Overview of osteoimmunology. Calcif Tissue Int. 2018;102(5):503–11.
29. Li JY, Tawfeek H, Bedi B, Yang X, Adams J, Gao KY, Zayzafoon M, Weitzmann MN, Pacifici R. Ovariectomy disregulates osteoblast and osteoclast formation through the T-cell receptor CD40 ligand. Proc Natl Acad Sci U S A. 2011;108:768–73.
30. Lee HW, Suh JH, Kim AY, Lee YS, Park SY, Kim JB. Histone deacetylase 1-mediated histone modification regulates osteoblast differentiation. Mol Endocrinol. 2006;20:2432–43.
31. Katono T, Kawato T, Tanabe N, Suzuki N, Iida T, Morozumi A, Ochiai K, Maeno M. Sodium butyrate stimulates mineralized nodule formation and osteoprotegerin expression by human osteoblasts. Arch Oral Biol. 2008;53:903–9.
32. Albenberg LG, Wu GD. Diet and the intestinal microbiome: associations, functions, and implications for health and disease. Gastroenterology. 2014;146:1564–72.
33. Rowland I, Gibson G, Heinken A, Scott K, Swann J, Thiele I, Tuohy K. Gut microbiota functions: metabolism of nutrients and other food components. Eur J Nutr. 2018;57:1–24.
34. Ammann P, Rizzoli R, Fleisch H. Influence of the disaccharide lactitol on intestinal absorption and body retention of calcium in rats. J Nutr. 1988;118:793–5.
35. Weaver CM. Diet, gut microbiome, and bone health. Curr Osteoporos Rep. 2015;13:125–30.
36. Rizzoli R, Bonjour JP. Physiology of calcium and phosphate homeostasis. In: Seibel MJ, Robins SP, Bilezikian JP, editors. Dynamics of bone and cartilage metabolism: principles and clinical applications. San Diego: Academic; 2006. p. 345–60.
37. Yadav VK, Ryu JH, Suda N, et al. Lrp5 controls bone formation by inhibiting serotonin synthesis in the duodenum. Cell. 2008;135:825–37.
38. Yan J, Herzog JW, Tsang K, Brennan CA, Bower MA, Garrett WS, Sartor BR, Aliprantis AO, Charles JF. Gut microbiota induce IGF-1 and promote bone formation and growth. Proc Natl Acad Sci U S A. 2016;113:E7554–e7563.
39. Schwarzer M, Strigini M, Leulier F. Gut microbiota and host juvenile growth. Calcif Tissue Int. 2017;102(4):387–405.
40. Cromwell GL. Why and how antibiotics are used in swine production. Anim Biotechnol. 2002;13:7–27.
41. Cho I, Yamanishi S, Cox L, et al. Antibiotics in early life alter the murine colonic microbiome and adiposity. Nature. 2012;488:621–6.
42. Cox LM, Yamanishi S, Sohn J, et al. Altering the intestinal microbiota during a critical developmental window has lasting metabolic consequences. Cell. 2014;158:705–21.
43. Williams S, Wakisaka A, Zeng QQ, Barnes J, Martin G, Wechter WJ, Liang CT. Minocycline prevents the decrease in bone mineral density and trabecular bone in ovariectomized aged rats. Bone. 1996;19:637–44.

44. Pytlik M, Folwarczna J, Janiec W. Effects of doxycycline on mechanical properties of bones in rats with ovariectomy-induced osteopenia. Calcif Tissue Int. 2004;75:225–30.
45. Cox-York KA, Sheflin AM, Foster MT, Gentile CL, Kahl A, Koch LG, Britton SL, Weir TL. Ovariectomy results in differential shifts in gut microbiota in low versus high aerobic capacity rats. Physiol Rep. 2015;3:e12488.
46. Clavel T, Fallani M, Lepage P, et al. Isoflavones and functional foods alter the dominant intestinal microbiota in postmenopausal women. J Nutr. 2005;135:2786–92.
47. Druart C, Alligier M, Salazar N, Neyrinck AM, Delzenne NM. Modulation of the gut microbiota by nutrients with prebiotic and probiotic properties. Adv Nutr. 2014;5:624s–33s.
48. Smith MI, Yatsunenko T, Manary MJ, et al. Gut microbiomes of Malawian twin pairs discordant for kwashiorkor. Science. 2013;339:548–54.
49. Blanton LV, Charbonneau MR, Salih T, et al. Gut bacteria that prevent growth impairments transmitted by microbiota from malnourished children. Science. 2016;351:aad3311.
50. Denou E, Marcinko K, Surette MG, Steinberg GR, Schertzer JD. High-intensity exercise training increases the diversity and metabolic capacity of the mouse distal gut microbiota during diet-induced obesity. Am J Phys Endocrinol Metab. 2016;310:E982–93.
51. Suez J, Korem T, Zeevi D, et al. Artificial sweeteners induce glucose intolerance by altering the gut microbiota. Nature. 2014;514:181–6.
52. Mitsou EK, Kakali A, Antonopoulou S, Mountzouris KC, Yannakoulia M, Panagiotakos DB, Kyriacou A. Adherence to the Mediterranean diet is associated with the gut microbiota pattern and gastrointestinal characteristics in an adult population. Br J Nutr. 2017;117:1645–55.
53. De Filippis F, Pellegrini N, Vannini L, et al. High-level adherence to a Mediterranean diet beneficially impacts the gut microbiota and associated metabolome. Gut. 2016;65:1812–21.
54. Tosti V, Bertozzi B, Fontana L. Health benefits of the mediterranean diet: metabolic and molecular mechanisms. J Gerontol A Biol Sci Med Sci. 2018;73:318–26.
55. Byberg L, Bellavia A, Larsson SC, Orsini N, Wolk A, Michaelsson K. Mediterranean diet and hip fracture in Swedish men and women. J Bone Miner Res. 2016;31:2098–105.
56. Haring B, Crandall CJ, Wu C, et al. Dietary patterns and fractures in postmenopausal women: results from the women's health initiative. JAMA Intern Med. 2016;176:645–52.
57. Whisner CM, Castillo LF. Prebiotics, bone and mineral metabolism. Calcif Tissue Int. 2018;102:443–79.
58. Roberfroid M, Gibson GR, Hoyles L, et al. Prebiotic effects: metabolic and health benefits. Br J Nutr. 2010;104(Suppl 2):S1–63.
59. Garcia-Vieyra MI, Del Real A, Lopez MG. Agave fructans: their effect on mineral absorption and bone mineral content. J Med Food. 2014;17:1247–55.
60. Weaver CM, Martin BR, Nakatsu CH, Armstrong AP, Clavijo A, McCabe LD, McCabe GP, Duignan S, Schoterman MH, van den Heuvel EG. Galactooligosaccharides improve mineral absorption and bone properties in growing rats through gut fermentation. J Agric Food Chem. 2011;59:6501–10.
61. Lee C, Kim BG, Kim JH, Chun J, Im JP, Kim JS. Sodium butyrate inhibits the NF-kappa B signaling pathway and histone deacetylation, and attenuates experimental colitis in an IL-10 independent manner. Int Immunopharmacol. 2017;51:47–56.
62. Langlands SJ, Hopkins MJ, Coleman N, Cummings JH. Prebiotic carbohydrates modify the mucosa associated microflora of the human large bowel. Gut. 2004;53:1610–6.
63. Nakatsu CH, Armstrong A, Clavijo AP, Martin BR, Barnes S, Weaver CM. Fecal bacterial community changes associated with isoflavone metabolites in postmenopausal women after soy bar consumption. PLoS One. 2014;9:e108924.
64. Bindels LB, Delzenne NM, Cani PD, Walter J. Towards a more comprehensive concept for prebiotics. Nat Rev Gastroenterol Hepatol. 2015;12:303–10.
65. Roberfroid MB, Cumps J, Devogelaer JP. Dietary chicory inulin increases whole-body bone mineral density in growing male rats. J Nutr. 2002;132:3599–602.
66. Chonan O, Matsumoto K, Watanuki M. Effect of galactooligosaccharides on calcium absorption and preventing bone loss in ovariectomized rats. Biosci Biotechnol Biochem. 1995;59:236–9.

67. Legette LL, Lee W, Martin BR, Story JA, Campbell JK, Weaver CM. Prebiotics enhance magnesium absorption and inulin-based fibers exert chronic effects on calcium utilization in a postmenopausal rodent model. J Food Sci. 2012;77:H88–94.
68. Macfarlane S, Macfarlane GT, Cummings JH. Review article: prebiotics in the gastrointestinal tract. Aliment Pharmacol Ther. 2006;24:701–14.
69. Scholz-Ahrens KE, Ade P, Marten B, Weber P, Timm W, Acil Y, Gluer CC, Schrezenmeir J. Prebiotics, probiotics, and synbiotics affect mineral absorption, bone mineral content, and bone structure. J Nutr. 2007;137:838s–46s.
70. Mitamura R, Hara H. Ingestion of difructose anhydride III partially restores calcium absorption impaired by vitamin D and estrogen deficiency in rats. Eur J Nutr. 2006;45:242–9.
71. Ohta A, Uehara M, Sakai K, Takasaki M, Adlercreutz H, Morohashi T, Ishimi Y. A combination of dietary fructooligosaccharides and isoflavone conjugates increases femoral bone mineral density and equol production in ovariectomized mice. J Nutr. 2002;132:2048–54.
72. Zafar TA, Weaver CM, Zhao Y, Martin BR, Wastney ME. Nondigestible oligosaccharides increase calcium absorption and suppress bone resorption in ovariectomized rats. J Nutr. 2004;134:399–402.
73. Ammann P, Rizzoli R, Fleisch H. Calcium absorption in rat large intestine in vivo: availability of dietary calcium. Am J Phys. 1986;251:G14–8.
74. Takahara S, Morohashi T, Sano T, Ohta A, Yamada S, Sasa R. Fructooligosaccharide consumption enhances femoral bone volume and mineral concentrations in rats. J Nutr. 2000;130:1792–5.
75. Mathey J, Puel C, Kati-Coulibaly S, Bennetau-Pelissero C, Davicco MJ, Lebecque P, Horcajada MN, Coxam V. Fructooligosaccharides maximize bone-sparing effects of soy isoflavone-enriched diet in the ovariectomized rat. Calcif Tissue Int. 2004;75:169–79.
76. Yang LC, Wu JB, Lu TJ, Lin WC. The prebiotic effect of Anoectochilus formosanus and its consequences on bone health. Br J Nutr. 2013;109:1779–88.
77. Shiga K, Nishimukai M, Tomita F, Hara H. Ingestion of difructose anhydride III, a non-digestible disaccharide, improves postgastrectomy osteopenia in rats. Scand J Gastroenterol. 2006;41:1165–73.
78. Bryk G, Coronel MZ, Pellegrini G, Mandalunis P, Rio ME, de Portela ML, Zeni SN. Effect of a combination GOS/FOS(R) prebiotic mixture and interaction with calcium intake on mineral absorption and bone parameters in growing rats. Eur J Nutr. 2015;54:913–23.
79. Muhlbauer RC, Li F. Effect of vegetables on bone metabolism. Nature. 1999;401:343–4.
80. Muhlbauer RC, Lozano A, Reinli A. Onion and a mixture of vegetables, salads, and herbs affect bone resorption in the rat by a mechanism independent of their base excess. J Bone Miner Res. 2002;17:1230–6.
81. Chaplin A, Parra P, Laraichi S, Serra F, Palou A. Calcium supplementation modulates gut microbiota in a prebiotic manner in dietary obese mice. Mol Nutr Food Res. 2016;60:468–80.
82. Charbonneau MR, O'Donnell D, Blanton LV, et al. Sialylated milk oligosaccharides promote microbiota-dependent growth in models of infant under nutrition. Cell. 2016;164:859–71.
83. Underwood MA, German JB, Lebrilla CB, Mills DA. Bifidobacterium longum subspecies infantis: champion colonizer of the infant gut. Pediatr Res. 2015;77:229–35.
84. Sjogren YM, Tomicic S, Lundberg A, Bottcher MF, Bjorksten B, Sverremark-Ekstrom E, Jenmalm MC. Influence of early gut microbiota on the maturation of childhood mucosal and systemic immune responses. Clin Exp Allergy. 2009;39:1842–51.
85. He Y, Liu S, Leone S, Newburg DS. Human colostrum oligosaccharides modulate major immunologic pathways of immature human intestine. Mucosal Immunol. 2014;7:1326–39.
86. Peng L, Li ZR, Green RS, Holzman IR, Lin J. Butyrate enhances the intestinal barrier by facilitating tight junction assembly via activation of AMP-activated protein kinase in Caco-2 cell monolayers. J Nutr. 2009;139:1619–25.
87. Abrams SA, Griffin IJ, Hawthorne KM, Liang L, Gunn SK, Darlington G, Ellis KJ. A combination of prebiotic short- and long-chain inulin-type fructans enhances calcium absorption and bone mineralization in young adolescents. Am J Clin Nutr. 2005;82:471–6.

88. Rizzoli R, Bianchi ML, Garabedian M, McKay HA, Moreno LA. Maximizing bone mineral mass gain during growth for the prevention of fractures in the adolescents and the elderly. Bone. 2010;46:294–305.
89. van den Heuvel EG, Muys T, van Dokkum W, Schaafsma G. Oligofructose stimulates calcium absorption in adolescents. Am J Clin Nutr. 1999;69:544–8.
90. Whisner CM, Martin BR, Schoterman MH, Nakatsu CH, McCabe LD, McCabe GP, Wastney ME, van den Heuvel EG, Weaver CM. Galacto-oligosaccharides increase calcium absorption and gut bifidobacteria in young girls: a double-blind cross-over trial. Br J Nutr. 2013;110:1292–303.
91. Whisner CM, Martin BR, Nakatsu CH, McCabe GP, McCabe LD, Peacock M, Weaver CM. Soluble maize fibre affects short-term calcium absorption in adolescent boys and girls: a randomised controlled trial using dual stable isotopic tracers. Br J Nutr. 2014;112:446–56.
92. Walton GE, van den Heuvel EG, Kosters MH, Rastall RA, Tuohy KM, Gibson GR. A randomised crossover study investigating the effects of galacto-oligosaccharides on the faecal microbiota in men and women over 50 years of age. Br J Nutr. 2012;107:1466–75.
93. van den Heuvel EG, Schoterman MH, Muijs T. Transgalactooligosaccharides stimulate calcium absorption in postmenopausal women. J Nutr. 2000;130:2938–42.
94. Holscher HD, Faust KL, Czerkies LA, Litov R, Ziegler EE, Lessin H, Hatch T, Sun S, Tappenden KA. Effects of prebiotic-containing infant formula on gastrointestinal tolerance and fecal microbiota in a randomized controlled trial. JPEN J Parenter Enteral Nutr. 2012;36:95s–105s.
95. Holscher HD, Bauer LL, Gourineni V, Pelkman CL, Fahey GC Jr, Swanson KS. Agave inulin supplementation affects the fecal microbiota of healthy adults participating in a randomized, double-blind, placebo-controlled, crossover trial. J Nutr. 2015;145:2025–32.
96. Griffin IJ, Davila PM, Abrams SA. Non-digestible oligosaccharides and calcium absorption in girls with adequate calcium intakes. Br J Nutr. 2002;87(Suppl 2):S187–91.
97. Holloway L, Moynihan S, Abrams SA, Kent K, Hsu AR, Friedlander AL. Effects of oligofructose-enriched inulin on intestinal absorption of calcium and magnesium and bone turnover markers in postmenopausal women. Br J Nutr. 2007;97:365–72.
98. Van den Heuvel EG, Muijs T, Van Dokkum W, Schaafsma G. Lactulose stimulates calcium absorption in postmenopausal women. J Bone Miner Res. 1999;14:1211–6.
99. Slevin MM, Allsopp PJ, Magee PJ, Bonham MP, Naughton VR, Strain JJ, Duffy ME, Wallace JM, Mc Sorley EM. Supplementation with calcium and short-chain fructo-oligosaccharides affects markers of bone turnover but not bone mineral density in postmenopausal women. J Nutr. 2014;144:297–304.
100. Whisner CM, Martin BR, Nakatsu CH, Story JA, MacDonald-Clarke CJ, McCabe LD, McCabe GP, Weaver CM. Soluble corn fiber increases calcium absorption associated with shifts in the gut microbiome: a randomized dose-response trial in free-living pubertal females. J Nutr. 2016;146:1298–306.
101. McCabe LR, Parameswaran N. Advances in probiotic regulation of bone and mineral metabolism. Calcif Tissue Int. 2018;102:480–8.
102. Abdelqader A, Irshaid R, Al-Fataftah AR. Effects of dietary probiotic inclusion on performance, eggshell quality, cecal microflora composition, and tibia traits of laying hens in the late phase of production. Trop Anim Health Prod. 2013;45:1017–24.
103. Mutus R, Kocabagli N, Alp M, Acar N, Eren M, Gezen SS. The effect of dietary probiotic supplementation on tibial bone characteristics and strength in broilers. Poult Sci. 2006;85:1621–5.
104. McCabe LR, Irwin R, Schaefer L, Britton RA. Probiotic use decreases intestinal inflammation and increases bone density in healthy male but not female mice. J Cell Physiol. 2013;228:1793–8.
105. Britton RA, Irwin R, Quach D, Schaefer L, Zhang J, Lee T, Parameswaran N, McCabe LR. Probiotic *L. reuteri* treatment prevents bone loss in a menopausal ovariectomized mouse model. J Cell Physiol. 2014;229:1822–30.

106. Zhang J, Motyl KJ, Irwin R, MacDougald OA, Britton RA, McCabe LR. Loss of bone and Wnt10b expression in male type 1 diabetic mice is blocked by the probiotic *Lactobacillus reuteri*. Endocrinology. 2015;156:3169–82.
107. Ohlsson C, Engdahl C, Fak F, Andersson A, Windahl SH, Farman HH, Moverare-Skrtic S, Islander U, Sjogren K. Probiotics protect mice from ovariectomy-induced cortical bone loss. PLoS One. 2014;9:e92368.
108. Chiang SS, Pan TM. Antiosteoporotic effects of lactobacillus-fermented soy skim milk on bone mineral density and the microstructure of femoral bone in ovariectomized mice. J Agric Food Chem. 2011;59:7734–42.
109. Narva M, Rissanen J, Halleen J, Vapaatalo H, Vaananen K, Korpela R. Effects of bioactive peptide, valyl-prolyl-proline (VPP), and lactobacillus helveticus fermented milk containing VPP on bone loss in ovariectomized rats. Ann Nutr Metab. 2007;51:65–74.
110. Rodrigues FC, Castro AS, Rodrigues VC, Fernandes SA, Fontes EA, de Oliveira TT, Martino HS, de Luces Fortes Ferreira CL. Yacon flour and bifidobacterium longum modulate bone health in rats. J Med Food. 2012;15:664–70.
111. Parvaneh K, Ebrahimi M, Sabran MR, Karimi G, Hwei AN, Abdul-Majeed S, Ahmad Z, Ibrahim Z, Jamaluddin R. Probiotics (*Bifidobacterium longum*) increase bone mass density and Upregulate Sparc and Bmp-2 genes in rats with bone loss resulting from ovariectomy. Biomed Res Int. 2015;2015:897639.
112. Amdekar S, Singh V, Singh R, Sharma P, Keshav P, Kumar A. Lactobacillus casei reduces the inflammatory joint damage associated with collagen-induced arthritis (CIA) by reducing the pro-inflammatory cytokines: lactobacillus casei: COX-2 inhibitor. J Clin Immunol. 2011;31:147–54.
113. Foureaux RDC, Messora MR, de Oliveira LF, Napimoga MH, Pereira AN, Ferreira MS, Pereira LJ. Effects of probiotic therapy on metabolic and inflammatory parameters of rats with ligature-induced periodontitis associated with restraint stress. J Periodontol. 2014;85: 975–83.
114. Garcia VG, Knoll LR, Longo M, Novaes VC, Assem NZ, Ervolino E, de Toledo BE, Theodoro LH. Effect of the probiotic *Saccharomyces cerevisiae* on ligature-induced periodontitis in rats. J Periodontal Res. 2016;51:26–37.
115. Rizzoli R, Biver E. Effects of fermented milk products on bone. Calcif Tissue Int. 2018;102:489–500.
116. Alvaro E, Andrieux C, Rochet V, Rigottier-Gois L, Lepercq P, Sutren M, Galan P, Duval Y, Juste C, Dore J. Composition and metabolism of the intestinal microbiota in consumers and non-consumers of yogurt. Br J Nutr. 2007;97:126–33.
117. Sahni S, Tucker KL, Kiel DP, Quach L, Casey VA, Hannan MT. Milk and yogurt consumption are linked with higher bone mineral density but not with hip fracture: the Framingham offspring study. Arch Osteoporos. 2013;8:119.
118. Giver E, Durosier-Izart C, Merminod F, Chevalley T, van Rietbergen B, Fewari SL, Rizzoli R. Fermented dairy products consumption is associated with attenuated cortical bone loss independently of total calcium, protein, and energy intakes in healthy postmenopausal women. Osteoporos Int. 2018;29:1771–82.
119. Michaelsson K, Wolk A, Lemming EW, Melhus H, Byberg L. Intake of milk or fermented milk combined with fruit and vegetable consumption in relation to hip fracture rates: a cohort study of Swedish women. J Bone Miner Res. 2018;33:449457.
120. Michaëlsson K, Wolk A, Langenskiöld S, Basu S, Warensjö Lemming E, Melhus H, Byberg L. Milk intake and risk of mortality and fractures in women and men: cohort studies. BMJ. 2014;349:g6015.
121. Laird E, Molloy AM, McNulty H, Ward M, McCarroll K, Hoey L, Hughes CF, Cunningham C, Strain JJ, Casey MC. Greater yogurt consumption is associated with increased bone mineral density and physical function in older adults. Osteoporos Int. 2017;28:2409–19.
122. Radavelli-Bagatini S, Zhu K, Lewis JR, Prince RL. Dairy food intake, peripheral bone structure, and muscle mass in elderly ambulatory women. J Bone Miner Res. 2014;29:1691–700.

123. Biver E, Durosier-Izart C, Merminod F, Chevalley T, van Rietbergen B, Ferrari SL, Rizzoli R. Fermented dairy products consumption is associated with attenuated cortical bone loss independently of total calcium, protein and energy intakes in healthy postmenopausal women. Osteoporos Int. 2018; https://doi.org/10.1007/s00198-018-4535-4.
124. Jones ML, Martoni CJ, Prakash S. Oral supplementation with probiotic *L. reuteri* NCIMB 30242 increases mean circulating 25-hydroxyvitamin D: a post hoc analysis of a randomized controlled trial. J Clin Endocrinol Metab. 2013;98:2944–51.
125. Agustina R, Bovee-Oudenhoven IM, Lukito W, et al. Probiotics *Lactobacillus reuteri* DSM 17938 and lactobacillus casei CRL 431 modestly increase growth, but not iron and zinc status, among Indonesian children aged 1-6 years. J Nutr. 2013;143:1184–93.
126. McNulty NP, Yatsunenko T, Hsiao A, et al. The impact of a consortium of fermented milk strains on the gut microbiome of gnotobiotic mice and monozygotic twins. Sci Transl Med. 2011;3:106ra106.
127. Mika A, Fleshner M. Early-life exercise may promote lasting brain and metabolic health through gut bacterial metabolites. Immunol Cell Biol. 2016;94:151–7.
128. Clarke SF, Murphy EF, O'Sullivan O, et al. Exercise and associated dietary extremes impact on gut microbial diversity. Gut. 2014;63:1913–20.
129. Barton W, Penney NC, Cronin O, Garcia-Perez I, Molloy MG, Holmes E, Shanahan F, Cotter PD, O'Sullivan O. The microbiome of professional athletes differs from that of more sedentary subjects in composition and particularly at the functional metabolic level. Gut. 2018;67:625–33.
130. Allen JM, Mailing LJ, Niemiro GM, Moore R, Cook MD, White BA, Holscher HD, Woods JA. Exercise alters gut microbiota composition and function in lean and obese humans. Med Sci Sports Exerc. 2018;50:747–57.
131. Kong J, Zhang Z, Musch MW, Ning G, Sun J, Hart J, Bissonnette M, Li YC. Novel role of the vitamin D receptor in maintaining the integrity of the intestinal mucosal barrier. Am J Physiol Gastrointest Liver Physiol. 2008;294:G208–16.
132. Jin D, Wu S, Zhang YG, Lu R, Xia Y, Dong H, Sun J. Lack of vitamin D receptor causes Dysbiosis and changes the functions of the murine intestinal microbiome. Clin Ther. 2015;37:996–1009.e7.
133. Luthold RV, Fernandes GR, Franco-de-Moraes AC, Folchetti LG, Ferreira SR. Gut microbiota interactions with the immunomodulatory role of vitamin D in normal individuals. Metab Clin Exp. 2017;69:76–86.
134. Wu S, Yoon S, Zhang YG, Lu R, Xia Y, Wan J, Petrof EO, Claud EC, Chen D, Sun J. Vitamin D receptor pathway is required for probiotic protection in colitis. Am J Physiol Gastrointest Liver Physiol. 2015;309:G341–9.
135. Bashir M, Prietl B, Tauschmann M, Mautner SI, Kump PK, Treiber G, Wurm P, Gorkiewicz G, Hogenauer C, Pieber TR. Effects of high doses of vitamin D3 on mucosa-associated gut microbiome vary between regions of the human gastrointestinal tract. Eur J Nutr. 2016;55:1479–89.
136. Clooney AG, Bernstein CN, Leslie WD, Vagianos K, Sargent M, Laserna-Mendieta EJ, Claesson MJ, Targownik LE. A comparison of the gut microbiome between long-term users and non-users of proton pump inhibitors. Aliment Pharmacol Ther. 2016;43:974–84.
137. Leonard J, Marshall JK, Moayyedi P. Systematic review of the risk of enteric infection in patients taking acid suppression. Am J Gastroenterol. 2007;102:2047–56. quiz 2057.
138. Jackson MA, Goodrich JK, Maxan ME, et al. Proton pump inhibitors alter the composition of the gut microbiota. Gut. 2016;65:749–56.
139. Imhann F, Bonder MJ, Vich Vila A, et al. Proton pump inhibitors affect the gut microbiome. Gut. 2016;65:740–8.
140. Forslund K, Hildebrand F, Nielsen T, et al. Disentangling type 2 diabetes and metformin treatment signatures in the human gut microbiota. Nature. 2015;528:262–6.
141. Brommage R, Binacua C, Antille S, Carrie AL. Intestinal calcium absorption in rats is stimulated by dietary lactulose and other resistant sugars. J Nutr. 1993;123:2186–94.

142. Bueno-Vargas P, Manzano M, Diaz-Castro J, Lopez-Aliaga I, Rueda R, Lopez-Pedrosa JM. Maternal dietary supplementation with oligofructose-enriched inulin in gestating/lactating rats preserves maternal bone and improves bone microarchitecture in their offspring. PLoS One. 2016;11:e0154120.
143. Coudray C, Rambeau M, Feillet-Coudray C, Tressol JC, Demigne C, Gueux E, Mazur A, Rayssiguier Y. Dietary inulin intake and age can significantly affect intestinal absorption of calcium and magnesium in rats: a stable isotope approach. Nutr J. 2005;4:29.
144. Delzenne N, Aertssens J, Verplaetse H, Roccaro M, Roberfroid M. Effect of fermentable fructo-oligosaccharides on mineral, nitrogen and energy digestive balance in the rat. Life Sci. 1995;57:1579–87.
145. Hirama Y, Morohashi T, Sano T, Maki K, Ohta A, Sakai N, Yamada S, Sasa R. Fructooligosaccharides prevent disorders of the femoral neck following gastrectomy in growing rats. J Bone Miner Metab. 2003;21:294–8.
146. Ohta A, Motohashi Y, Sakai K, Hirayama M, Adachi T, Sakuma K. Dietary fructooligosaccharides increase calcium absorption and levels of mucosal calbindin-D9k in the large intestine of gastrectomized rats. Scand J Gastroenterol. 1998;33:1062–8.
147. Scholz-Ahrens KE, Acil Y, Schrezenmeir J. Effect of oligofructose or dietary calcium on repeated calcium and phosphorus balances, bone mineralization and trabecular structure in ovariectomized rats. Br J Nutr. 2002;88:365–77.
148. Tousen Y, Matsumoto Y, Matsumoto C, Nishide Y, Nagahata Y, Kobayashi I, Ishimi Y. The combined effects of soya isoflavones and resistant starch on equol production and trabecular bone loss in ovariectomised mice. Br J Nutr. 2016;116:247–57.
149. Varley PF, McCarney C, Callan JJ, O'Doherty JV. Effect of dietary mineral level and inulin inclusion on phosphorus, calcium and nitrogen utilisation, intestinal microflora and bone development. J Sci Food Agric. 2010;90:2447–54.
150. Younes H, Coudray C, Bellanger J, Demigne C, Rayssiguier Y, Remesy C. Effects of two fermentable carbohydrates (inulin and resistant starch) and their combination on calcium and magnesium balance in rats. Br J Nutr. 2001;86:479–85.
151. Abrams SA, Griffin IJ, Hawthorne KM. Young adolescents who respond to an inulin-type fructan substantially increase total absorbed calcium and daily calcium accretion to the skeleton. J Nutr. 2007;137:2524s–6s.
152. Abrams SA, Hawthorne KM, Aliu O, Hicks PD, Chen Z, Griffin IJ. An inulin-type fructan enhances calcium absorption primarily via an effect on colonic absorption in humans. J Nutr. 2007;137:2208–12.
153. Boler BM, Serao MC, Bauer LL, Staeger MA, Boileau TW, Swanson KS, Fahey GC Jr. Digestive physiological outcomes related to polydextrose and soluble maize fibre consumption by healthy adult men. Br J Nutr. 2011;106:1864–71.
154. Coudray C, Bellanger J, Castiglia-Delavaud C, Remesy C, Vermorel M, Rayssignuier Y. Effect of soluble or partly soluble dietary fibres supplementation on absorption and balance of calcium, magnesium, iron and zinc in healthy young men. Eur J Clin Nutr. 1997;51:375–80.
155. Dahl WJ, Whiting SJ, Isaac TM, Weeks SJ, Arnold CJ. Effects of thickened beverages fortified with inulin on beverage acceptance, gastrointestinal function, and bone resorption in institutionalized adults. Nutrition. 2005;21:308–11.
156. Hicks PD, Hawthorne KM, Berseth CL, Marunycz JD, Heubi JE, Abrams SA. Total calcium absorption is similar from infant formulas with and without prebiotics and exceeds that in human milk-fed infants. BMC Pediatr. 2012;12:118.
157. Jakeman SA, Henry CN, Martin BR, McCabe GP, McCabe LD, Jackson GS, Peacock M, Weaver CM. Soluble corn fiber increases bone calcium retention in postmenopausal women in a dose-dependent manner: a randomized crossover trial. Am J Clin Nutr. 2016;104:837–43.
158. Tahiri M, Tressol JC, Arnaud J, et al. Five-week intake of short-chain fructo-oligosaccharides increases intestinal absorption and status of magnesium in postmenopausal women. J Bone Miner Res. 2001;16:2152–60.

159. Tahiri M, Tressol JC, Arnaud J, et al. Effect of short-chain fructooligosaccharides on intestinal calcium absorption and calcium status in postmenopausal women: a stable-isotope study. Am J Clin Nutr. 2003;77:449–57.
160. Teuri U, Karkkainen M, Lamberg-Allardt C, Korpela R. Addition of inulin to breakfast does not acutely affect serum ionized calcium and parathyroid hormone concentrations. Ann Nutr Metab. 1999;43:356–64.
161. van den Heuvel EG, Schaafsma G, Muys T, van Dokkum W. Nondigestible oligosaccharides do not interfere with calcium and nonheme-iron absorption in young, healthy men. Am J Clin Nutr. 1998;67:445–51.
162. van den Heuvel EG, Muijs T, Brouns F, Hendriks HF. Short-chain fructo-oligosaccharides improve magnesium absorption in adolescent girls with a low calcium intake. Nutr Res. 2009;29:229–37.
163. Kimoto-Nira H, Suzuki C, Kobayashi M, Sasaki K, Kurisaki J, Mizumachi K. Anti-ageing effect of a lactococcal strain: analysis using senescence-accelerated mice. Br J Nutr. 2007;98:1178–86.

13 Therapeutic Targeting of Gut-Bone Signaling to Treat Osteoporosis

Laura R. McCabe and Narayanan Parameswaran

Introduction

Intestinal microbiota refers to microorganisms present in the intestine, including bacteria, viruses, protozoa, and fungi. Microbiome refers to their collective genome. The intestinal microbiota accounts for ~90% of the cells in the host. Bacteria have been a key focus with over ~100 trillion microbes with ~1000 different bacterial species in 28 different phyla found in the microbiota [1]. Thus, they not only outnumber the host cells but also express ~100-fold more genes compared to the host genome. Bacterial numbers increase from proximal to the distal end of the GI tract, with the colon consisting of ~10^{12} CFU of bacteria. Although majority of the bacteria are in the lumen, there are also microbes that are associated with the top mucus layer. Different regions of the gut colonize different types of bacteria, an effect that is determined by environmental factors such as pH and nutrient availability [2]. A healthy balance of bacterial species (eubiosis) is critical for intestinal health. Imbalance in the bacterial composition (dysbiosis) can lead to negative outcomes to the host intestinal physiology. Most studies to date have focused on the gut bacteria and their physiological and pathophysiological roles in host physiology and disease (Fig. 13.1). Here, we will discuss the microbiota impact on the host intestine, the effect of intestinal inflammation on skeletal health, the role of probiotics in mediating bone health, and the benefits of probiotics to bone health in a disease model, type 1 diabetes (T1D).

L. R. McCabe (✉)
Department of Physiology, Michigan State University, East Lansing, MI, USA

Department of Radiology, Michigan State University, East Lansing, MI, USA
e-mail: mccabel@msu.edu

N. Parameswaran
Department of Physiology, Michigan State University, East Lansing, MI, USA
e-mail: narap@msu.edu

© Springer Nature Switzerland AG 2019
C. M. Weaver et al. (eds.), *Nutritional Influences on Bone Health*,
https://doi.org/10.1007/978-3-319-98464-3_13

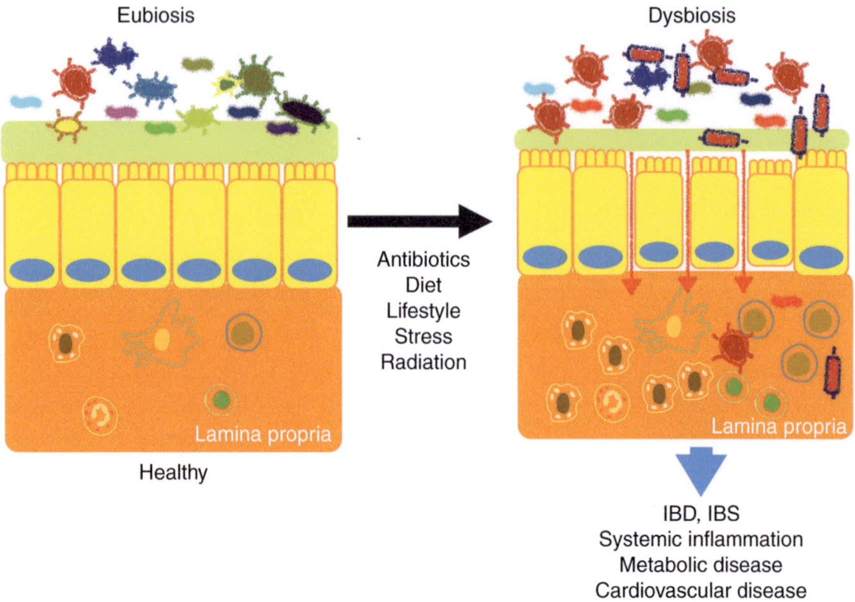

Fig. 13.1 Importance of microbiota in health and disease: eubiosis (healthy composition of gut bacteria) is essential for normal physiological functions of the gut. Perturbation to eubiosis by factors including antibiotic treatment, diet, lifestyle, stress, etc., leads to dysbiosis (unhealthy composition of gut bacteria). Dysbiosis has negative consequences to host physiology including reduced mucus secretion, disrupted intestinal barrier, dysregulated immune response, etc. This has now been shown to be associated with a number of disease processes

Microbiome and Intestine

Intestinal bacteria are in a symbiotic relationship with their host. Specifically, bacteria survive on foods ingested by the host, while they also contribute to the nutritional support of the host through a variety of mechanisms including processing of some foods into absorbable energy and synthesizing certain vitamins [2, 3]. Gut microbiota are essential and most well-known for fermentation of dietary fibers [4] which are a key source of energy for bacteria and provide metabolic end products, such as acetate, propionate, and butyrate. Short-chain fatty acids are efficiently absorbed in the colon and can benefit the host physiology. For example, butyrate is an important source of energy for intestinal epithelial cells, and acetate is important for lipogenesis in the liver (reviewed in [4]).

In addition to nutritional support, the gut microbiota is also an important modulator of the mucosal immune system. While the immune system has the ability to defend against microbial invasion, it is clear that the presence of commensal gut bacteria shapes the mucosal immune system, one of the largest in the body. Early studies using germ-free mice indicated that the microbiota is an important source of regulatory signals that influence host physiology [5]. Importantly, these studies show that the development of mucosal immune system is aberrant in the absence of microbiota. Germ-free mice exhibit decreased intestinal lymphocytes and antimicrobial peptides as well as reduced immunoglobulin A levels. Interestingly, many of these effects on the germ-free mouse immune system are reversed by colonization with commensal microbes, demonstrating that microbiota indeed shape the gut mucosal immune system [6–8]. Recent studies indicate that specific microbes are involved in shaping the immune responses in the gut as well as in modulating different intestinal functions including mucus secretion, permeability, and immune cell activation [9–12]. Together, studies to date underscore the importance of gut microbiota in the regulation of host intestinal physiology and pathophysiology.

The human microbiota consists of phyla *Firmicutes*, *Bacterioides*, *Actinobacteria*, *Proteobacteria*, *Fusobacteria*, *Cyanobacteria*, and *Verrucomicrobia* [1]. The most abundant phyla are *Firmicutes*, *Bacterioides*, and *Actinobacteria*. However, the composition of the microbiome changes over the course of a lifetime and is influenced by exposure to factors such as diet composition and medications (reviewed in [13]). During the natural aging process, involving changes in diet and sex hormones, the composition of microbiome changes to reach a peak of "core microbiome" [13]. This peaking in richness and complexity is thought to afford flexibility and avoid vulnerability to various challenges. Microbial richness or bacterial diversity is considered a surrogate for the health status of the microbiota. Reduced diversity is linked to diseases such as obesity and inflammatory diseases (reviewed in [14]). The *Firmicutes* to *Bacterioides* ratio has also been used as a surrogate for dysbiosis (imbalance in gut microbiota) and has been correlated with a number of diseases. The process of aging (over 65) reduces richness of *Proteobacteria* and *Lentisphaerae* (reviewed in [13]). These changes affect a number of gut physiological processes including bowel contractility, mucus secretion, and barrier integrity. This can lead to translocation of bacterial products and metabolites into the systemic circulation leading to a number of systemic pathophysiological conditions (Fig. 13.1). Similar mechanisms have also been suggested in other metabolic diseases.

Recent studies are focusing on the role of gut microbiota in influencing extra-intestinal organ physiology. These studies have shed light on previously less understood role of microbiota in regulating physiological functions such as behavior, blood pressure, and, important to this chapter, bone physiology. In this context, dysregulated microbiota (dysbiosis) has also been attributed to the pathogenesis of several diseases outside of the gut. These include metabolic, allergic, and neurological diseases as well as osteoporosis [3, 9, 14].

Inflammatory Bowel Disease and Bone

Inflammatory bowel disease, of which there are two main forms, ulcerative colitis (which targets the colon) and Crohn's disease (which can affect both the small and large intestine), affects more than 1.3% of Americans. It is characterized by intestinal microbial dysbiosis, damage to the intestinal epithelial barrier, inflammation, and increased intestinal permeability. Commensal bacteria have been shown to be a key factor in the pathogenesis of intestinal inflammation [15]. Intestinal dysbiosis or deficiency has been shown to also affect bone density [16–20].

Consistent with a role for the microbiome and intestinal permeability in regulating bone health, IBD negatively impacts bone [21–24] (Fig. 13.2). Patients with IBD have a 40% higher risk of developing osteoporosis than the general population [25]. Studies in mice demonstrate that ingestion of detergent (dextran sodium sulfate, DSS) is sufficient to promote intestinal barrier breaks, increase permeability, promote intestinal inflammation, and cause bone loss [23]. The DSS-treated mice display decreased osteoblast markers (serum osteocalcin, osteoblast surface, and mineral apposition rate (MAR)) as well as suppressed osteoclast and chondrocyte markers. Early on, serum IGF-1 levels were suppressed; however, cessation of DSS treatment led to restoration of the bone parameters and serum IGF-1 at 38 days post treatment [23].

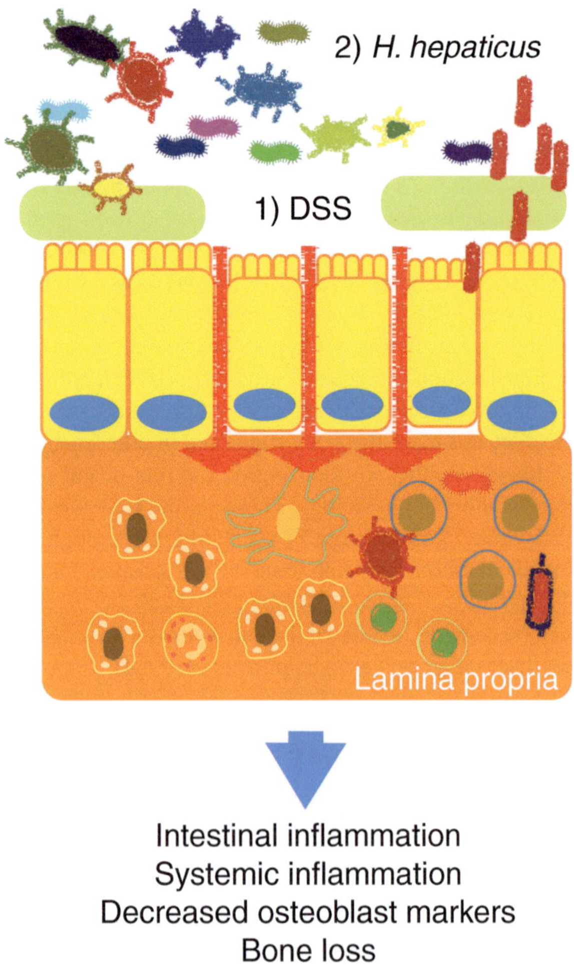

Fig. 13.2 Detergent (dextran sodium sulfate, DSS) and pathogenic bacteria (*H. hepaticus*) promote intestinal barrier breaks and increase intestinal and systemic inflammation which ultimately leads to bone loss. Intestinal barrier breaks, a reduced mucus layer, and increased intestinal inflammation can contribute to systemic inflammation, decreased osteoblast markers (as a result of decreased lineage selection, maturation, and/or viability), and ultimately bone loss

To address if this response could occur in another model of colitis, we treated mice with the pathogenic bacteria, *H. hepaticus* [24]. For these studies, IL-10 knockout mice were used to enhance the inflammatory response to *H. hepaticus*. Similar to the DSS studies, at 6 weeks post infection, male mice displayed increased intestinal inflammation and significantly decreased trabecular bone density. This was apparent in both long bone (femur) and vertebrae. Intestinal disease score correlated with bone loss in male mice. Interestingly, females did not lose bone in response to the infection. Intestinal *H. hepaticus* levels were lower in female compared to male mice, suggesting decreased survival in female intestine [24], suggesting a sex-dependent difference in response in this model.

To address if the weight loss observed in the DSS and *H. hepaticus* models contributed to the bone loss, we treated mice with a low dose of DSS that caused intestinal inflammation but did not cause weight loss [26]. Despite not losing weight, the mice still lost a significant amount of trabecular bone volume fraction and displayed decreased bone formation, osteoblast numbers, and serum osteocalcin. This indicates that weight loss is not required for bone loss as a consequence to intestinal inflammation. In addition, intestinal pathology score and colon TNFα levels were reciprocally related to bone density ($p < 0.003$; $r > -0.075$). This is consistent with other studies showing that inflammatory cytokine levels increase in IBD [27], that bone marrow expression levels of pro-inflammatory cytokine genes increase in colitic mice [24, 28, 29], and that colitis can influence bone marrow cell composition [30]. The increase in pro-inflammatory cytokines, such as TNFα, can cause bone loss via a pro-osteoclastogenic and anti-osteoblastic effects.

Probiotics and Bone

Given that gut inflammation is tightly linked with reduced measures of trabecular bone density, it follows that factors that reduce intestinal inflammation would benefit bone health. Probiotics have been consumed by humans for their health benefits (preventing and treating diseases) for thousands of years [31–33]. A typical dose of naturally ingested probiotic bacteria can range from 10^8 to 10^{12} CFU/day [34]. This amount can lead to a 1:1 ratio of ingested/endogenous bacteria in the small intestine, but the ingested bacteria are far outnumbered by the resident bacteria in the colon (by more than 1:10,000) [34, 35]. Thus, probiotics can influence the microbiome composition (especially of the small intestine), and they can also modify composition through secreting lactic acid, bacteriocins (antimicrobial peptides), and hydrogen peroxide [36]. These changes can beneficially affect the intestinal environment [3].

Our laboratory has focused on studying the probiotic *Lactobacillus reuteri* since this probiotic is a commensal bacteria found in the human gut and milk, is used to treat colic in babies, produces antimicrobials, and has reported anti-inflammatory activity [37]. Treatment of healthy male mice with *L. reuteri* results in decreased TNFα and, as hypothesized, increased trabecular bone volume in male mice [19]. Further analyses indicated that bone formation rate was markedly increased in the treated mice. Interestingly, we did not see a similar response in healthy female mice.

However, when female mice deficient in estrogen were treated with *L. reuteri*, bone density was increased (and bone loss was prevented) compared to untreated mice, suggesting that estrogen negatively influences *L. reuteri* effects on bone [16]. *L. reuteri* treatment of estrogen-deficient female mice reduced osteoclastogenesis signals, like RANKL, and decreased isolated bone marrow osteoclastogenesis [16]. Later studies showed that the probiotic increases bone density in intact females (estrogen sufficient) only in the presence of mild inflammatory stimuli [17]. *L. reuteri* treatment also caused shifts in the small intestinal microbiome composition, suggesting that the probiotic could work by modifying the microbiota. It is known that probiotic treatment can induce changes in microbiota composition in a beneficial manner which are suggested to account for bone health benefits in both mice and humans [38]. Several studies indicate the probiotic ingestion can modify bone density, though links with specific microbiota components have not been fully determined [18–20, 39]. Dysbiosis has been shown to decrease GI barrier integrity and therefore increased leakage of bacterial factors (e.g., endotoxin), and this correlates with bone loss [3, 18, 23, 24, 26, 40]. Thus, probiotic prevention of dysbiosis may benefit bone health through enhancement of intestinal barrier function [41–45] (Fig. 13.3). Supporting evidence for this includes studies where probiotic treatments (*Lactobacillus*

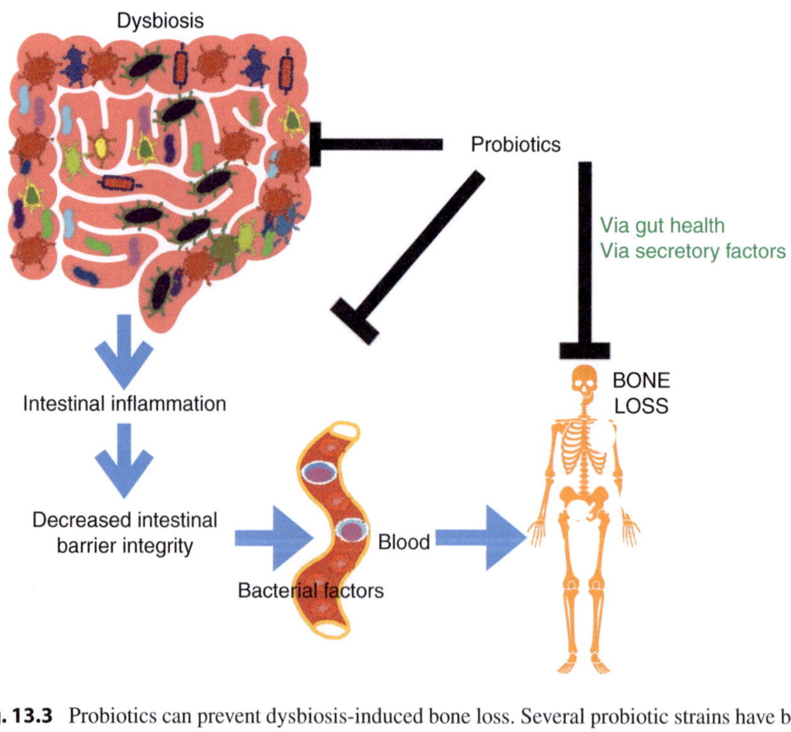

Fig. 13.3 Probiotics can prevent dysbiosis-induced bone loss. Several probiotic strains have been demonstrated to prevent dysbiosis and subsequent bone loss. Probiotics reduce dysbiosis, intestinal inflammation, and barrier breaks. Enhancing intestinal health promotes bone health. Probiotics also secrete factors that may directly benefit bone health

rhamnosus GG and VSL#3) prevent intestinal permeability and bone loss in estrogen-deficient female mice [18]. However, in addition to probiotic effects on the microbiota and intestinal permeability, there are also studies supporting direct effects of probiotics on bone cell activity (Fig. 13.3). For example, conditioned media (secretory products) from *L. reuteri* can prevent osteoclastogenesis in vitro [16].

Type 1 Diabetes and Osteoporosis Therapies

Type 1 diabetes (T1D) is a metabolic disease that affects over one million children and adults in the United States and is characterized by autoimmune destruction of insulin-producing pancreatic β-cells. Because of this, patients are required to use insulin injections to control their blood glucose levels. While patients have a longer lifespan due to exogenous insulin therapy, maintaining euglycemia remains difficult, even under therapeutic vigilance [46]. Therefore, patients continue to suffer from secondary complications of metabolic dysregulation, including osteoporosis and increased fracture risk [47]. Bone loss (trabecular and cortical) is seen in patients [48] as well as in genetic and chemically induced T1D animal models. Decreased osteoblast activity is the key contributor to decreased bone mineral density observed in T1D children and adults [49–54]. Consistent with a decrease in bone mineral density, serum osteocalcin levels are typically lower in diabetic patients compared to nondiabetic subjects [49, 55–71] and are inversely proportional to glycosylated hemoglobin levels, a measure of metabolic control [72, 73]. T1D reduction in osteoblast activity is thought to result from decreased osteoblast linage selection, maturation, and viability and therefore causes reduced bone volume and increased bone marrow adiposity [57, 74–80]. With increasing lifespan, the effects of T1D in postmenopausal women are also of concern. Mouse studies show that bone loss is compounded (greater) in estrogen-deficient-T1D mice which display greater decreases in osteoblast markers, and increases in osteoclast activity lead to bone volume fractions significantly lower than estrogen-deficient or T1D mice alone [81]. Diabetic mouse models exhibit elevated TNFα levels in serum and increased TNFα mRNA level/expression in bone [69, 82] and the TNF level in T1D-estrogen-deficient mice is markedly higher than T1- or estrogen-deficient mice alone. Furthermore, the level of TNF expression (RNA and protein) in bone is correlated ($p = 0.0003$; $r = 0.522$) with femur bone volume fraction. Accordingly, inhibition of TNF with pegsunercept treatment, a TNFα antibody that suppresses serum TNFα levels, benefits bone health in diabetic mice [83].

The gut microbiome is also thought to be involved in the development of T1D as suggested in a variety of mouse studies. In non-obese diabetic (NOD) mice, a requirement for commensal microbes in protection from diabetes was demonstrated using germ-free NOD mice. These germ-free animals develop severe diabetes, whereas bacterial colonization attenuates T1D [84]. Similarly, antibiotic use (which depletes the microbiome) early in life accelerates T1D in NOD mice [85]. Based on the above information, we and others have examined the role of the microbiota in T1D bone loss.

In the streptozotocin-induced T1D bone loss model, our lab demonstrated that treatment with probiotic *L. reuteri 6475* can prevent the 35% trabecular bone loss seen in T1D male mice [20]. T1D reduction of osteoblast activity, characterized by decreased serum osteocalcin and decreases in mineral apposition rate (MAR), was prevented by treatment with *L. reuteri* suggesting that this probiotic, in this model, has an anabolic effect on bone [20]. Additionally, T1D induction of bone marrow adiposity [86] was also prevented [85]. Wnt10b signaling which in mesenchymal precursor cells stimulates osteoblastogenesis and inhibits adipogenesis was decreased in T1D mouse bone and restored with *L. reuteri* treatment [85]. These findings suggest that probiotic use can prevent T1D bone loss by modulation of expression of Wnt10b in bone. In an elegant study, Xiao et al. demonstrated that transfer of diabetic mouse oral microbiota into germ-free mice leads to inflammation and periodontal bone loss [87] (Motyl 2011 #6275). This indicates the transferability of bone loss with microbiome transfer. Furthermore, this response was prevented by blocking IL-17 levels, suggesting a role for IL-17 in diabetic periodontal bone loss. Together, these data suggest that the microbiota plays a key role in diabetic bone loss, and accordingly the microbiota can be targeted to prevent diabetic bone loss. Interestingly, while these effects can be mediated through changes within the gut, our studies with *Lactobacillus reuteri*-secreted factors indicate the possibility that probiotics can also secrete factors that directly impact bone cells to benefit skeletal health.

Summary

The gut and microbiota are critical for the health of the host. Existing studies from our lab and others suggest that the gut-bone signaling pathway represents a viable therapeutic target for treating osteoporosis. Studies also demonstrate that modulation of microbiota composition by probiotic ingestion could be an effective and readily available treatment strategy. Mechanisms likely include probiotic-induced changes to the microbiome and intestine (barrier and immune cells) but likely also involve bacterial-secreted factors and their effects on bone cells. This is an exciting and rapidly expanding area of research that holds great future promise for human health.

Acknowledgments The authors thank their trainees and the funding received from the National Institutes of Health, grants RO1 DK101050 and RO1 AT007695.

References

1. Qin J, Li R, Raes J, Arumugam M, Burgdorf KS, Manichanh C, Nielsen T, Pons N, Levenez F, Yamada T, Mende DR, Li J, Xu J, Li S, Li D, Cao J, Wang B, Liang H, Zheng H, Xie Y, Tap J, Lepage P, Bertalan M, Batto JM, Hansen T, Le Paslier D, Linneberg A, Nielsen HB, Pelletier E, Renault P, Sicheritz-Ponten T, Turner K, Zhu H, Yu C, Li S, Jian M, Zhou Y, Li Y, Zhang X, Li S, Qin N, Yang H, Wang J, Brunak S, Dore J, Guarner F, Kristiansen K, Pedersen O,

Parkhill J, Weissenbach J, Meta HITC, Bork P, Ehrlich SD, Wang J. A human gut microbial gene catalogue established by metagenomic sequencing. Nature. 2010;464:59–65.
2. Schepper JD, Irwin R, Kang J, Dagenais K, Lemon T, Shinouskis A, Parameswaran N, McCabe LR. Probiotics in gut-bone signaling. Adv Exp Med Biol. 2017;1033:225–47.
3. McCabe LR, Parameswaran N. Advances in probiotic regulation of bone and mineral metabolism. Calcif Tissue Int. 2018;102:480–8.
4. Janssen AW, Kersten S. The role of the gut microbiota in metabolic health. FASEB J. 2015;29:3111–23.
5. Grover M, Kashyap PC. Germ-free mice as a model to study effect of gut microbiota on host physiology. Neurogastroenterol Motil. 2014;26:745–8.
6. Hapfelmeier S, Lawson MA, Slack E, Kirundi JK, Stoel M, Heikenwalder M, Cahenzli J, Velykoredko Y, Balmer ML, Endt K, Geuking MB, Curtiss R 3rd, McCoy KD, Macpherson AJ. Reversible microbial colonization of germ-free mice reveals the dynamics of IgA immune responses. Science. 2010;328:1705–9.
7. Umesaki Y. Use of gnotobiotic mice to identify and characterize key microbes responsible for the development of the intestinal immune system. Proc Jpn Acad Ser B Phys Biol Sci. 2014;90:313–32.
8. Chung H, Pamp SJ, Hill JA, Surana NK, Edelman SM, Troy EB, Reading NC, Villablanca EJ, Wang S, Mora JR, Umesaki Y, Mathis D, Benoist C, Relman DA, Kasper DL. Gut immune maturation depends on colonization with a host-specific microbiota. Cell. 2012;149:1578–93.
9. Collins FL, Schepper JD, Rios-Arce ND, Steury MD, Kang HJ, Mallin H, Schoenherr D, Camfield G, Chishti S, McCabe LR, Parameswaran N. Immunology of gut-bone signaling. Adv Exp Med Biol. 2017;1033:59–94.
10. Kabat AM, Srinivasan N, Maloy KJ. Modulation of immune development and function by intestinal microbiota. Trends Immunol. 2014;35:507–17.
11. McDermott AJ, Huffnagle GB. The microbiome and regulation of mucosal immunity. Immunology. 2014;142:24–31.
12. Thaiss CA, Zmora N, Levy M, Elinav E. The microbiome and innate immunity. Nature. 2016;535:65–74.
13. Kundu P, Blacher E, Elinav E, Pettersson S. Our gut microbiome: the evolving inner self. Cell. 2017;171:1481–93.
14. D'Argenio V, Salvatore F. The role of the gut microbiome in the healthy adult status. Clin Chim Acta. 2015;451:97–102.
15. Bamias G, Okazawa A, Rivera-Nieves J, Arseneau KO, De La Rue SA, Pizarro TT, Cominelli F. Commensal bacteria exacerbate intestinal inflammation but are not essential for the development of murine ileitis. J Immunol. 2007;178:1809–18.
16. Britton RA, Irwin R, Quach D, Schaefer L, Zhang J, Lee T, Parameswaran N, McCabe LR. Probiotic L. reuteri treatment prevents bone loss in a menopausal ovariectomized mouse model. J Cell Physiol. 2014;229(11):1822–30.
17. Collins FL, Irwin R, Bierhalter H, Schepper J, Britton RA, Parameswaran N, McCabe LR. Lactobacillus reuteri 6475 increases bone density in intact females only under an inflammatory setting. PLoS One. 2016;11:e0153180.
18. Li JY, Chassaing B, Tyagi AM, Vaccaro C, Luo T, Adams J, Darby TM, Weitzmann MN, Mulle JG, Gewirtz AT, Jones RM, Pacifici R. Sex steroid deficiency-associated bone loss is microbiota dependent and prevented by probiotics. J Clin Invest. 2016;126:2049–63.
19. McCabe LR, Irwin R, Schaefer L, Britton RA. Probiotic use decreases intestinal inflammation and increases bone density in healthy male but not female mice. J Cell Physiol. 2013;228:1793–8.
20. Zhang J, Motyl KJ, Irwin R, MacDougald OA, Britton RA, McCabe LR. Loss of bone and Wnt10b expression in male type 1 diabetic mice is blocked by the probiotic Lactobacillus reuteri. Endocrinology. 2015;156:3169–82.
21. Bianchi ML. Inflammatory bowel diseases, celiac disease, and bone. Arch Biochem Biophys. 2010;503:54–65.

22. Ghishan FK, Kiela PR. Advances in the understanding of mineral and bone metabolism in inflammatory bowel diseases. Am J Physiol Gastrointest Liver Physiol. 2011;300:G191–201.
23. Harris L, Senagore P, Young VB, McCabe LR. Inflammatory bowel disease causes reversible suppression of osteoblast and chondrocyte function in mice. Am J Physiol Gastrointest Liver Physiol. 2009;296:G1020–9.
24. Irwin R, Lee T, Young VB, Parameswaran N, McCabe LR. Colitis-induced bone loss is gender dependent and associated with increased inflammation. Inflamm Bowel Dis. 2013;19:1586–97.
25. Compston JE, Judd D, Crawley EO, Evans WD, Evans C, Church HA, Reid EM, Rhodes J. Osteoporosis in patients with inflammatory bowel disease. Gut. 1987;28:410–5.
26. Irwin R, Raehtz S, Parameswaran N, McCabe LR. Intestinal inflammation without weight loss decreases bone density and growth. Am J Physiol Regul Integr Comp Physiol. 2016;311:R1149–57.
27. Nielsen OH, Vainer B, Madsen SM, Seidelin JB, Heegaard NH. Established and emerging biological activity markers of inflammatory bowel disease. Am J Gastroenterol. 2000;95:359–67.
28. Kobayashi K, Kambe F, Kurokouchi K, Sakai T, Ishiguro N, Iwata H, Koga K, Gruener R, Seo H. TNF-α-dependent activation of NF-κB in human osteoblastic HOS-TE85 cells is repressed in vector-averaged gravity using clinostat rotation. Biochem Biophys Res Commun. 2000;279:258–64.
29. Kudo O, Fujikawa Y, Itonaga I, Sabokbar A, Torisu T, Athanasou NA. Proinflammatory cytokine (TNFalpha/IL-1alpha) induction of human osteoclast formation. J Pathol. 2002;198:220–7.
30. Trottier MD, Irwin R, Li Y, McCabe LR, Fraker PJ. Enhanced production of early lineages of monocytic and granulocytic cells in mice with colitis. Proc Natl Acad Sci U S A. 2012;109:16594–9.
31. Gasbarrini G, Bonvicini F, Gramenzi A. Probiotics history. J Clin Gastroenterol. 2016;50(Suppl 2):S116–9. Proceedings from the 8th Probiotics, Prebiotics & New Foods for Microbiota and Human Health meeting held in Rome, Italy on September 13-15, 2015.
32. Gogineni V. Probiotics: history and evolution. J Anc Dis Prev Remedies. 2013;1:1–7.
33. Anukam KC, Reid G. Organisms associated with bacterial vaginosis in Nigerian women as determined by PCR-DGGE and 16S rRNA gene sequence. Afr Health Sci. 2007;7:68–72.
34. Derrien M, van Hylckama Vlieg JE. Fate, activity, and impact of ingested bacteria within the human gut microbiota. Trends Microbiol. 2015;23:354–66.
35. Loh G, Blaut M. Role of commensal gut bacteria in inflammatory bowel diseases. Gut Microbes. 2012;3:544–55.
36. Lebeer S, Vanderleyden J, De Keersmaecker SC. Genes and molecules of lactobacilli supporting probiotic action. Microbiol Mol Biol Rev. 2008;72:728–64. Table of Contents.
37. Thomas CM, Hong T, van Pijkeren JP, Hemarajata P, Trinh DV, Hu W, Britton RA, Kalkum M, Versalovic J. Histamine derived from probiotic Lactobacillus reuteri suppresses TNF via modulation of PKA and ERK signaling. PLoS One. 2012;7:e31951.
38. Whisner CM, Weaver CM. Prebiotics and bone. Adv Exp Med Biol. 2017;1033:201–24.
39. Ohlsson C, Engdahl C, Fak F, Andersson A, Windahl SH, Farman HH, Moverare-Skrtic S, Islander U, Sjogren K. Probiotics protect mice from ovariectomy-induced cortical bone loss. PLoS One. 2014;9:e92368.
40. Collins F, Rios-Arce N, Atkinson N, Bierhalter H, Schoenherr D, Bazil J, McCabe L, Parameswaran N. Temporal and regional intestinal change in permeability, tight junction and cytokine gene expression following ovariectomy-induced estrogen deficiency. Physiol Rep. 2017;5(9):e13263.
41. Rosenfeldt V, Benfeldt E, Valerius NH, Paerregaard A, Michaelsen KF. Effect of probiotics on gastrointestinal symptoms and small intestinal permeability in children with atopic dermatitis. J Pediatr. 2004;145:612–6.
42. Stratiki Z, Costalos C, Sevastiadou S, Kastanidou O, Skouroliakou M, Giakoumatou A, Petrohilou V. The effect of a bifidobacter supplemented bovine milk on intestinal permeability of preterm infants. Early Hum Dev. 2007;83:575–9.

43. Madsen K, Cornish A, Soper P, McKaigney C, Jijon H, Yachimec C, Doyle J, Jewell L, De Simone C. Probiotic bacteria enhance murine and human intestinal epithelial barrier function. Gastroenterology. 2001;121:580–91.
44. Zareie M, Johnson-Henry K, Jury J, Yang PC, Ngan BY, McKay DM, Soderholm JD, Perdue MH, Sherman PM. Probiotics prevent bacterial translocation and improve intestinal barrier function in rats following chronic psychological stress. Gut. 2006;55:1553–60.
45. Bron PA, Kleerebezem M, Brummer RJ, Cani PD, Mercenier A, MacDonald TT, Garcia-Rodenas CL, Wells JM. Can probiotics modulate human disease by impacting intestinal barrier function? Br J Nutr. 2017;117:93–107.
46. Huang ES, Brown SES, Ewigman BG, Foley EC, Meltzer DO. Patient perceptions of quality of life with diabetes-related complications and treatments. Diabetes Care. 2007;30: 2478–83.
47. Atkinson MA, Eisenbarth GS, Michels AW. Type 1 diabetes. Lancet. 2014;383:69–82.
48. Hofbauer LC, Brueck CC, Singh SK, Dobnig H. Osteoporosis in patients with diabetes mellitus. J Bone Miner Res. 2007;22:1317–28.
49. Kemink SAG, Hermus A, Swinkels L, Lutterman JA, Smals AGH. Osteopenia in insulin-dependent diabetes mellitus; prevalence and aspects of pathophysiology. J Endocrinol Investig. 2000;23:295–303.
50. MunozTorres M, Jodar E, EscobarJimenez F, LopezIbarra PJ, Luna JD. Bone mineral density measured by dual X-ray absorptiometry in Spanish patients with insulin-dependent diabetes mellitus. Calcif Tissue Int. 1996;58:316–9.
51. Inzerillo AM, Epstein S. Osteoporosis and diabetes mellitus. Rev Endocr Metab Disord. 2004;5:261–8.
52. Rix M, Andreassen H, Eskildsen P. Impact at peripheral neuropathy an bone density in patient with type 1 diabetes. Diabetes Care. 1999;22:827–31.
53. Forst T, Pfutzner A, Kann P, Schehler B, Lobmann R, Schafer H, Andreas J, Bockisch A, Beyer J. Peripheral osteopenia in adult patients with insulin-dependent diabetes-mellitus. Diabet Med. 1995;12:874–9.
54. Ivers RQ, Cumming RG, Mitchell P, Peduto AJ. Diabetes and risk of fracture – The Blue Mountains Eye Study. Diabetes Care. 2001;24:1198–203.
55. Bouillon R, Bex M, Vanherck E, Laureys J, Dooms L, Lesaffre E, Ravussin E. Influence of age, sex, and insulin on osteoblast function – osteoblast dysfunction in diabetes-mellitus. J Clin Endocrinol Metab. 1995;80:1194–202.
56. McCabe LR. Understanding the pathology and mechanisms of type I diabetic bone loss. J Cell Biochem. 2007;102:1343–57.
57. Botolin S, McCabe LR. Bone loss and increased bone adiposity in spontaneous and pharmacologically induced diabetic mice. Endocrinology. 2007;148:198–205.
58. Bain S, Ramamurthy NS, Impeduglia T, Scolman S, Golub LM, Rubin C. Tetracycline prevents cancellous bone loss and maintains near-normal rates of bone formation in streptozotocin diabetic rats. Bone. 1997;21:147–53.
59. Botolin S, Faugere MC, Malluche H, Orth M, Meyer R, McCabe LR. Increased bone adiposity and peroxisomal proliferator-activated receptor-gamma 2 expression in type I diabetic mice. Endocrinology. 2005;146:3622–31.
60. Epstein S, Takizawa M, Stein B, Katz IA, Joffe II, Romero DF, Liang XG, Li M, Ke HZ, Jee WSS, Jacobs TW, Berlin J. Effect of cyclosporine-a on bone-mineral metabolism in experimental diabetes-mellitus in the rat. J Bone Miner Res. 1994;9:557–66.
61. Glajchen N, Epstein S, Ismail F, Thomas S, Fallon M, Chakrabarti S. Bone-mineral metabolism in experimental diabetes-mellitus – osteocalcin as a measure of bone remodeling. Endocrinology. 1988;123:290–5.
62. Verhaeghe J, Suiker AMH, Visser WJ, Vanherck E, Vanbree R, Bouillon R. The effects of systemic insulin, insulin-like growth factor-I and growth-hormone on bone-growth and turnover in spontaneously diabetic BB rats. J Endocrinol. 1992;134:485–92.

63. Shires R, Teitelbaum SL, Bergfeld MA, Fallon MD, Slatopolsky E, Avioli LV. The effect of streptozotocin-induced chronic diabetes-mellitus on bone and mineral homeostasis in the rat. J Lab Clin Med. 1981;97:231–40.
64. Motyl K, McCabe LR. Streptozotocin, type I diabetes severity and bone. Biol Proced Online. 2009;11:296–315.
65. Lumachi F, Camozzi V, Tombolan V, Luisetto G, Karsenty G. Bone mineral density, osteocalcin, and bone-specific alkaline phosphatase in patients with insulin-dependent diabetes mellitus. Integr Physiol. 2009;1173:E64–7.
66. Cakatay U, Telci A, Kayali R, Akcay T, Sivas A, Aral F. Changes in bone turnover on deoxypyridinoline levels in diabetic patients. Diabetes Res Clin Pract. 1998;40:75–9.
67. Verhaeghe J, Oloumi G, VanHerck E, vanBree R, Dequeker J, Einhorn TA, Bouillon R. Effects of long-term diabetes and/or high-dose 17 beta-estradiol on bone formation, bone mineral density, and strength in ovariectomized rats. Bone. 1997;20:421–8.
68. Ishida H, Seino Y, Taminato T, Usami M, Takeshita N, Seino Y, Tsutsumi C, Moriuchi S, Akiyama Y, Hara K, Imura H. Circulating levels and bone contents of bone gamma-carboxyglutamic acid-containing protein are decreased in streptozocin-induced diabetes – possible marker for diabetic osteopenia. Diabetes. 1988;37:702–6.
69. Motyl KJ, Botolin S, Irwin R, Appledorn DM, Kadakia T, Amalfitano A, Schwartz RC, McCabe LR. Bone inflammation and altered gene expression with type I diabetes early onset. J Cell Physiol. 2009;218:575–83.
70. Motyl KJ, McCabe LR. Leptin treatment prevents type I diabetic marrow adiposity but not bone loss in mice. J Cell Physiol. 2009;218:376–84.
71. Verhaeghe J, Vanherck E, Visser WJ, Suiker AMH, Thomasset M, Einhorn TA, Faierman E, Bouillon R. Bone and mineral metabolism in bb rats with long-term diabetes – decreased bone turnover and osteoporosis. Diabetes. 1990;39:477–82.
72. Pater A, Sypniewska G, Pilecki O. Biochemical markers of bone cell activity in children with type 1 diabetes mellitus. J Pediatr Endocrinol Metab. 2010;23:81–6.
73. Peters AL, Davidson MB, Schriger DL, Hasselblad V. A clinical approach for the diagnosis of diabetes mellitus – an analysis using glycosylated hemoglobin levels. JAMA. 1996;276:1246–52.
74. Kajkenova O, LeckaCzernik B, Gubrij I, Hauser SP, Takahashi K, Parfit AM, Jilka RL, Manolagas SC, Lipschitz DA. Increased adipogenesis and myelopoiesis in the bone marrow of SAMP6, a murine model of defective osteoblastogenesis and low turnover osteopenia. J Bone Miner Res. 1997;12:1772–9.
75. Verma S, Rajaratnam JH, Denton J, Hoyland JA, Byers RJ. Adipocytic proportion of bone marrow is inversely related to bone formation in osteoporosis. J Clin Pathol. 2002;55:693–8.
76. Moerman EJ, Teng K, Lipschitz DA, Lecka-Czernik B. Aging activates adipogenic and suppresses osteogenic programs in mesenchymal marrow stroma/stem cells: the role of PPAR-gamma 2 transcription factor and TGF-beta/BMP signaling pathways. Aging Cell. 2004;3:379–89.
77. Nuttall ME, Gimble JM. Controlling the balance between osteoblastogenesis and adipogenesis and the consequent therapeutic implications. Curr Opin Pharmacol. 2004;4:290–4.
78. Martin LM, McCabe LR. Type I diabetic bone phenotype is location but not gender dependent. Histochem Cell Biol. 2007;128:125–33.
79. McCabe LR. Switching fat from the periphery to bone marrow: why in type I diabetes? Expert Rev Endocrinol Metab. 2009;4(3):203–7.
80. Weinberg E, Maymon T, Moses O, Weinreb M. Streptozotocin-induced diabetes in rats diminishes the size of the osteoprogenitor pool in bone marrow. Diabetes Res Clin Pract. 2014;103:35–41.
81. Raehtz S, Bierhalter H, Schoenherr D, Parameswaran N, McCabe LR. Estrogen deficiency exacerbates type 1 diabetes induced bone loss in female mice. Endocrinology. 2017;158(7):2086–101.
82. Coe LM, Irwin R, Lippner D, McCabe LR. The bone marrow microenvironment contributes to type I diabetes induced osteoblast death. J Cell Physiol. 2011;226:477–83.

83. Ko KI, Coimbra LS, Tian C, Alblowi J, Kayal RA, Einhorn TA, Gerstenfeld LC, Pignolo RJ, Graves DT. Diabetes reduces mesenchymal stem cells in fracture healing through a TNFalpha-mediated mechanism. Diabetologia. 2015;58:633–42.
84. Wen L, Ley RE, Volchkov PY, Stranges PB, Avanesyan L, Stonebraker AC, Hu C, Wong FS, Szot GL, Bluestone JA, Gordon JI, Chervonsky AV. Innate immunity and intestinal microbiota in the development of type 1 diabetes. Nature. 2008;455:1109–13.
85. Livanos AE, Greiner TU, Vangay P, Pathmasiri W, Stewart D, McRitchie S, Li H, Chung J, Sohn J, Kim S, Gao Z, Barber C, Kim J, Ng S, Rogers AB, Sumner S, Zhang XS, Cadwell K, Knights D, Alekseyenko A, Backhed F, Blaser MJ. Antibiotic-mediated gut microbiome perturbation accelerates development of type 1 diabetes in mice. Nat Microbiol. 2016;1:16140.
86. Botolin S, Faugere MC, Malluche H, Orth M, Meyer R, McCabe LR. Increased bone adiposity and peroxisomal proliferator-activated receptor-gamma2 expression in type I diabetic mice. Endocrinology. 2005;146:3622–31.
87. Xiao E, Mattos M, Vieira GHA, Chen S, Correa JD, Wu Y, Albiero ML, Bittinger K, Graves DT. Diabetes enhances IL-17 expression and alters the oral microbiome to increase its pathogenicity. Cell Host Microbe. 2017;22:120–8.e124.

14 Meeting Calcium Needs in Asia and Prebiotic Study Protocol

Winnie Chee, Kanimolli Arasu, Chang Chung Yuan, Soon Yee Wong, Ong Shu Hwa, Wai Yew Yang, Megan Chong, Meenal Mavinkurve, and Jia Yuan Khoo

Introduction

While the burden of hip fractures is increasing markedly throughout the world, the greatest impact is expected to be felt in Asia; specifically, the percentage of hip fractures in Asia is expected to rise from 26% in 1990 to 37% in 2025 [1]. By the year 2050, half of all hip fractures in the world are projected to occur in Asia [2]. Diet and lifestyle factors have been shown to be modifiable risk factors associated with the osteoporosis risk in Asia [3].

Optimization of diet and lifestyle factors known to influence peak bone mass (PBM) is an important strategy aimed at reducing risk of osteoporosis and fractures later in life. Epidemiological studies have shown that it is possible to predict that a 10% increase (about 1 SD) in PBM could reduce the risk of fracture by 50% in women after the menopause [4, 5]. The distribution of bone mass may vary across populations due to differences in the attainment of skeletal dimensions, peak bone mineral accretion timing, and lifestyle factors. Nevertheless, addressing modifiable risk factors that may predispose to allow bone mass during this critical window for bone accrual is an opportunity for optimizing peak bone mass and prevent osteoporosis.

A recent systematic review by Weaver et al. [6] demonstrated that the best evidence currently available is ensuring adequate calcium intake and physical activity during peak bone mass development and the next level of evidence supported a role for vitamin D adequacy and consumption of dairy products. Calcium is needed for

W. Chee (✉) · K. Arasu · C. C. Yuan · S. Y. Wong · O. S. Hwa · W. Y. Yang · M. Chong
Department of Nutrition and Dietetics, School of Health Sciences, International Medical University, Kuala Lumpur, Malaysia
e-mail: winnie_chee@imu.edu.my

M. Mavinkurve · J. Y. Khoo
Department of Paediatrics, School of Medicine, International Medical University, Kuala Lumpur, Malaysia

© Springer Nature Switzerland AG 2019

C. M. Weaver et al. (eds.), *Nutritional Influences on Bone Health*,
https://doi.org/10.1007/978-3-319-98464-3_14

normal mineralization of the bone and cartilage matrix. Once calcium intake is adequate to prevent rickets or osteomalacia, provision of additional calcium may increase bone density by affecting bone turnover and the size of the remodeling space [7, 8]. Calcium absorption efficiency is optimized by adequate vitamin D status.

Calcium Intakes of Asian Children and Adolescents

The IOF (International Osteoporosis Foundation) published a systematic review of global intakes of calcium in adults [9]. Most surveyed countries in South, East, and Southeast Asia have low dietary calcium intake (<400 mg/day). However, calcium intakes in Asian children and adolescents lack good published data, and reports are mainly available from individual country cross-sectional studies and national nutrition surveys. Table 14.1 shows the mean calcium intakes extracted from various surveys in recent 5 years. It seems that there is a universal phenomenon of large gaps between actual calcium intakes and requirement levels set by national bodies in most Asian countries, similar to the scenario reported in adults. Calcium intakes which are too low have been shown to have a negative impact on growth and attainment of adult height in Asian children and correlated with low bone mineral density [10, 11].

Sources of Calcium Intake and Bioavailability

One of the factors contributing to the low calcium intakes in Asia is the lack of dairy food consumption and poor dietary habits. In a systematic assessment of beverage intake conducted in 187 countries, countries in Asia have the lowest servings of milk averaging 0.05–0.30 servings a day only [18].

Milk and dairy products contain other essential nutrient besides calcium such as protein; vitamins A, D, and B12; riboflavin; and niacin. When dairy intakes are low, nondairy or plant-based calcium sources can contribute to as much as two-thirds of total calcium intakes in the diets of Asian children and adolescents [13, 19]. While it has been shown that plant-based foods such as green vegetables are a good source

Table 14.1 Calcium intakes versus requirement levels among children and adolescents in selected countries in Asia

Country	Age groups (years)	Mean intake (mg/day)	RDA/RNI (mg/day)	Percentage consuming below RDA/RNI	References
China	4–17	355–426	800–1000	>96%	[12]
Korea	1–18	431–510	670–800	75%	[13]
Malaysia	0.5–12	400–700	1300	>50%	[14]
Vietnam	1–18	506	1000	–	[15]
Thailand	0.5–12	350–600	800–1000	>70%	[16]
Indonesia	0.5–12	180–230	1300	>90%	[17]

of bioavailable calcium [20], the quantity of vegetables required to meet daily requirements is substantial, making it difficult to attain dietary calcium requirements with vegetables alone. Certain cereals (e.g., whole bran cereals) contain phytates, which also reduce calcium bioavailability. It is also widely reported that the young population do not meet the recommended servings of fruits and vegetables in many Asian countries [21].

Strategies to Improve Calcium Intakes

A holistic approach is needed to promote adequate calcium intakes in the younger population. These strategies may include promoting public health awareness on the importance of calcium intakes, food fortification, or enrichment as well as conducting studies on bioavailability of local or indigenous food sources. For example, fermented soybean cake/tempeh has been reported to be equally bioavailable as milk and can be a good source of calcium for the Malaysian population [22]. Functional foods or ingredients such as prebiotic fibers that enhance calcium absorption and can be incorporated into foods may also be a useful strategy to ensure adequate calcium intake in Asian countries.

Prebiotic Fibers to Enhance Calcium Intake

Dietary fibers and oligosaccharides are being investigated for their potential to improve bone health largely through their influence on mineral metabolism. These carbohydrate ingredients are considered to be nondigestible because of the lack of appropriate intestinal enzymes to hydrolyze them or structural hindrances that prevent enzyme access (i.e., high crystallinity). Bacteria in the lower gut can ferment these carbohydrates, but the rate and degree of fermentation in the colon for various fibers can be from approximately 5% for cellulose to nearly complete for pectin [23]. The resulting short-chain fatty acids (SCFA), including butyrate and propionate, are thought to solubilize minerals, thereby improving their absorption and subsequent utilization [24–27].

Prebiotic fibers have been shown to improve calcium absorption and net bone balance during growth. Fructo-oligosaccharides (FOS), galacto-oligosaccharides (GOS), and other prebiotic fibers such as soluble corn fiber (SCF) have resulted in increased calcium absorption in animal and human models. A landmark clinical study in this area showed that pubertal adolescents assigned to 8 g/day mixed short- and long-chain inulin-type fructans increased calcium absorption at 8 weeks and whole-body bone mineral density at 1 year [28].

In a 3-week, randomized, double-blind, placebo-controlled crossover study of 24 adolescents, calcium absorption was increased by 12% when 12 g/day of soluble corn fiber was consumed, compared to a control, in conjunction with a background diet that contained 600 mg/day of calcium [29]. In addition, researchers found that consumption of the soluble corn fiber increased specific beneficial gut bacteria—namely, bifidobacteria, parabacteroidetes, and alistipes—which correlated with the observed increase in calcium absorption and may be a mechanism that enables greater calcium absorption [30]. While the results of this human study only assessed calcium metabolism, a 12-week study conducted in rats investigated the impact of soluble corn fiber on bone indices as well as calcium metabolism [31]. Compared to a cellulose control, soluble corn fiber improved total bone mineral content (BMC), total bone mineral density (BMD), trabecular BMC and BMD, cortical BMC, and cortical area and thickness in the distal femur. Bone strength of the distal femur was also significantly improved by the ingestion of soluble corn fiber. Additional long-term studies in humans are needed to assess potential impact on bone indices.

Prebiotic Study Design Among Preadolescents

Rationale

In view that Malaysian children and adolescents habitually consume low calcium intake, there is merit to study if addition of soluble corn fiber (SCF) to the usual diet will lead to greater calcium absorption and improve bone density accrual at the critical period of peak bone mass attainment. The current studies with SCF are short term, and longer-term studies to track improvements in BMD and BMC are needed.

Abrams et al. [32] had reported that despite an increased in calcium absorption, a deficit of up to 80 g/year of bone calcium deposit still occurs when calcium intake is below 450 mg/day (similar to current calcium intakes among Malaysian children). Hence, the other hypothesis was to test the effects SCF on habitual low calcium intake and when supplemented with adequate calcium intake and their concomitant placebo groups.

Design and Methods

The prebiotic study is a double-blind, randomized, parallel trial where the SCF is consumed in the form of fruit-flavored beverage powder (orange or blackcurrant) to be mixed into a drink with water, with or without calcium and placebo powder. Subjects are randomized into four groups: placebo, 12 g soluble corn fiber (SCF), 600 mg calcium lactate gluconate, and 12 g SCF fiber added with 600 mg calcium lactate gluconate. The intervention period is 12 months, and subjects are healthy preadolescent boys and girls aged 9–11 years.

The inclusion criteria are healthy as determined by standard medical assessment on physical and mental health, Tanner stage 2 based on breast development for girls, and pubic hair in boys, premenarcheal for girls, and having obtained his/her informed consent and parents' or legal guardians' consent. Subjects are excluded if they present with history of serious medical conditions, taking medications on a regular basis which are known to interfere with bone metabolism such as steroids (e.g., asthmatics), practice strict dietary restrictions, and participate in competitive sports such as gymnastics.

The primary outcomes of the study are bone mineral content (BMC) and bone mineral density (BMD) at the total body and lumbar spine, while the secondary outcomes are bone biomarkers of serum CTX1, P1NP, BAP, and osteocalcin. The sample size was calculated based on the minimum clinically significant difference expected to be similar to the effects of inulin on BMC and BMD in preadolescents [28]. The total sample size needed was calculated to be 240 (120 boys and 120 girls).

Participants on the intervention arm will be provided with the supplement in the form of fruit-flavored beverage powder (mix with 200 mL water) containing SCF with/without calcium to be taken in divided doses of 6 g fiber from SCF and/or 300 mg Ca in the morning and evening (to total 12 g fiber from SCF per day and 600 mg Ca/day according to treatment groups). Participants will consume these daily for 12 months. Placebo groups will consume fruit-flavored beverage powder (mix with 200 mL water) with/without added calcium twice a day also in divided doses of 300 mg twice per day to total 600 mg Ca/day according to treatment groups.

Compliance

Compliance is calculated based on percentage of sachets consumed. Compliance is set at 80% as a threshold. Subjects will receive a booklet to fill out each day to note the number of powder sachet drank and timing. Subjects keep all sachet packs after they had consumed the powder and return them to the researchers every month along with their booklet and any uneaten sachets. Compliant days and the number of fruit-flavored beverage packs consumed are counted. Participants can be given a small gift if they returned their calendars and sachets.

Subjects compliance are also enhanced through a rewards system upon fulfilling a minimum of 80% compliance each month, frequent contacts and activities to engage participation such as weekly telephone calls and use of social media to stay in touch with subjects' parents. School talks and activities for children to educate on importance of bone health and nutrition are organized periodically.

Conclusion

A positive calcium balance is mandatory to achieve maximum peak bone mass. Asian children and adolescents have calcium intakes below 500 mg/day. Prebiotic fibers have been shown to improve calcium absorption, and our Malaysian study will add scientific evidence on the role of soluble corn fiber to improve bone accretion in preadolescent children with habitual low calcium intakes.

References

1. Cooper C, Campion G, Melton L. Hip fractures in the elderly: a world-wide projection. Osteoporos Int. 2001;2:285–9.
2. Cooper C, Cole ZA, Holroyd CR, et al. Secular trends in the incidence of hip and other osteoporotic fractures. Osteoporos Int. 2011;22:1277–88.
3. Lau EMC, Lee JK, Suriwongpaisal P, et al. The incidence of hip fracture in four Asian countries. The Asian Osteoporosis Study (AOS). Osteoporos Int. 2001;12:239–43.
4. Cummings SR, Black DM, Nevitt MC, et al. Bone density at various sites for prediction of hip fractures. The Study of Osteoporotic Fractures Research Group. Lancet. 1993;341(8837):72–5.
5. Marshall D, Johnell O, Wedel H. Meta-analysis of how well measures of bone mineral density predict occurrence of osteoporotic fractures. Br Med J. 1996;312(7041):1254–9.
6. Weaver CM, Gordon CM, Janz KF, et al. Osteoporos Int. 2016;27:1281.
7. Riggs BL, Melton LJ, Robb RA, et al. A population-based assessment of rates of bone loss at multiple skeletal sites: evidence for substantial trabecular bone loss in young adult women and men. J Bone Miner Res. 2008;23:205–14.
8. Berger C, Goltzman D, Langsetmo L, et al. Peak bone mass from longitudinal data: implications for the prevalence, pathophysiology, and diagnosis of osteoporosis. J Bone Miner Res. 2010;25:1948–57.
9. Balk EM, Adam GP, Langberg VN, Earley A, Clark P, Ebeling PR, Mithal A, Rizzoli R, Zerbini CAF, Pierroz DD, Dawson-Hughes B, International Osteoporosis Foundation Calcium Steering Committee. Global dietary calcium intake among adults: a systematic review. Osteoporos Int. 2017;28(12):3315–24.
10. Fang A, Li K, Li H, Guo M, He J, Shen X, Song J. Low habitual dietary calcium and linear growth from adolescence to young adulthood: results from the China Health and Nutrition Survey. Sci Rep. 2017;7:9111.
11. Burrow M, Baxter-Jones A, Mirwald R, Macdonald H, McKay H. Bone mineral accrual across growth in a mixed-ethnic group of children: are Asian children disadvantaged from an early age? Calcif Tissue Int. 2009;84:366–78.
12. Wang H, Wang D, Ouyang Y, Huang F, Ding G, Zhang B. Do Chinese children get enough micronutrients? Nutrients. 2017;9:397.
13. Im JG, Kim SH, Lee G-Y, Joung H, Park M-J. Inadequate calcium intake is highly prevalent in Korean children and adolescents: the Korean National Health and Nutrition Examination Survey (KNHANES) 2007–2010. Public Health Nutr. 2013;17(11):2489–95.
14. Poh BK, Ng BK, Haslinda MDS, Shanita SN, Wong JE, Budin SB, Ruzita AT, Ng LO, Khouw I, Karim Norimah A. Nutritional status and dietary intakes of children aged 6 months to 12 years: findings of the Nutrition Survey of Malaysian Children (SEANUTS Malaysia). Br J Nutr. 2013;110:S21–35.
15. Thuyen LD, Hien VT, Binh PT, Yamamoto S. Calcium and vitamin D deficiency in Vietnamese: recommendations for an intervention strategy. J Nutr Sci Vitaminol. 2016;62:1–5.
16. Rojroongwasinkul N, Kijboonchoo K, Wimonpeerapattana W, Purttiponthanee S, Yamborisut U, Boonpraderm A, Kunapan P, Thasanasuwan W, Khouw I. SEANUTS: the nutritional status and dietary intakes of 0.5–12-year-old Thai children. Br J Nutr. 2013;110:S36–44.
17. Sandjaja S, Budiman B, Harahap H, Ernawati F, Soekatri M, Widodo Y, Sumedi E, Rustan E, Sofia G, Syarief SN, Khouw I. Food consumption and nutritional and biochemical status of 0·5–12-year-old Indonesian children: the SEANUTS study. Br J Nutr. 2013;110:S11–20.
18. Singh GM, Micha R, Khatibzadeh S, et al. Global, regional, and national consumption of sugar-sweetened beverages, fruit juices, and milk: a systematic assessment of beverage intake in 187 countries. PLoS One. 10(8):e0124845. https://doi.org/10.1371/journal.pone.0124845.
19. Hayase S, Kumagai Y, Shoji R, Nakahashi S, Tokudome Y, et al. Consumption of bone mineral density-associated nutrients, and their food sources in pre-school Japanese Children. Vitam Miner. 2016;4:133.

20. Weaver CM, Plawecki KL. Dietary calcium: adequacy of a vegetarian diet. Am J Clin Nutr. 1994;59(suppl):1238S–41S.
21. Peltzer K, Pengpid S. Fruits and vegetables consumption and associated factors among in-school adolescents in five Southeast Asian countries. Int J Environ Res Public Health. 2012;9:3575–87.
22. Haron H, Ismail A, Shahar S, Azlan A, Peng LS. Apparent bioavailability of isoflavones in urinary excretions of postmenopausal Malay women consuming tempeh compared with milk. Int J Food Sci Nutr. 2011;62(6):642–50.
23. Cook SI, Sellin JH. Review article: short chain fatty acids in health and disease. Ailment Pharmacol Ther. 1998;12:499–507.
24. Topping DL, Clifton PM. Short-chain fatty acids and human colonic function: roles of resistant starch and nonstarch polysaccharides. Physiol Rev. 2001;81:1031–64.
25. Morohashi T, Sano T, Ohta A, Yamada S. True calcium absorption in the intestine is enhanced by fructooligosaccharide feeding in rats. J Nutr. 1998;128:1815–8.
26. Perrin P, Pierre F, Patry Y, et al. Only fibres promoting a stable butyrate producing colonic ecosystem decrease the rate of aberrant crypt foci in rats. Gut. 2001;48:53–61.
27. Weaver CM. Inulin, oligofructose and bone health: experimental approaches and mechanisms. Br J Nutr. 2005;93(1):S99–S103.
28. Abrams SA, Griffin IJ, Hawthorne KM, et al. A combination of prebiotic short- and long-chain inulin type fructans enhances calcium absorption and bone mineralization in young adolescents. Am J Clin Nutr. 2005;82:471–6.
29. Whisner CM, Martin BR, McCabe GP, et al. Soluble corn fiber effects on calcium absorption and retention in adolescent girls and boys. FASEB J. 2012;26:373.4.25.
30. Nakatsu CH, Clavijo A, Armstrong A, et al. Impact of diet on human gut microbial communities. In: 14th international symposium on microbial ecology (ISME14). Copenhagen, Denmark; 2012.
31. Weaver CM, Martin BR, Story JA, et al. Novel fibers increase bone calcium content and strength beyond efficiency of large intestine fermentation. J Agric Food Chem. 2010;58:8952–7.
32. Abrams SA, Griffin IJ, Hicks PD, Gunn SK. Pubertal girls only partially adapt to low dietary calcium intakes. J Bone Miner Res. 2004;19:759–63.

Part V

Bioactives/Functional Foods

15 Effect of Dried Plum on Bone Biomarkers in Men

Shirin Hooshmand

Introduction

Osteoporosis in men is an overlooked yet increasingly important clinical problem that, historically, has not received the same degree of awareness as with women. Epidemiologic studies demonstrate that male osteoporosis contributes significantly to the burden of osteoporotic fractures, especially among the aging population. In particular, men have higher morbidity and mortality associated with osteoporotic fractures compared with women [1]. Typically thought of as a disease impacting women, increasing attention is being paid to osteoporosis in men; however, little research has been conducted to address the situation. About 47% of men older than 50 years have osteopenia [1], and as many as one in four men over the age of 50 years will develop at least one osteoporosis-related fracture in their lifetime [2, 3]. Each year, about 80,000 men in the USA will break their hip [2]; of these, one in three will die in the first year after a hip fracture, and another one-third will fracture again [4]. In light of these statistics, male osteoporosis is recognized as a growing public health concern, and many clinical guidelines now address the evaluation and treatment of osteoporosis in males. Despite this guidance, male osteoporosis remains an underdiagnosed and undertreated condition [5]. Overall, treatments for osteoporosis in men are less defined than in women, mainly due to (a) the fact that there are fewer randomized clinical trials performed in male populations, (b) the relatively smaller sample sizes in the few studies available, and (c) the lack of long-term studies [6].

S. Hooshmand
School of Exercise and Nutritional Sciences, San Diego State University, San Diego, CA, USA
e-mail: shooshmand@sdsu.edu

© Springer Nature Switzerland AG 2019
C. M. Weaver et al. (eds.), *Nutritional Influences on Bone Health*, https://doi.org/10.1007/978-3-319-98464-3_15

Effects of Dried Plum on Bone

Dried plum is the most effective fruit in both preventing and reversing bone loss. Bone-protective properties of dried plum have been shown in ovariectomized [7, 8] and orchidectomized [9, 10] animal models of osteoporosis and in postmenopausal women [11, 12]. The beneficial effects of dried plum were also tested on male young adult with normal bones vs. old mice with bone loss. The results demonstrated that dried plum increased bone volume above basal levels by nearly 50% in the young adults and 40% in the old mice. Dietary dried plum not only prevented bone loss but also replaced bone that had already been lost due to aging. The magnitude of the changes in bone volume was similar to those in gonadal hormone-deficient male (+36%) and female (+50%) rats fed diets supplemented with dried plum [9]. The effects of the dried plum diet were greatest in the young adult mice, suggesting that although both adult and old mice can respond to dried plum, the effects are somewhat blunted in the aged mice. In almost all cases, the response of adult mice to lower doses of dried plum was similar to the response to higher doses of dried plum, whereas old mice showed little or no response to lower doses of dried plum [13]. Although several animal studies have demonstrated bone-protective effects of dried plum, no human study has evaluated the effect of dried plum on bone metabolism in men.

Dried Plum Improves Bone Biomarkers in Men

To determine whether the addition of 100 g dried plum to the diets of men, regardless of their bone status, can positively influences their indices of bone turnover in comparison with their corresponding baseline values and the control regimen, we conducted a controlled randomized trial in which 66 men (50–79 years of age) received either 100 g dried plum/day or a control regimen for 6 months. All participants received 500 mg of calcium carbonate plus 10 μg (400 IU) of vitamin D_3 (cholecalciferol) daily. The rationale for choosing the dried plum dose (100 g/day) was that this amount has been used in previous studies [11, 12] and has been found effective in preventing bone loss in postmenopausal women. Even though we recently showed that 50 g/day dried plum is as effective as 100 g/day dried plum in preventing bone loss in postmenopausal women [14], we proposed to use 100 g/day dose for this study: (1) because men on average have a bigger body size and (2) because this is the first human study evaluating the bone-protective properties of dried plum in men; therefore, starting with a higher dose increases the probability of detecting significant effects. Subjects treated with any prescription medications known to alter bone and calcium metabolism such as calcitonin, bisphosphonates, raloxifene, and/or anabolic agents such as parathyroid hormone, growth hormone, or steroids within 3 months before the start of the study were excluded. In addition, subjects with metabolic bone disease, renal disease, cancer, cardiovascular disease, diabetes mellitus, respiratory disease, gastrointestinal disease, liver disease or other chronic diseases, and heavy smokers (>20 cigarettes/day) were excluded. Men who regularly consumed dried plum or prune juice were not included in the study. A complete medical history and a dietary vitamin D and calcium questionnaire (SCQ2002) were obtained from the subjects before initiating the treatments. The subjects were advised to maintain their usual physical activity and diet pattern throughout the duration of the study. The subjects completed a 3-day food record and physical activity (IPAQ) questionnaire at baseline, 3 months, and 6 months. Anthropometric data were collected at baseline and 6 months, and height and weight were used to calculate BMI (kg/m^2). Characteristics of study participants are displayed in Table 15.1. Bone density was assessed at the beginning and at the end of the treatment by dual-energy X-ray absorptiometry (LUNAR Prodigy Advanced, GE Healthcare Lunar, Madison, WI, USA) equipped with appropriate software for whole-body, lumbar spine, hip, and forearm BMD. To better understand bone structure changes and to differentiate between cortical and trabecular bone changes, bone structure was assessed using high-resolution peripheral quantitative computed tomography (pQCT, Stratec XCT3000 scanner, Bone Diagnostics, Inc.). The distal tibia was scanned at baseline and final visits. Venous blood samples were obtained after an overnight fast from each subject at baseline, 3 months, and 6 months of the study for various analyses. Blood samples were centrifuged at 1200 × *g* for 15 min at 4 °C, and serum samples were separated, divided into aliquots, and stored at −80 °C until analyses. Changes in bone-specific alkaline phosphatase (BAP) and tartrate-resistant acid phosphatase 5b (TRAP-5b) were analyzed at baseline, 3 months, and 6 months using ELISA kits from Quidel Corporation (San Diego, CA, USA).

Forty men (21 on 0 g/day dried plum and 19 on 100 g/day dried plum) completed the baseline, 3-month, and 6-month visits so far (Fig. 15.1). As expected, baseline characteristics were not significantly different by group for men enrolled in the study (Table 15.1). Age, height, body weight, and BMI were similar at baseline and between the two treatment groups. The 40 participants who completed the study so far adhered to the regimens, as indicated by a self-monitoring calendar provided to them on a monthly basis. Overall, the dried plum treatment was well accepted and considered to be palatable, as stated by the subjects. Mean serum concentrations of biomarkers of bone metabolism, BAP, and TRAP-5b are presented in Table 15.2. Dried plum consumption resulted in a reduction in serum TRAP-5b levels, a marker of bone resorption, at 3 months compared to baseline, while there were no significant changes in serum TRAP-5b levels in the control group (0 g/day dried plum). BAP, a marker of bone formation, did not change after 3 months in either group.

Table 15.1 Characteristics of study participants

	Control	Dried plum	*P* value
Age (years)	64 ± 6	63 ± 7	0.713
Height (cm)	178 ± 7	175 ± 6	0.081
Weight (kg)	88.5 ± 15	88.5 ± 13	0.469
BMI (kg/m^2)	27.5 ± 3.6	27.8 ± 3.6	0.743

Values are mean ± standard deviations, there were no statistically significant differences observed between baseline values of two groups. *BMI* body mass index

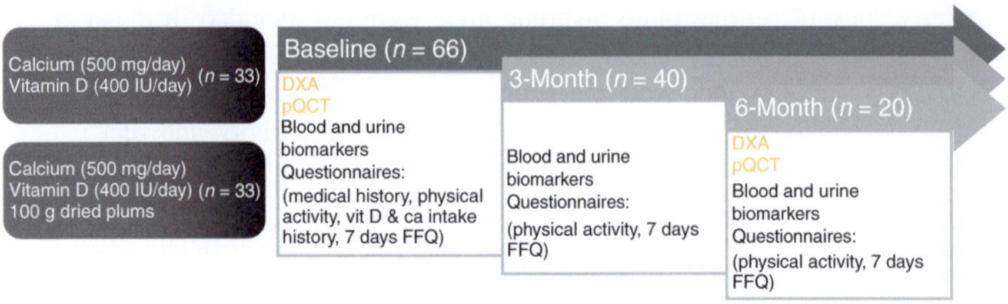

Fig. 15.1 Flowchart of the study design and study participant

Table 15.2 Effect of dried plum on bone biomarkers

	Control (n = 21)			Dried plum (n = 19)			P value
Biomarkers	Baseline	3-month	P value	Baseline	3-month	P value	(group × time)
BAP (U/L)	24.9 ± 4.1	23.9 ± 4.0	0.12	25.5 ± 8.1	24.3 ± 8.1	0.29	0.08
TRAP5b (U/L)	3.2 ± 1.4	2.9 ± 0.9	0.1	2.7 ± 0.9	2.4 ± 0.7	0.006	0.8

Values are mean ± SD. *BAP* bone-specific alkaline phosphatase, *TRAP-5b* tartrate-resistant acid phosphatase-5b

Conclusions

Dried plum has potent effects on bone in terms of bone mass, microarchitecture, and strength in osteopenic male rats. In our clinical study we have seen suppression of bone resorption marker, TRAP5b, after 3 months of dried plum consumption in men. These findings suggest that dried plum bone-protective effects mediated in part through suppression of bone resorption.

References

1. Lambert JK, Zaidi M, Mechanick JI. Male osteoporosis: epidemiology and the pathogenesis of aging bones. Curr Osteoporos Rep. 2011;9(4):229–36.
2. National Osteoporosis Foundation [webpage on the Internet] Just for Men. Accessed 10 Dec 2017. http://nof.org/articles/236.
3. Johnell O, Kanis JA. An estimate of the worldwide prevalence and disability associated with osteoporotic fractures. Osteoporos Int. 2006;17(12):1726–33.
4. von Friesendorff M, McGuigan FE, Besjakov J, Akesson K. Hip fracture in men-survival and subsequent fractures: a cohort study with 22-year follow-up. J Am Geriatr Soc. 2011;59(5):806–13.
5. Willson T, Nelson SD, Newbold J, Nelson RE, LaFleur J. The clinical epidemiology of male osteoporosis: a review of the recent literature. Clin Epidemiol. 2015;7:65–76.
6. Giusti A, Bianchi G. Treatment of primary osteoporosis in men. Clin Interv Aging. 2014;30(10):105–15.
7. Deyhim F, Stoecker BJ, Brusewitz GH, Devareddy L, Arjmandi BH. Dried plum reverses bone loss in an osteopenic rat model of osteoporosis. Menopause. 2005;12(6):755–62.
8. Arjmandi BH, Lucas EA, Juma S, Soliman A, Stoecker BJ, Khalil DA, Smith BJ, Wang C. Dried plums prevent ovariectomy-induced bone loss in rats. JANA. 2001;4(1):50–6.

9. Bu SY, Lucas EA, Franklin M, Marlow D, Brackett DJ, Boldrin EA, Devareddy L, Arjmandi BH, Smith BJ. Comparison of dried plum supplementation and intermittent PTH in restoring bone in osteopenic orchidectomized rats. Osteoporos Int. 2007;18(7):931–42.
10. Franklin M, et al. Dried plum prevents bone loss in a male osteoporosis model via IGF-I and the RANK pathway. Bone. 2006;39(6):1331–42.
11. Arjmandi BH, Khalil DA, Lucas EA, Georgis A, Stoecker BJ, Hardin C, Payton ME, Wild RA. Dried plums improve indices of bone formation in postmenopausal women. J Womens Health Gend Based Med. 2002;11(1):61–8.
12. Hooshmand S, Chai SC, Saadat RL, Payton ME, Brummel-Smith K, Arjmandi BH. Comparative effects of dried plum and dried apple on bone in postmenopausal women. Br J Nutr. 2011;106(06):923–30.
13. Halloran BP, Wronski TJ, VonHerzen DC, Chu V, Xia X, Pingel JE, Williams AA, Smith BJ. Dietary dried plum increases bone mass in adult and aged male mice. J Nutr. 2010;40(10):1781–7.
14. Hooshmand S, Kern M, Metti D, Shamloufard P, Chai SC, Johnson SA, Payton ME, Arjmandi BH. The effect of two doses of dried plum on bone density and bone biomarkers in osteopenic postmenopausal women: a randomized, controlled trial. Osteoporos Int. 2016;27(7):2271–9.

Bone-Protective Chinese Herbs: The Story of Fructus Ligustri Lucidi

16

Sisi Cao, Xiao-Li Dong, Yan Zhang, and Man-Sau Wong

Introduction

Fructus Ligustri Lucidi (FLL, Chinese name *Nuzhenzi*, 女貞子), the fruit of *Ligustrum lucidum Ait*, has been used in traditional Chinese medicine (TCM) for over 1000 years to treat age-related disease such as menopausal problems. FLL was first described in *Shen Nong Ben Cao Jing*, the ancient Chinese material medica. In TCM theory, FLL could effectively preserve healthy energy through nourishing the kidneys and liver. Therefore, it is known as a kidney-tonifying herbal medicine and is commonly prescribed in formulae to treat symptoms such as tinnitus, backache, insomnia, blurred vision, and other symptoms that occur with aging [1].

There are several types of chemical constituents isolated from FLL, including 40 triterpenoids, 48 iridoids, 10 flavones, 10 phenylethanoid glycosides, and other components such as amino acid, polysaccharide, fatty acid, pigment, volatile components, and minor elements [2]. Triterpenoids, which take up 5.61% of the total content of FLL, are a major type of components found in FLL [3]. There are 40 triterpenoids identified in FLL during the past 40 years. They belong to four skeleton types: oleanane (I), ursane (II), lupine (III), and dammarane (IV) (Fig. 16.1) [4]. Among the triterpenoids found in FLL, oleanolic acid (OA) and ursolic acid (UA) are the two most abundant, and they are two of the major active ingredients found in FLL (Fig. 16.1).

S. Cao · X.-L. Dong · Y. Zhang
Department of Applied Biology and Chemical Technology, The Hong Kong Polytechnic University, Kowloon, Hong Kong

M.-S. Wong (✉)
Department of Applied Biology and Chemical Technology, The Hong Kong Polytechnic University, Kowloon, Hong Kong

State Key Laboratory of Chinese Medicine and Molecular Pharmacology (Incubation), The Hong Kong Polytechnic University Shenzhen Research Institute, Shenzhen, China
e-mail: man-sau.wong@polyu.edu.hk

© Springer Nature Switzerland AG 2019

C. M. Weaver et al. (eds.), *Nutritional Influences on Bone Health*,
https://doi.org/10.1007/978-3-319-98464-3_16

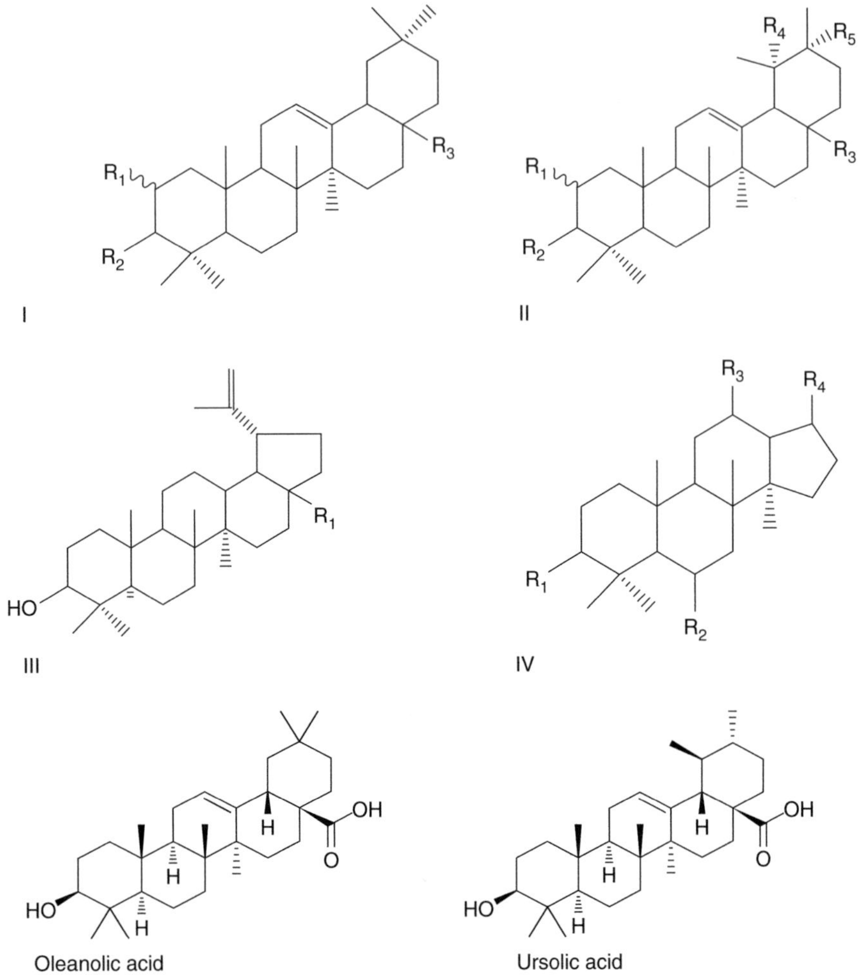

Fig. 16.1 Skeleton structures of the triterpenoids identified in *Fructus Ligustri Lucidi*. Triterpenoids backbone: oleanane (I), ursane (II), lupine (III), and dammarane (IV) as well as the chemical structure of oleanolic acid (OA) and ursolic acid (UA)

Oleanolic acid (3β-hydroxyolean-12-en-28-oic acid) is a biologically active pentacyclic triterpenoid compound that has been identified in over 1620 plant species [5, 6]. The compound is named after olive (*Olea europaea*), which contains a large amount of OA [7]. Ursolic acid (3β-hydroxyurs-12-en-28-oic acid) is the isomer of OA. They are usually present in combination and share most of the pharmacological properties [8]. OA and UA are the two compounds used in the quality control of FLL extract [9]. In our group, we determined the content of both OA and UA in the ethanol extract of FLL to confirm its quality (Fig. 16.2). The reverse-phase HPLC was used to qualitatively analyze the OA and UA content in FLL as previously reported [1].

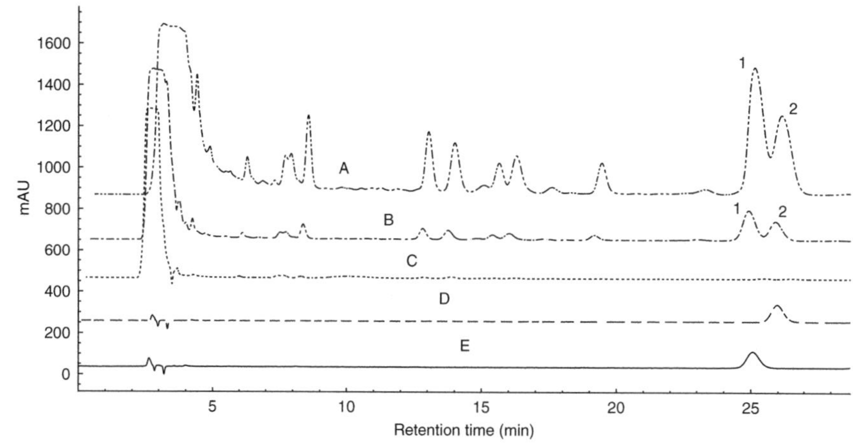

Fig. 16.2 Reverse-phase HPLC chromatograms for quantitative analysis of OA and UA in FLL ethanol extract and its subfractions. The chromatographs of ethyl acetate fraction of FLL (**A**), 70% ethanol extract of FLL (**B**), and water fraction of FLL (**C**) are shown in the upper graph, and the standards of OA (**D**) and UA (**E**) are shown in the lower graph. OA (peak 1) and UA (peak 2) can be clearly resolved from other miscellaneous compounds and identified by retention time. The quality of FLL ethanol extract is confirmed by the identification of OA and UA. (From Dong et al. [24])

FLL Regulated Bone Turnover and Improved Calcium Balance in Mature OVX Rat Model

FLL has been used in TCM formula for bone health since ancient times. Studies on the anti-osteoporotic effect of FLL using evidence-based methods were first reported by our group. Zhang et al. [1] first demonstrated the positive effect of ethanol extract of FLL on enhancing calcium balance and suppressing bone turnover markers such as serum osteocalcin and urinary deoxypyridinoline in 3-month-old ovariectomized (OVX) rats. FLL extract could significantly prevent OVX-induced calcium loss by suppressing urinary calcium excretion, increasing intestinal calcium absorption rate, and increasing bone calcium content in mature OVX rats.

FLL Improved Bone Properties via Increasing Calcium Balance and Regulating Calciotropic Hormone Levels in Aged Normal and OVX Rat Models

The subsequent study was designed to study whether the bone-protective effect of FLL ethanol extract acts through the estrogen axis or the calcium-vitamin D axis. Eleven-month-old sham and OVX rats were orally administered FLL or its vehicle and pair-fed with diets containing three different calcium levels: low-calcium diet (LCD, 0.1% Ca), medium-calcium diet (MCD, 0.6% Ca), and high-calcium diet (HCD, 1.2% Ca) for 12 weeks. The ethanol extract of FLL significantly improved bone mineral density and bone mineral content at multiple bone sites including tibial and femoral diaphyses as well as the lumbar vertebra (LV-2) in aged OVX rats fed with LCD or MCD. The action of FLL might be mediated by its direct action on enhancing bone mineralization process [10]. FLL also exerted positive effects on calcium retention by significantly reducing urinary and fecal calcium loss in both normal and OVX rats fed with MCD or HCD [11, 12]. The results on calciotropic hormone levels indicated that FLL improved bone health via its action on the vitamin D-PTH axis by stimulating the production of $1,25(OH)_2D_3$ in aged rats and such actions are independent of the estrogen status in the female rats [11]. In addition, vitamin-D-dependent duodenal CaBP9k and renal CaBP28k mRNA expressions in aged female rat were increased by FLL [12]. Therefore, improvement of calcium balance by FLL was found to be associated, at least in part, with increase in the levels of circulating $1,25(OH)_2D_3$ in both aged normal and OVX rats.

FLL Increased Circulating 1,25D Levels via Modulating CYP27B1 Expressions and Activities

The increased circulating $1,25(OH)_2D_3$ levels in aged normal and OVX rats after FLL treatment were further demonstrated to be via its action on inducing renal 25-hydroxyvitamin D 1α-hydroxylase (CYP27B1) mRNA and protein expressions. The direct effect of FLL on increasing renal CYP27B1 mRNA expression and enzymatic activity was confirmed by using primary cultures of rat renal proximal tubule cells [13]. At the same time, the increase in $1,25(OH)_2D_3$ levels by FLL might also be associated with its action to suppress renal mRNA expression of 25-hydroxyvitamin D 24-hydroxylase (CYP24A1) both in vivo [11] and in vitro [14].

OA and UA Are the Bioactives in FLL Accounting for Its Actions on Bone, Calcium Balance, and Calciotropic Hormone (1,25D and PTH) Levels in Aged Female Rats

In the present study, we aimed at identifying the active ingredients in FLL extract that accounts for its positive actions. We focused on OA and UA as their direct effects on bone protection had already been extensively studied. Studies by Li et al. showed that OA glucosides and their derivatives reduced the formation of osteoclast-like multinucleated cells in a primary co-culture system [15–17]. Bian et al. demonstrated that oral consumption of 20 mg/kg/day OA for 3 months protected OVX rats against bone loss and induced osteoblastic differentiation of bone mesenchymal stem cells (MSCs) [18]. A mechanistic study by Xu et al. demonstrated that the inhibitory effects of OA on osteoclastogenesis were mediated by the RANKL signaling pathway in RAW264.7 cells [19], while by Shu et al. reported the stimulatory effects of OA on human MSCs toward osteoprogenitor cells involving the inhibition of Notch signaling pathway [20]. On the other hand, the bone-protective effect of UA was shown to stimulate osteoblast differentiation through activating mitogen-activated protein (MAP) kinases and transcription factors in mouse osteoblastic MC3T3-E1 cells [21]. Studies by Tan et al. [22] demonstrated an UA-rich herb

(*Eriobotrya japonica*) significantly improved the ovariectomy-induced deterioration of bone mineral density in OVX mice. The mechanism involved in the inhibitory effect of UA on osteoclastogenesis might be via inhibiting RANKL-induced osteoclastogenesis via c-Jun N-terminal kinase (JNK) and NF-κB signaling pathway [23]. Therefore, as the two most abundant compounds found in FLL, OA and UA were employed to determine if they are the active ingredients that account for the positive actions of FLL on bone, calcium balance, and vitamin D-PTH axis.

Aged (13-month-old) female rats were randomly divided into five groups ($n = 8$/group) with oral administration of drug or vehicle treatment for 3 months. The five groups were medium-calcium diet (MCD, 0.6% calcium), high-calcium diet (HCD, 1.2% calcium), MCD + FLL (700 mg/kg/day), MCD + OA (25 mg/kg/day), and MCD + OA (25 mg/kg/day) + UA (8.3 mg/kg/day). There was also a group of mature (3-month-old) female rats fed with MCD to act as the positive control. The dosages of OA (25 mg) and UA (8.3 mg) used were the naturally occurring amounts in FLL (700 mg). Bone properties were measured by micro-CT (viva-CT40; Scanco Medical, Switzerland); bone calcium was determined by atomic absorption spectrophotometer (PerkinElmer, AAnalyst 100 Spectrometer, Norwalk, CT, USA); calcium balance was calculated by calcium intake minus urinary and fecal calcium excretion; serum PTH (Immutopics, Inc., San Clemente, CA, USA) and 1,25$(OH)_2D_3$ (Immundiagnostik AG, Bensheim, Germany) were measured by commercial kits.

The effects of FLL, OA, and OA + UA on the proximal tibia of aged rats are illustrated by their representative three-dimensional images obtained from micro-CT analysis (Fig. 16.3). Compared with mature rats, aged rats had significant bone loss

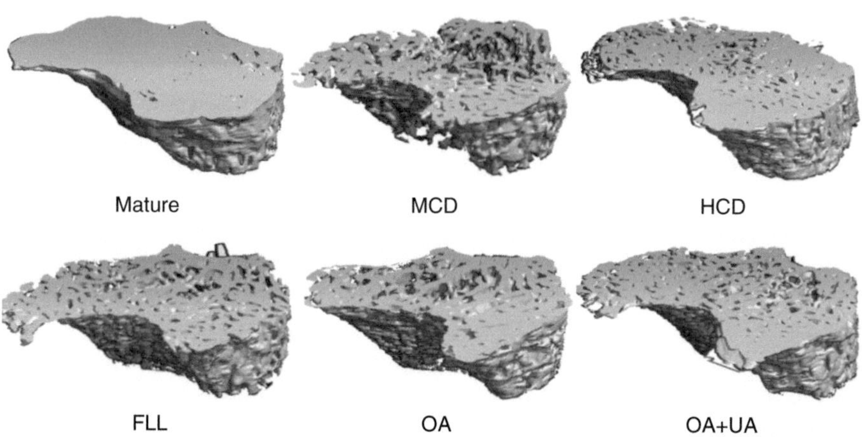

Fig. 16.3 Representative micro-CT three-dimensional images of the trabecular bone microarchitecture of proximal tibia in mature and aged female rats. Thirteen-month-old aged female Sprague Dawley rats were randomly divided into five groups ($n = 8$/group) with oral administration of drug or vehicle treatment for 3 months. The five groups were medium-calcium diet (MCD, 0.6% calcium), high-calcium diet (HCD, 1.2% calcium), MCD + FLL (FLL, 700 mg/kg/day), MCD + OA (OA, 25 mg/kg/day), and MCD + OA (25 mg/kg/day) + UA (8.3 mg/kg/day) (OA + UA). There was also a group of 3-month-old mature female rats fed with MCD (mature, $n = 8$) to act as the positive control group. Left tibia was collected upon sacrifice and scanned at proximal tibia head by micro-CT system (viva-CT40, Scanco Medical, Switzerland). A constant threshold of 300 was used to generate three-dimensional images for all samples

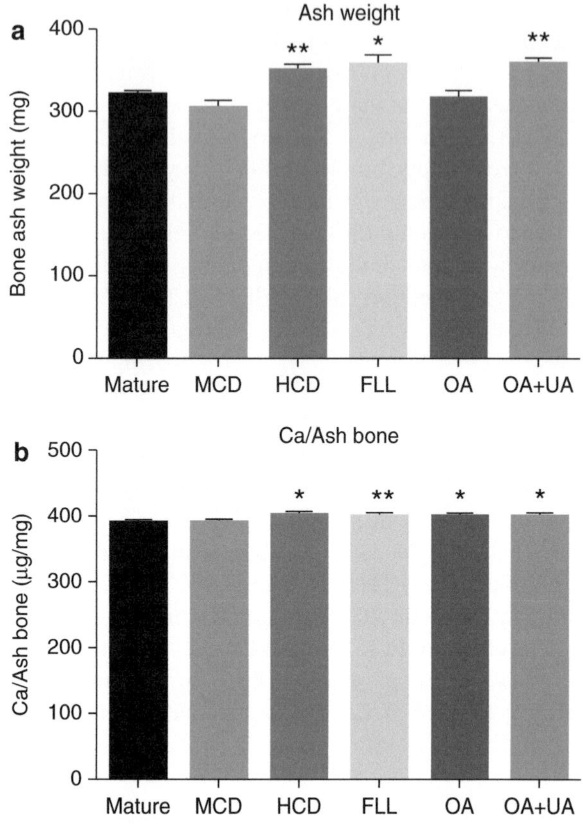

Fig. 16.4 Effect of FLL, OA, and OA + UA on bone calcium content in aged female rats. A group of 3-month-old mature rats were fed with MCD, and five groups of 13-month-old aged female rats were orally administrated with drug (FLL, OA, and OA + UA) or vehicle for 3 months. (**a**) Ash weight of rat tibia (mg); (**b**) calcium content of rat tibia. Data were presented by mean ± SEM and analyzed by one-way ANOVA followed by Tukey's multiple comparison tests. * $P < 0.05$ and ** $P < 0.01$, vs. MCD

at the proximal tibia. The bone deterioration in aged female rats was to some degree prevented by treatment with high-calcium diet as well as treatment with FLL, OA, or OA + UA. Consistent with micro-CT result, bone ash weight was significantly increased by FLL and OA + UA (Fig. 16.4a), and bone calcium content was significantly increased by all treatment with FLL and in aged female rats (Fig. 16.4b).

In addition to the bone-protective effect, the action of FLL on enhancing calcium balance in aged female rats was also confirmed (Fig. 16.5a). Without altering serum calcium levels, treatment with OA and OA + UA also significantly increased net calcium balance by suppressing urinary calcium loss in aged female rats (data not shown). Taken together, this study confirmed that FLL, as well as its active constituents OA and OA + UA, improved calcium balance by increasing the utilization of dietary calcium without mobilizing calcium in the bone of aged female rats.

Unlike our previous study [13], the serum $1{,}25(OH)_2D_3$ level remained unaltered by the treatments in the present study. The mechanism involved in the unaltered $1{,}25(OH)_2D_3$ level needs further investigation. On the other hand, FLL and OA + UA treatments significantly suppressed the age-induced secondary hyperparathyroidism in aged female rats (data not shown). This is in agreement with our previous report that FLL managed to maintain serum PTH level within a normal and narrow range in aged OVX rats fed with different levels of dietary calcium [11].

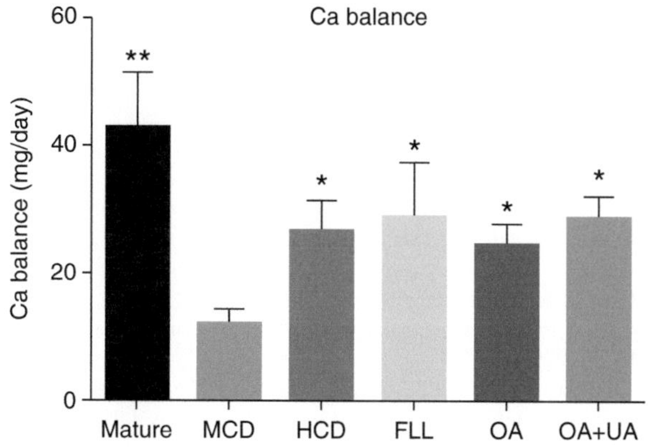

Fig. 16.5 Effect of FLL, OA, and OA + UA on calcium balance in aged female rats. A group of 3-month-old mature rats were fed with MCD, and five groups of 13-month-old aged female rats were orally administrated with drug (FLL, OA, and OA + UA) or vehicle for 3 months. Ca balance = Ca intake − (urinary Ca − fecal Ca). Data were presented by mean ± SEM and analyzed by one-way ANOVA followed by Tukey's multiple comparison tests. $*P < 0.05$ and $**P < 0.01$, vs. MCD

In the present study, more evidence was provided for the effectiveness of using FLL, OA, and OA + UA for bone protection and improving calcium balance using an aged female rat model. OA + UA could be considered as the active ingredient of FLL ethanol extract that accounts for its positive action on improving bone properties through enhancing calcium balance and modulating PTH level in aged female rats.

Conclusion

FLL is an herbal mixture that exerts osteoprotective effects via multiple in vivo targets. Apart from the reported direct anabolic effects of FLL on bone, studies of our group provided strong evidence that the osteoprotective effects of FLL were also associated with its actions on improving calcium balance and modulating the vitamin D-PTH axis. OA and UA, and especially their combination in their naturally occurring ratio, can be regarded as the active constituents of FLL. It is hoped that our study could provide some mechanistic basis for the developing of FLL and its bioactive constituents OA + UA into an alternative, low-cost, and orally administrated regimen for prevention and treatment of osteoporosis.

Acknowledgment We thank the State Key Laboratory of Chinese Medicine and Molecular Pharmacology (Incubation) Shenzhen and PolyU Food Safety and Technology Research Center for their support. This work was supported by the University Grants Committee of the Hong Kong Special Administrative Region, China (POLYU 5402/04M), National Natural Science Foundation of China (81528024), and Research Studentship of the Hong Kong Polytechnic University for Dr. Xiaoli Dong and Dr. Sisi Cao.

References

1. Zhang Y, Lai WP, Leung PC, Wu CF, et al. Effects of Fructus Ligustri Lucidi extract on bone turnover and calcium balance in ovariectomized rats. Biol Pharm Bull. 2006;29:291–6.
2. Gao L, Li C, Wang Z, Liu X, et al. Ligustri lucidi fructus as a traditional Chinese medicine: a review of its phytochemistry and pharmacology. Nat Prod Res. 2015;29:493–510.
3. Tan W, Liu W, Lu F, Liu J, et al. Extraction and content determination of triterpenoids in Fructus ligustri lucidi. Food Sci. 2006;11:057.
4. Wu L, Yin S, Wang S, Tian Y, et al. Study on the chemical constituents of the fruits of Ligustrum lucidum Ait. Chin J Med Chem. 1995;6:117–28.
5. Fai YM, Tao CC. A review of presence of oleanolic acid in natural products. Natura Proda Medica. 2009;2:77–290.
6. Fukushima EO, Seki H, Ohyama K, Ono E, et al. CYP716A subfamily members are multifunctional oxidases in triterpenoid biosynthesis. Plant Cell Physiol. 2011;52:2050–61.
7. Simonsen JL, Ross W. The terpenes: the triterpenes and their derivatives. Cambridge: Cambridge University Press; 1957.
8. Liu J. Pharmacology of oleanolic acid and ursolic acid. J Ethnopharmacol. 1995;49:57–68.
9. China Pharmacopoeia Committee. Chinese pharmacopoeia. Beijing: China Medica Science Press; 2010. p. 276.
10. Zhang Y, Leung PC, Che CT, Chow HK, et al. Improvement of bone properties and enhancement of mineralization by ethanol extract of Fructus Ligustri Lucidi. Br J Nutr. 2008;99: 494–502.
11. Zhang Y, Dong XL, Leung PC, Che CT, et al. Fructus ligustri lucidi extract improves calcium balance and modulates the calciotropic hormone level and vitamin D-dependent gene expression in aged ovariectomized rats. Menopause. 2008;15:558–65.
12. Zhang Y, Lai WP, Leung PC, Che CT, et al. Improvement of Ca balance by Fructus Ligustri Lucidi extract in aged female rats. Osteoporos Int. 2008;19:235–42.
13. Dong XL, Zhang Y, Favus MJ, Che CT, et al. Ethanol extract of Fructus Ligustri Lucidi increases circulating 1,25-dihydroxyvitamin D3 by inducing renal 25-hydroxyvitamin D-1alpha hydroxylase activity. Menopause. 2010;17:1174–81.
14. Dong XL, Cao SS, Zhou LP, Denney L, et al. Ethanol extract of Fructus ligustri lucidi increased circulating 1,25(OH)2D3 levels, but did not improve calcium balance in mature ovariectomized rats. Am J Chin Med. 2016;44:1237–53.
15. Li J-X, Hareyama T, Tezuka Y, Zhang Y, et al. Five new oleanolic acid glycosides from Achyranthes bidentata with inhibitory activity on osteoclast formation. Planta Med. 2005;71:673–9.
16. Zhang Y, Li J, Zhao J, Wang S, et al. Synthesis and activity of oleanolic acid derivatives, a novel class of inhibitors of osteoclast formation. Bioorg Med Chem Lett. 2005;15:1629–32.
17. Li JF, Zhao Y, Cai MM, Li XF, et al. Synthesis and evaluation of a novel series of heterocyclic oleanolic acid derivatives with anti-osteoclast formation activity. Eur J Med Chem. 2009;44:2796–806.
18. Bian Q, Liu SF, Huang JH, Yang Z, et al. Oleanolic acid exerts an osteoprotective effect in ovariectomy-induced osteoporotic rats and stimulates the osteoblastic differentiation of bone mesenchymal stem cells in vitro. Menopause. 2012;19:225–33.
19. Xu D, Lyu Y, Chen X, Zhu X, et al. Fructus Ligustri Lucidi ethanol extract inhibits osteoclastogenesis in RAW264.7 cells via the RANKL signaling pathway. Mol Med Rep. 2016;14:4767–74.
20. Shu B, Zhao Y, Wang Y, Wang G, et al. Oleanolic acid enhances mesenchymal stromal cell osteogenic potential by inhibition of notch signaling. Sci Rep. 2017;7:7002.
21. Lee SU, Park SJ, Kwak HB, Oh J, et al. Anabolic activity of ursolic acid in bone: stimulating osteoblast differentiation in vitro and inducing new bone formation in vivo. Pharmacol Res. 2008;58:290–6.

22. Tan H, Furuta S, Nagata T, Ohnuki K, et al. Inhibitory effects of the leaves of loquat (Eriobotrya japonica) on bone mineral density loss in ovariectomized mice and osteoclast differentiation. J Agric Food Chem. 2014;62:836–41.
23. Jiang C, Xiao F, Gu X, Zhai Z, et al. Inhibitory effects of ursolic acid on osteoclastogenesis and titanium particle-induced osteolysis are mediated primarily via suppression of NF-kappaB signaling. Biochimie. 2015;111:107–18.
24. Dong XL, Zhao M, Wong KK, Che CT, et al. Improvement of calcium balance by Fructus Ligustri Lucidi extract in mature female rats was associated with the induction of serum parathyroid hormone levels. Br J Nutr. 2012;108:92–101.

Part VI

Diet Patterns/Micronutrients

The Relationship Between Dietary Fat and Sarcopenia, Skeletal Muscle Loss, Osteoporosis and Risk of Fractures in Aging

17

Ailsa A. Welch and Richard P. G. Hayhoe

Introduction

The Rationale for Understanding the Relationship Between Dietary Fat Intake and Skeletal Muscle Mass and Bone Health

This chapter provides an overview of dietary fat intake and the research into its importance to musculoskeletal health. We focus on the available evidence concerning total fat, saturated fatty acids, monounsaturated fatty acids, total polyunsaturated fatty acids (PUFA), n-6 PUFA, n-3 PUFA and the polyunsaturated to saturated fatty acid (P:S) ratio.

We review the evidence in relation to dietary fat and aging of the musculoskeletal system for middle and older age populations. In particular, we focus on the relevance of fat in the diet to risk of osteoporosis and fractures as well as to loss of skeletal muscle mass with aging and sarcopenia.

Overall, there is a large body of scientific research associating the importance of dietary fat to cardiovascular and metabolic conditions but very little research on its relevance to the health of the musculoskeletal system [1].

Fat in the Diet

Fat intake in the diet is highly variable both in the total amount consumed and the amount of the different types of fatty acids consumed within it.

A. A. Welch (✉) · R. P. G. Hayhoe
Department of Public Health and Primary Care, Norwich Medical School,
The University of East Anglia, Norwich, Norfolk, UK
e-mail: a.welch@uea.ac.uk

© Springer Nature Switzerland AG 2019

C. M. Weaver et al. (eds.), *Nutritional Influences on Bone Health*,
https://doi.org/10.1007/978-3-319-98464-3_17

Fat consists of the main types or classes of fatty acids: saturated (SFA) and polyunsaturated fatty acids (PUFA) which are further divided into omega 6 (from herein referred to as n-6 PUFA) and omega-3 PUFA (referred to as n-3 PUFA). These fatty acids are classified according to the number of double bonds (also referred to unsaturated fatty acids) that form their structure. Saturated fatty acids (SFA) have no double bonds, monounsaturated fatty acids (MUFA) have one double bond and polyunsaturated fatty acids (PUFA) have two or more double bonds.

It is important to realise that all sources of fat are mixtures of these different classes of fatty acids, for instance, olive oil is composed of 14.3% saturated fatty acids, 73% monounsaturated fatty acids and 8.2% polyunsaturated fatty acids whereas butter contains 63% saturated fatty acids, 25.4% monounsaturated fatty acids and 3.4% polyunsaturated fatty acids [2].

Dietary intake of fat is extremely variable within and between populations. This is largely attributable to the different sources of fat used in food preparation, added to meals and used in food manufacturing. There is regional variation within Europe. Two studies that estimated fat intakes across the ten countries in the EPIC-Europe Study (European Prospective Investigation into Cancer and Nutrition Study) found large variations in the amounts and types of fats, oils and margarines consumed [3]. For example, the contribution of fat to total energy intake ranged between 29.7% in men in Italy and 42% in women in Italy [3]. Average MUFA intake ranged between 10% and 13% of energy, with a high proportion derived from animal sources. SFA intake ranged from 9% to 16% of energy with PUFA intake ranging 4% to 8% of energy. There were also substantial differences in food sources of dietary lipids and in added fats (vegetable oils, margarines and butter varied across the countries) [3].

Worldwide, the variations in fat intake are even greater. Micha et al. in their comprehensive review of the variation of the different types of fatty acid intake at a global level found saturated fat ranged from 4% to 10% in large parts of Africa, South America and East Asia [4]. On the other hand, in northern America intakes of SFA ranged from 10.0% to 12.9%, and in Europe and Russia, these were above 14.5% of energy. Overall there was a 5.5-fold variation in intake [4]. Overall variation in n-6 PUFA was approximately threefold, and for trans fatty acid intake this was fivefold. Long-chain n-3 PUFA intakes, of seafood origin, ranged from 5 to 3886 mg/d, and plant-based ALA range was tenfold (from 302 to 3205 mg/day) [4].

Fat is relevant for dietary prevention strategies as the type and proportion of fat in the diet is modifiable firstly by food manufacturers, through changing the formulation of products by using fats or oils with preferable profiles of fatty acids in food production, and secondly by individuals within populations who can modify fats used in cooking and consumed with meals. Total fat as a proportion of intake can also be modified. Thirdly, government policy for food consumption (dietary guidelines) can recommend types and amounts of fat in the diet for individuals and manufacturers.

Given the variability in fat and fatty acid intake, the potential for modifications of fat intake by individuals and governments for population prevention strategies of skeletal muscle, bone health and risk of fractures could be important.

The Importance of Maintaining Good Skeletal Muscle and Bone in Aging for Prevention of Fractures

Bone is a metabolically active organ which is continuously undergoing remodelling through a dynamic equilibrium of osteoclast-mediated bone resorption and osteoblast-mediated bone deposition, with little net change in total bone mass. Indeed, it is estimated that the whole skeleton is replaced by new bone every 10 years [5]. However, beyond the age of 40 years, when peak bone mass has been achieved, the balance undergoes a shift resulting in a relative increase in bone resorption and thus a net loss of bone mass. Where there is significant loss of bone mass and density, this may manifest as osteoporosis. Osteoporosis thus represents a major public health concern for our aging population [6]. Indeed, the relevance of an aging population is highlighted by study of the global variation of osteoporotic fractures which shows that Europe, followed by the Western Pacific, Southeast Asia and the Americas, has the greatest number of fractures, with just 3% of total fractures worldwide accounted for by other regions [7]. Women are at particular risk, with 1 in 2 women over 50 expected to sustain an osteoporotic fracture, compared to 1 in 5 men [8]. Osteoporotic fracture may have significant detrimental effects for an individual, ranging from chronic pain to loss of mobility and independence leading to institutionalisation and death. For example, hip fracture inevitably requires hospitalisation, only 50% of patients return to their previous level of mobility and there is a 30% mortality rate at 1 year post fracture [9]. This is also reflected in study of the global health burden, which demonstrates that despite hip fractures representing only 18.2% of total fractures, due to their high risk of disability and mortality, they account for 40% of the total global health burden of fractures [7]. The Global Burden of Diseases project estimated that in the year 2000 there were nine million osteoporotic fractures in the world. Of these, 1.6 million were hip fractures, 1.7 million were forearm fractures, and 1.4 million were vertebral fractures [7].

The huge burden of fractures on health and social care is predicted to increase with our aging populations. The cost of fractures to health and social care is £2.3 billion per year in the UK (and $17 billion in the USA).

Bone Health and Osteoporosis

Osteoporosis is a systemic bone disorder characterised by deterioration of bone microarchitecture which results in decreased bone density and strength [10]. As a direct consequence of this, there is a significant risk that relatively low velocity force, which would not be expected to fracture non-osteoporotic bone, may cause fracture of osteoporotic bone. Indeed, the terms ‘fragility fracture’ and ‘low-level trauma fracture’ are often used to signify osteoporotic fracture resulting from forces equivalent to a fall from standing height or less [11]. The majority of fragility fractures occur in the hip (proximal femur), spine (vertebrae) or wrist (distal radius), although other sites can also be affected [11]. The World Health Organisation working definition for osteoporosis is a bone mineral density (BMD) more than 2.5

standard deviations (SD) lower than the mean of a population of healthy young adults [12]. In the same way, osteopenia is defined as a BMD between 1 and 2.5 SD below the mean and is indicative of greater risk of developing osteoporosis [12].

Estimates for the prevalence of osteoporosis in the community are 22.1% and 5.5% in European women and men, aged 50 years and over [2]. In the USA 77.1% of women and 10.0% of men over the age of 65 years have either osteoporosis or low bone density [13].

Sarcopenia

Sarcopenia is defined as the age-associated low skeletal muscle mass with low muscle strength and/or low physical performance [14]. Definitions of sarcopenia are still under development. However, the consequences of sarcopenia are the increased risk of frailty, falls and fractures. Sarcopenia and its risk factors (the reduction in skeletal muscle mass and strength or function with age) are also associated with osteoporosis.

Skeletal muscle mass or free mass can be measured using a number of techniques which include DXA, bioelectrical impedance and PCT [13, 15]. The proportion of lean mass or fat-free mass is calculated according to body size [16, 17].

Sarcopenia has been identified in between 1% and 29% in community-dwelling people over the age of 60 years, with estimates for those living in long-term care of between 14% and 33% [18, 19]. Recent predictions for Europe estimate that the prevalence of sarcopenia will almost double overall in the elderly population to 22.3% by 2045 [18, 19]. Pre-sarcopenia occurs (the presence of low skeletal muscle mass according to specific cut points, but not strength) (EWGSOP) before sarcopenia occurs. The newly recognised conditions of osteosarcopenia (the co-existence of osteoporosis and sarcopenia) and sarcopenic obesity (the presence of sarcopenia as well as obesity) also exist. Sarcopenic obesity leads to weakness and mobility problems, even in those who appear to be adequately nourished and of normal body weight.

The prevalence of frailty is estimated to be 25% in those over the age of 80 [20–22].

There are no recent estimates of the costs of sarcopenia available, but estimates of the costs of sarcopenia in 2004 were $US18.5B [23]. These estimates are set to rise [23].

The Interactions Between Skeletal Muscle, Bone Health, Osteoporosis and Risk of Fractures

It is increasingly recognised that the interactions between the skeletal muscle and bone compartments in the body are important and synergistic. The mechanical force of skeletal muscle contraction has a stimulatory effect on bone, increasing both mass and strength [24]. Skeletal muscle mass is positively correlated with bone mineral content and density [25]. Skeletal muscles secrete a collection of cytokine and growth factors known as myokines. These signalling molecules stimulate bone formation and inhibit osteoclast differentiation. A reduction in muscle mass with age may thus reduce myokine secretion and have negative effects on bone [26]. Overall, the interactions between the skeletal muscle and bone maintain postural balance [27, 28].

In this chapter, we review the potential for dietary fat to influence both skeletal muscle and bone health and the physiology of these body tissues. In the next section, we detail the relevance of dietary fat and fatty acids to the physiology and mechanisms of aging of the skeletal muscle and bone.

Dietary Fat and Skeletal Muscle Health and Function

Mechanisms of Age-Related Skeletal Muscle Loss and Sarcopenia

There are a number of mechanisms that lead to the onset of loss of skeletal muscle mass and function and sarcopenia [1, 29, 30]. These include the presence of low-grade inflammatory cytokines which increase with age such as TNF-α, C-reactive protein and IL-6 [29, 31, 32]; see also later in this chapter. They also include the reduction in sex hormones with age, smoking habit, physical inactivity and malnutrition [30, 33].

It is well established that dietary protein is important for maintaining skeletal muscle mass and function and the maintenance and balance between protein synthesis (anabolism) and breakdown (catabolism) is important [34–37]. However, although dietary fat can influence skeletal muscle composition, function and physiology, the importance of dietary fat has not been studied extensively, particularly in aging populations [1].

Dietary Fat Is a Source of Energy for Muscle and Can Influence Mechanisms of Loss of Skeletal Muscle Mass and Function

The fatty acids found in fat are the dominant substrate for production of ATP during aerobic exercise [38–41]. The relationship between fat and performance has been understudied even in sports exercise nutrition where carbohydrate has been the major focus [41]. In working muscle long-chain free fatty acids circulating in the blood are transported across muscle membrane (sarcolemma) by protein transporters which have recently been identified: fatty acid-binding protein into the plasma membrane (FABPpm), fatty acid translocase (FAT/CD36) and the fatty acid transport protein (FATP) [38–41]. Dietary fat has structural importance to skeletal muscle being integral to the sarcolemma. Additionally, the fat profile of the diet is reflected in fatty acid composition of skeletal muscle membranes although a limited amount of research suggests that physical activity also modifies the fatty acid composition of the skeletal muscle [42, 43].

The mechanisms by which dietary fat can modify skeletal muscle mass and function in aging have only recently begun to be elucidated with evidence mainly arising from cell and animal studies [40]. An overview of the potential mechanisms can be found in Lipina 2017.

The different types of fatty acids in the diet, as well as total fat, have the potential for interacting and modifying the mechanisms leading to skeletal muscle loss and sarcopenia with aging [1, 40]. Total fat and SFA may be detrimental to skeletal muscle health and the PUFA (total, n-3 PUFA, n-6 PUFA), MUFA and the P:S ratio may be beneficial [1, 40].

High intakes of total fat and SFA are considered risk factors for increased inflammatory cytokines, and PUFA, particularly n-3 PUFA, have the potential for reducing inflammatory cytokines as well as improving synthesis of protein [1, 40, 44–46].

Review of the Existing Evidence from Animal and Human Studies

Animal Studies and Total Dietary Fat

The effects of a diet high in fat as a percentage of energy (43% energy) on the amount of skeletal muscle during aging were studied in rats over a 10-month period. The investigators found a decline in the cross-sectional area of the quadriceps muscle in male rats but not in female rats fed the same high-fat diet over a longer period (of 12 and 16 months). In the group of female rats, the cross-sectional area of the quadriceps increased on the high-fat diet by the age of 16 months [47–49]. However, overall muscle loss in these aging rats was 22% greater in the male than in the female rats, and there was a greater weight gain over the course of the study in the female rats, which may explain the differences in the findings.

Human Cross-Sectional Studies

In our previous study in 2689 women aged 18–79 years, the range of dietary fat and fatty acid intake was investigated in relation to the proportion of skeletal muscle mass (measured as fat-free mass) [1]. Fat-free mass was measured with dual-energy X-ray absorptiometry and scaled for total body size by dividing by height^2. Dietary intake was assessed with a food frequency questionnaire and a detailed database of the fatty acid composition of foods to calculate intake of individual fatty acids [1].

In this study positive associations were found between a higher polyunsaturated fatty acid to saturated fatty acid ratio (P:S ratio) and fat-free mass with significant differences across quintiles of 0.25 kg/m^2, representing a difference of 1.7% between the highest and lowest intakes. There was a detrimental association with saturated fatty acids with those in the highest quintile of intake having a 1.9% lower fat-free mass than those in the lowest (16.0% energy vs 8.7%). There were also negative associations with the individual saturated fatty acids: lauric, myristic, pentadecanoic, palmitic, stearic and arachidic acids with the strongest associations found with myristic and pentadecanoic acids [1]. Unexpectedly, we found the associations with the n-3 PUFA, EPA, DHA and α-linolenic acid were not beneficial in this cohort. Total fat as a percentage energy intake was also negatively related to lower fat-free mass of 1.9%. At the time this observation was not expected, but subsequent cell and animal studies have confirmed this finding [40, 48].

Prior to this a study in men and women aged 50–79 years found a significant and negative association with intakes of SFA [50]. These investigators found a lower appendicular lean mass (fat-free mass in the arms and legs) of −0.05 kg per quartile of SFA [50].

Human Randomised Controlled Trials

There have only been randomised controlled trials with dietary fat for either total PUFA, n-3 PUFA or n-6 PUFA [51–53]. In our ongoing systematic review of either total PUFA, n-3 PUFA or n-6 PUFA on musculoskeletal health, sarcopenia and functional health, we have found a limited number of studies of mixed designs in older adult populations (Abdelhamid A, Hooper L, Sivakaran R, Hayhoe R and Welch A on behalf of the PUFAH group, in preparation of systematic review registration—PROSPERO 2017 CRD42017079211). We found 28 studies that reported on either the effects of long-chain n-3 PUFA, n-6 PUFA or mixed PUFA with only 20% of studies judged to be at risk of low bias. However, there were a limited number of studies on which to draw definitive conclusions, and further well-conducted trials would be needed in older adult populations to establish firm evidence of the effects of improving PUFA intake in older people.

Summary of the Evidence

Although dietary fat has the potential to modify skeletal muscle health, particularly skeletal muscle mass, during aging the evidence is very limited to date.

Dietary Fat and Bone Health and Risk of Fractures

Experimental studies, both in vitro and using animal models, have demonstrated dietary fats have significant importance to bone health. Although evidence from human studies is less definitive, recent epidemiological studies suggest that dietary fatty acid profiles may be important for human bone health. The mechanisms likely to be involved in the interaction between dietary fatty acid intakes and bone homeostasis or pathology are discussed below with particular reference to aging.

Inflammation and Fatty Acid Metabolites

Osteoclast and osteoblast activity is modulated by a range of cytokines and growth factors. For example, osteoclast formation is promoted by tumour necrosis factor-α (TNF-α) and the interleukins, IL-1α, IL-1β, IL-6 and IL-7, while their function is inhibited by interferon (IFN)-β and IFN-γ, IL-4, IL-10, IL-12 and IL-13. However, the function of these signalling molecules is complex, such that some may transition between functions, e.g. tumour growth factor β (TGF-β) can act as an inducer or a suppressor of both osteoblast and osteoclast activity [5]. There is growing evidence to support the concept that aging is associated with alteration in the profile of inflammatory cytokines and development of a chronic inflammatory state in the elderly, in a process now known as 'inflamm-aging'. Due to the delicate balance of inflammatory mediators which modulate osteoclast and osteoblast activity, this altered inflammatory profile may be partly responsible for detrimental outcomes on bone health. Both pro- and anti-inflammatory signalling molecules can influence osteoblast and osteoclast activity, upsetting the balance of which can cause osteoporosis. The acute phase reactant C-reactive protein (CRP) is a useful biomarker of systemic inflammation, and, although the evidence isn't entirely consistent, cross-sectional studies suggest that higher concentrations of CRP are found in older individuals and that it is negatively associated with BMD [54]. Furthermore, longitudinal analysis of a cohort of older women demonstrated that those with high CRP concentrations over a period of 5 years had higher rates of bone loss than women with low CRP concentrations [55], thus confirming the association of systemic inflammatory status with bone health.

The link between fatty acids and inflammation via metabolism of fatty acids to eicosanoids has been well established by previous research. The n-6 arachidonic acid (AA) is metabolised by cyclooxygenase (COX) to n-6 eicosanoids (prostaglandin E_2, PGE_2, and thromboxane A2, TXA_2) or by 5-lipoxygenase (5-LOX) to n-6 leukotrienes. The n-3 eicosapentaenoic acid (EPA) is metabolised to n-3 PGs and LTs by the same process, although due to EPA being a relatively poor substrate for COX, less n-3 PGs are produced. EPA and DHA competitively inhibit n-6 eicosanoid production (except PGI2), and an increase in dietary n-3 fatty acids consumption increases the incorporation of EPA in cell membranes, partly at the expense of AA incorporation. The combined effect of less production and the reduced inflammatory potency of n-3 eicosanoids compared to n-6 eicosanoids suggests that a higher n3:n6 ratio is likely to be less inflammatory and result in a net reduction in the bone loss.

In adults, there is a constant homeostatic process of bone renewal involving a balance of bone resorption by osteoclasts and bone formation by osteoblasts. Cytokines play an important role in regulating this balance by modulating the ratios of osteoprotegerin (OPG) and the receptor activator of nuclear factor-kB ligand (RANKL). While RANKL is present on osteoblasts and activates the RANK receptor on osteoclasts (suppressing their apoptosis and causing activation and formation of more osteoclasts), OPG is expressed by osteoblasts and acts to block RANKL activating RANK. Thus the ratio of these two signalling molecules is highly relevant to the pathogenesis of osteoporosis. In vitro experiments have shown that EPA can inhibit NF-kB by a variety of cell stimuli. For example, pretreating osteoclasts with the n-3 fatty acid EPA before stimulating the cells with TNF-α significantly reduced the resultant NF-κB expression compared with cells not pretreated with EPA [56]. As described above, n-3 fatty acids reduce the formation of prostaglandin E_2 derived from n-6 fatty acids by competing for COX. The resulting reduction in PGE_2 production has the effect of increasing OPG secretion from osteoblasts and thus the OPG:RANKL ratio is increased, tipping the balance in favour of bone formation and protection versus resorption.

In addition to metabolism of eicosanoids, a number of different lipid oxygenase pathways have been discovered recently which result in production of specialised pro-resolving lipid mediators (SPMs). These SPMs include the resolvins, lipoxins and protectins, which resolve inflammation as an active rather than passive process, through inhibiting both TNF-α and IL-1β production and the progression of leukocyte trans-endothelial migration [57]. In experimental models, resolvins and lipoxins inhibit inflammation-induced bone resorption [58, 59].

Another inflammatory mechanism independent of eicosanoid synthesis via COX is that mediated by nitric oxide (NO). NO is produced by NO synthase (NOS) and is released by osteoblasts to directly regulate osteoclast activity. Laboratory research has shown that the n-6 PUFA arachidonic acid (AA) significantly upregulates inducible NOS (iNOS) mRNA expression in human osteoblast-like cells via a mechanism mediated by intracellular signalling kinases (protein kinase C and tyrosine kinases) [60]. These effects were not replicated by either n-3 PUFA EPA or the MUFA oleic acid, and co-incubation of cells with these fatty acids caused a significant inhibition of AA-induced iNOS gene expression [60]. This work thus suggests the balance between different fatty acids is important for bone health.

Calcium Balance

Insufficient dietary calcium is well established as a risk factor for bone loss and osteoporosis. Despite an apparently adequate intake of calcium from the diet, some individuals may still be susceptible to insufficiency due to factors limiting the absorption of dietary calcium or enhancing its excretion. The primary factor affecting calcium absorption is vitamin D, and the essential fatty acids are important for optimal vitamin-D-dependent intestinal calcium absorption [61]. In particular the essential n-3 and n-6 fatty acids appear to be important for increasing calcium absorption and reducing calcium excretion when dietary availability is low: Experimental studies in vitro and using animal models have shown duodenal calcium absorption to be upregulated by the n-3 fatty acid, docosahexaenoic acid (DHA), acting to modulate calcium-ATPase when calcium levels are low [62, 63]; both DHA and another n-3 fatty acid, eicosapentaenoic acid (EPA), reduced urinary calcium excretion in a rat model of osteoporosis [64]; and fish oil supplementation in patients with calcium salt kidney stones ameliorated the problematic high calcium absorption and reduced urinary calcium excretion [65].

Growth Hormone and Effects on Insulin-Like Growth Factor

Insulin-like growth factor (IGF-1) is a hormone released mainly by the liver and acts as a mediator of pituitary-derived growth hormone but is also produced in smaller quantities by peripheral tissues, including muscle and bone, where it acts in an autocrine and paracrine fashion independently of systemic growth hormone [66]. IGF-1 is an important mediator of normal cell growth and proliferation and plays a critical role in skeletal growth and bone remodelling [66]. However, during aging there is a reduction in IGF-1 concentration alongside a reduction in muscle mass and bone mineral density [67]. IGF-1 concentrations in the body are known to be reduced by malnutrition, reduced protein intake and calorie restriction, and there is some evidence that dietary fatty acid profiles are also relevant to IGF-1: High dietary PUFA intakes of vegans were associated with low IGF-1 concentration [68], while low-fat diet with high n-3 fatty acids may increase circulating IGF-I concentrations without adversely affecting insulin sensitivity in healthy individuals [69].

Balance of Differentiation of Stem Cells to Adipocytes and Osteoblasts

Mesenchymal stem cells (MSCs or bone marrow stromal cells) are a morphologically heterogeneous population capable of differentiating into different cell types including fibroblasts, osteogenic cells and adipocytes, depending on the stimulus they receive [70]. For many years it has been known that the balance of bone resorption and formation is altered in older age, causing a net loss of bone tissue and an associated increase in marrow adipose tissue [71]. Indeed, early studies of osteoporosis identified the change in proportion of bone cells as the primary cause of osteoporosis. More recently, further insight has been gained into the underlying mechanisms and factors influencing the change in balance of cells. Evidence from in vitro experimentation has demonstrated fatty acids act to inhibit maturation of osteoblasts and enhance adipogenesis, and thus there is potential that dietary fatty acids may also exert some effect on the type of cells resulting from MSC differentiation [70]. This is supported by in vivo animal models, for example, when mice were fed an atherogenic diet (high in fat and cholesterol), their bone mineral content and density were reduced and the osteogenic differentiation of their stromal cells was inhibited [72, 73].

The likely mechanism of this hinges on the involvement of a nuclear transcription factor named peroxisome proliferator-activated receptor-gamma (PPAR-γ) in adipocyte differentiation. This receptor is expressed in osteoblasts, and activation by fatty acids, or their oxidation products, concomitantly induces adipogenesis and inhibits osteoblastogenesis in vitro [74].

Summary of Existing Human Evidence

Despite the evidence provided by animal models and in vitro studies suggesting dietary fatty acid profiles play an important role in determining skeletal outcomes, there have been very few studies addressing this in humans. Longitudinal cohort studies have demonstrated a detrimental effect of high total fatty acid intakes on BMD [75] and fractures [76] in postmenopausal women, and data from the National Health and Nutrition Examination Survey III (NHANES III) suggests SFA in particular has strong negative associations with bone density in both men and women

[77]. The role of MUFA is less clear, with conflicting cross-sectional study results showing MUFA intake associated with higher [78] or lower BMD [75] and a case-control study [79] reporting no significant trend in fracture risk across MUFA intake quartiles. In support of the evidence from animal studies, several human studies have suggested a beneficial role for n-3 FAs, including associations of dietary n-3 linolenic acid intake with higher BMD measures in elderly women [80], and n-3 serum phospholipid FAs with bone mineral accrual in young men [81]. However, in a cohort study investigating fracture risk, no associations were reported with total n-3 FA intake [82]. In terms of n-6 FA intakes and associations with bone, the majority of studies report negative effects, with higher n-6 FA intakes [75] associated with higher osteoporotic fracture risk. The proportions of different FAs within the diet are likely to be important in addition to absolute concentration values. Indeed, higher n-6 in proportion to n-3 has been associated with lower bone density [83], and higher PUFA:MUFA with greater risk of fracture [79].

Research Gaps and Suggestions for Future Work

Despite the relevance of dietary fat composition to skeletal muscle and bone physiology and metabolism, there is limited existing research evidence for the relationship between the importance of dietary fat and sarcopenia, skeletal muscle and osteoporosis and bone health in aging. Further work is needed to understand the relevance of dietary fat to skeletal muscle and bone health and its impact on the development of sarcopenia, osteoporosis and risk of fractures.

Particular gaps in the research include a lack of gender-specific data, especially for men, and limited information on different age groups in the population where this may be relevant. No studies to date have investigated the importance of biomarkers of fatty acids, such as circulating fatty acid concentration in blood on skeletal muscle and bone health and risk of fractures. In addition, a current failing is that research has not investigated associations in both muscle and bone at the same time so there is little appreciation of the interplay that may exist. There is also a need for better understanding of the relationship between the overall profiles of fatty acids in the diet as many previous studies have concentrated on investigating the effects of a particular type of fatty acids and less about the interaction and balance.

References

1. Welch AA, Macgregor AJ, Minihane AM, Skinner J, Valdes AA, Spector TD, Cassidy A. Dietary fat and fatty acid profile are associated with indices of skeletal muscle mass in women aged 18–79 years. J Nutr. 2014;144:327–34.
2. Agency FS. McCance and Widdowson's the composition of foods sixth summary edition. Cambridge: Royal Society of Chemistry; 2002.
3. Linseisen J, Welch AA, Ocke M, Amiano P, Agnoli C, Ferrari P, Sonestedt E, Chajes V, Bueno-de-Mesquita HB, Kaaks R, Weikert C, Dorronsoro M, Rodriguez L, Ermini I, Mattiello A, van der Schouw YT, Manjer J, Nilsson S, Jenab M, Lund E, Brustad M, Halkjaer J, Jakobsen MU,

Khaw KT, Crowe F, Georgila C, Misirli G, Niravong M, Touvier M, Bingham S, Riboli E, Slimani N. Dietary fat intake in the European prospective investigation into cancer and nutrition: results from the 24-h dietary recalls. Eur J Clin Nutr. 2009;63(Suppl 4):S61–80.

4. Michas G, Micha R, Zampelas A. Dietary fats and cardiovascular disease: putting together the pieces of a complicated puzzle. Atherosclerosis. 2014;234:320–8.
5. Boros K, Freemont T. Physiology of ageing of the musculoskeletal system. Best Pract Res Clin Rheumatol. 2017;31:203–17.
6. Rachner TD, Khosla S, Hofbauer LC. Osteoporosis: now and the future. Lancet. 2011;377:1276–87.
7. Johnell O, Kanis JA. An estimate of the worldwide prevalence and disability associated with osteoporotic fractures. Osteoporos Int. 2006;17:1726–33.
8. van Staa TP, Dennison EM, Leufkens HG, Cooper C. Epidemiology of fractures in England and Wales. Bone. 2001;29:517–22.
9. Lisk R, Yeong K. Reducing mortality from hip fractures: a systematic quality improvement programme. BMJ Qual Improv Rep. 2014;3:u205006.w2103. https://doi.org/10.1136/bmjquality.u205006.w2103.
10. World Health Organisation. Assessment of fracture risk and its application to screening for postmenopausal osteoporosis. World Health Organ Tech Rep Ser. 1994;843:1–129.
11. Kanis JA, Oden A, Johnell O, Jonsson B, De Laet C, Dawson A. The burden of osteoporotic fractures: a method for setting intervention thresholds. Osteoporos Int. 2001;12:417–27.
12. Kanis JA. Diagnosis of osteoporosis and assessment of fracture risk. Lancet. 2002;359:1929–36.
13. Cawthon PM. Assessment of lean mass and physical performance in sarcopenia. J Clin Densitom. 2015;18:467–71.
14. Cruz-Jentoft AJ, Baeyens JP, Bauer JM, Boirie Y, Cederholm T, Landi F, Martin FC, Michel JP, Rolland Y, Schneider SM, Topinkova E, Vandewoude M, Zamboni M. Sarcopenia: European consensus on definition and diagnosis: report of the European Working Group on sarcopenia in older people. Age Ageing. 2010;39:412–23.
15. Heymsfield SB, Adamek M, Gonzalez MC, Jia G, Thomas DM. Assessing skeletal muscle mass: historical overview and state of the art. J Cachexia Sarcopenia Muscle. 2014;5:9–18.
16. Heymsfield SB, Gonzalez MC, Lu J, Jia G, Zheng J. Skeletal muscle mass and quality: evolution of modern measurement concepts in the context of sarcopenia. Proc Nutr Soc. 2015;74:1–12.
17. Prado CM, Siervo M, Mire E, Heymsfield SB, Stephan BC, Broyles S, Smith SR, Wells JC, Katzmarzyk PT. A population-based approach to define body-composition phenotypes. Am J Clin Nutr. 2014;99:1369–77.
18. Cruz-Jentoft AJ, Landi F, Schneider SM, Zuniga C, Arai H, Boirie Y, Chen LK, Fielding RA, Martin FC, Michel JP, Sieber C, Stout JR, Studenski SA, Vellas B, Woo J, Zamboni M, Cederholm T. Prevalence of and interventions for sarcopenia in ageing adults: a systematic review. Report of the International Sarcopenia Initiative (EWGSOP and IWGS). Age Ageing. 2014;43:748–59.
19. Ethgen O, Beaudart C, Buckinx F, Bruyere O, Reginster JY. The future prevalence of sarcopenia in Europe: a claim for public health action. Calcif Tissue Int. 2017;100:229–34.
20. Gale CR, Cooper C, Sayer AA. Prevalence of frailty and disability: findings from the English longitudinal study of ageing. Age Ageing. 2015;44:162–5.
21. Kaehr E, Visvanathan R, Malmstrom TK, Morley JE. Frailty in nursing homes: the FRAIL-NH scale. J Am Med Dir Assoc. 2015;16:87–9.
22. Robinson SM, Reginster JY, Rizzoli R, Shaw SC, Kanis JA, Bautmans I, Bischoff-Ferrari H, Bruyere O, Cesari M, Dawson-Hughes B, Fielding RA, Kaufman JM, Landi F, Malafarina V, Rolland Y, van Loon LJ, Vellas B, Visser M, Cooper C, ESCEO Working Group. Does nutrition play a role in the prevention and management of sarcopenia? Clin Nutr. 2017;37(4): 1121–32.
23. Kilsby AJ, Sayer AA, Witham MD. Selecting potential pharmacological interventions in sarcopenia. Drugs Aging. 2017;34:233–40.

24. Russo CR. The effects of exercise on bone. Basic concepts and implications for the prevention of fractures. Clin Cases Miner Bone Metab. 2009;6:223–8.
25. Szulc P, Beck TJ, Marchand F, Delmas PD. Low skeletal muscle mass is associated with poor structural parameters of bone and impaired balance in elderly men--the MINOS study. J Bone Miner Res. 2005;20:721–9.
26. Hamrick MW. A role for myokines in muscle-bone interactions. Exerc Sport Sci Rev. 2011;39:43–7.
27. Curtis E, Litwic A, Cooper C, Dennison E. Determinants of muscle and bone aging. J Cell Physiol. 2015;230:2618–25.
28. Tagliaferri C, Wittrant Y, Davicco MJ, Walrand S, Coxam V. Muscle and bone, two interconnected tissues. Ageing Res Rev. 2015;21:55–70.
29. Dalle S, Rossmeislova L, Koppo K. The role of inflammation in age-related sarcopenia. Front Physiol. 2017;8:1045.
30. Welch AA. Nutritional influences on age-related skeletal muscle loss. Proc Nutr Soc. 2014;73:16–33.
31. Schaap LA, Pluijm SM, Deeg DJ, Harris TB, Kritchevsky SB, Newman AB, Colbert LH, Pahor M, Rubin SM, Tylavsky FA, Visser M. Higher inflammatory marker levels in older persons: associations with 5-year change in muscle mass and muscle strength. J Gerontol A Biol Sci Med Sci. 2009;64:1183–9.
32. Welch AA, Kelaiditi E, Jennings A, Steves CJ, Spector TD, Macgregor A. Dietary magnesium is positively associated with skeletal muscle power and indices of muscle mass and may attenuate the association between circulating C-reactive protein and muscle mass in women. J Bone Miner Res. 2016;31:317–25.
33. Szulc P, Duboeuf F, Marchand F, Delmas PD. Hormonal and lifestyle determinants of appendicular skeletal muscle mass in men: the MINOS study. Am J Clin Nutr. 2004;80:496–503.
34. Borsheim E, Bui QU, Tissier S, Kobayashi H, Ferrando AA, Wolfe RR. Effect of amino acid supplementation on muscle mass, strength and physical function in elderly. Clin Nutr. 2008;27:189–95.
35. Murton AJ. Muscle protein turnover in the elderly and its potential contribution to the development of sarcopenia. Proc Nutr Soc. 2015;74:1–10.
36. Wolfe RR. The underappreciated role of muscle in health and disease. Am J Clin Nutr. 2006;84:475–82.
37. Wolfe RR, Miller SL, Miller KB. Optimal protein intake in the elderly. Clin Nutr. 2008;27:675–84.
38. Frayn KN. Fat as a fuel: emerging understanding of the adipose tissue-skeletal muscle axis. Acta Physiol (Oxf). 2010;199:509–18.
39. Holloway GP, Luiken JJ, Glatz JF, Spriet LL, Bonen A. Contribution of FAT/CD36 to the regulation of skeletal muscle fatty acid oxidation: an overview. Acta Physiol (Oxf). 2008;194:293–309.
40. Lipina C, Hundal HS. Lipid modulation of skeletal muscle mass and function. J Cachexia Sarcopenia Muscle. 2017;8:190–201.
41. Spriet LL. Regulation of skeletal muscle fat oxidation during exercise in humans. Med Sci Sports Exerc. 2002;34:1477–84.
42. Andersson A, Nalsen C, Tengblad S, Vessby B. Fatty acid composition of skeletal muscle reflects dietary fat composition in humans. Am J Clin Nutr. 2002;76:1222–9.
43. Andersson A, Sjodin A, Hedman A, Olsson R, Vessby B. Fatty acid profile of skeletal muscle phospholipids in trained and untrained young men. Am J Physiol Metab. 2000;279: E744–51.
44. Calder PC, Albers R, Antoine JM, Blum S, Bourdet-Sicard R, Ferns GA, Folkerts G, Friedmann PS, Frost GS, Guarner F, Lovik M, Macfarlane S, Meyer PD, M'Rabet L, Serafini M, van Eden W, van Loo J, Vas Dias W, Vidry S, Winklhofer-Roob BM, Zhao J. Inflammatory disease processes and interactions with nutrition. Br J Nutr. 2009;101(Suppl 1):S1–45.
45. Da Boit M, Sibson R, Sivasubramaniam S, Meakin JR, Greig CA, Aspden RM, Thies F, Jeromson S, Hamilton DL, Speakman JR, Hambly C, Mangoni AA, Preston T, Gray SR. Sex

differences in the effect of fish-oil supplementation on the adaptive response to resistance exercise training in older people: a randomized controlled trial. Am J Clin Nutr. 2017;105:151–8.
46. Tachtsis B, Camera D, Lacham-Kaplan O. Potential roles of n-3 PUFAs during skeletal muscle growth and regeneration. Nutrients. 2018;10:E309.
47. Bollheimer LC, Buettner R, Pongratz G, Brunner-Ploss R, Hechtl C, Banas M, Singler K, Hamer OW, Stroszczynski C, Sieber CC, Fellner C. Sarcopenia in the aging high-fat fed rat: a pilot study for modeling sarcopenic obesity in rodents. Biogerontology. 2012;13:609–20.
48. Kob R, Fellner C, Bertsch T, Wittmann A, Mishura D, Sieber CC, Fischer BE, Stroszczynski C, Bollheimer CL. Gender-specific differences in the development of sarcopenia in the rodent model of the ageing high-fat rat. J Cachexia Sarcopenia Muscle. 2015;6:181–91.
49. Pongratz G, Lowin T, Kob R, Buettner R, Bertsch T, Bollheimer LC. A sustained high fat diet for two years decreases IgM and IL-1 beta in ageing Wistar rats. Immun Ageing. 2015;12:12.
50. Scott D, Blizzard L, Fell J, Giles G, Jones G. Associations between dietary nutrient intake and muscle mass and strength in community-dwelling older adults: the Tasmanian Older Adult Cohort Study. J Am Geriatr Soc. 2010;58:2129–34.
51. Smith GI, Atherton P, Reeds DN, Mohammed BS, Rankin D, Rennie MJ, Mittendorfer B. Dietary omega-3 fatty acid supplementation increases the rate of muscle protein synthesis in older adults: a randomized controlled trial. Am J Clin Nutr. 2010;93:402–12.
52. Smith GI, Atherton P, Reeds DN, Mohammed BS, Rankin D, Rennie MJ, Mittendorfer B. Omega-3 polyunsaturated fatty acids augment the muscle protein anabolic response to hyperinsulinaemia-hyperaminoacidaemia in healthy young and middle-aged men and women. Clin Sci (Lond). 2010;121:267–78.
53. Yoshino J, Smith GI, Kelly SC, Julliand S, Reeds DN, Mittendorfer B. Effect of dietary n-3 PUFA supplementation on the muscle transcriptome in older adults. Physiol Rep. 2016;4:e12785.
54. De Pablo P, Cooper MS, Buckley CD. Association between bone mineral density and C-reactive protein in a large population-based sample. Arthritis Rheum. 2012;64:2624–31.
55. Berglundh S, Malmgren L, Luthman H, Mcguigan F, Akesson K. C-reactive protein, bone loss, fracture, and mortality in elderly women: a longitudinal study in the OPRA cohort. Osteoporos Int. 2015;26:727–35.
56. Zwart SR, Pierson D, Mehta S, Gonda S, Smith SM. Capacity of omega-3 fatty acids or eicosapentaenoic acid to counteract weightlessness-induced bone loss by inhibiting NF-kappaB activation: from cells to bed rest to astronauts. J Bone Miner Res. 2010;25:1049–57.
57. Basil MC, Levy BD. Specialized pro-resolving mediators: endogenous regulators of infection and inflammation. Nat Rev Immunol. 2016;16:51–67.
58. Hasturk H, Kantarci A, Ohira T, Arita M, Ebrahimi N, Chiang N, Petasis NA, Levy BD, Serhan CN, Van Dyke TE. RvE1 protects from local inflammation and osteoclast-mediated bone destruction in periodontitis. FASEB J. 2006;20:401–3.
59. Herrera BS, Ohira T, Gao L, Omori K, Yang R, Zhu M, Muscara MN, Serhan CN, Van Dyke TE, Gyurko R. An endogenous regulator of inflammation, resolvin E1, modulates osteoclast differentiation and bone resorption. Br J Pharmacol. 2008;155:1214–23.
60. Priante G, Musacchio E, Pagnin E, Calo LA, Baggio B. Specific effect of arachidonic acid on inducible nitric oxide synthase mRNA expression in human osteoblastic cells. Clin Sci (Lond). 2005;109:177–82.
61. Hay AW, Hassam AG, Crawford MA, Stevens PA, Mawer EB, Jones FS. Essential fatty acid restriction inhibits vitamin D-dependent calcium absorption. Lipids. 1980;15:251–4.
62. Haag M, Kruger MC. Upregulation of duodenal calcium absorption by poly-unsaturated fatty acids: events at the basolateral membrane. Med Hypotheses. 2001;56:637–40.
63. Haag M, Magada ON, Claassen N, Bohmer LH, Kruger MC. Omega-3 fatty acids modulate ATPases involved in duodenal Ca absorption. Prostaglandins Leukot Essent Fatty Acids. 2003;68:423–9.
64. Sun L, Tamaki H, Ishimaru T, Teruya T, Ohta Y, Katsuyama N, Chinen I. Inhibition of osteoporosis due to restricted food intake by the fish oils DHA and EPA and perilla oil in the rat. Biosci Biotechnol Biochem. 2004;68:2613–5.

65. Baggio B, Budakovic A, Nassuato MA, Vezzoli G, Manzato E, Luisetto G, Zaninotto M. Plasma phospholipid arachidonic acid content and calcium metabolism in idiopathic calcium nephrolithiasis. Kidney Int. 2000;58:1278–84.
66. Guntur AR, Rosen CJ. IGF-1 regulation of key signaling pathways in bone. Bonekey Rep. 2013;2:437.
67. Toogood AA. The somatopause: an indication for growth hormone therapy? Treat Endocrinol. 2004;3:201–9.
68. Allen NE, Appleby PN, Davey GK, Kaaks R, Rinaldi S, Key TJ. The associations of diet with serum insulin-like growth factor I and its main binding proteins in 292 women meat-eaters, vegetarians, and vegans. Cancer Epidemiol Biomark Prev. 2002;11:1441–8.
69. Young LR, Kurzer MS, Thomas W, Redmon JB, Raatz SK. Low-fat diet with omega-3 fatty acids increases plasma insulin-like growth factor concentration in healthy postmenopausal women. Nutr Res. 2013;33:565–71.
70. Nuttall ME, Patton AJ, Olivera DL, Nadeau DP, Gowen M. Human trabecular bone cells are able to express both osteoblastic and adipocytic phenotype: implications for osteopenic disorders. J Bone Miner Res. 1998;13:371–82.
71. Meunier P, Aaron J, Edouard C, Vignon G. Osteoporosis and the replacement of cell populations of the marrow by adipose tissue. A quantitative study of 84 iliac bone biopsies. Clin Orthop Relat Res. 1971;80:147–54.
72. Parhami F, Jackson SM, Tintut Y, Le V, Balucan JP, Territo M, Demer LL. Atherogenic diet and minimally oxidized low density lipoprotein inhibit osteogenic and promote adipogenic differentiation of marrow stromal cells. J Bone Miner Res. 1999;14:2067–78.
73. Parhami F, Tintut Y, Beamer WG, Gharavi N, Goodman W, Demer LL. Atherogenic high-fat diet reduces bone mineralization in mice. J Bone Miner Res. 2001;16:182–8.
74. Lecka-Czernik B, Moerman EJ, Grant DF, Lehmann JM, Manolagas SC, Jilka RL. Divergent effects of selective peroxisome proliferator-activated receptor-gamma 2 ligands on adipocyte versus osteoblast differentiation. Endocrinology. 2002;143:2376–84.
75. Macdonald HM, New SA, Golden MH, Campbell MK, Reid DM. Nutritional associations with bone loss during the menopausal transition: evidence of a beneficial effect of calcium, alcohol, and fruit and vegetable nutrients and of a detrimental effect of fatty acids. Am J Clin Nutr. 2004;79:155–65.
76. Kato I, Toniolo P, Zeleniuch-Jacquotte A, Shore RE, Koenig KL, Akhmedkhanov A, Riboli E. Diet, smoking and anthropometric indices and postmenopausal bone fractures: a prospective study. Int J Epidemiol. 2000;29:85–92.
77. Corwin RL, Hartman TJ, Maczuga SA, Graubard BI. Dietary saturated fat intake is inversely associated with bone density in humans: analysis of NHANES III. J Nutr. 2006;136:159–65.
78. Trichopoulou A, Georgiou E, Bassiakos Y, Lipworth L, Lagiou P, Proukakis C, Trichopoulos D. Energy intake and monounsaturated fat in relation to bone mineral density among women and men in Greece. Prev Med. 1997;26:395–400.
79. Martinez-Ramirez MJ, Palma S, Martinez-Gonzalez MA, Delgado-Martinez AD, de la Fuente C, Delgado-Rodriguez M. Dietary fat intake and the risk of osteoporotic fractures in the elderly. Eur J Clin Nutr. 2007;61:1114–20.
80. Jarvinen R, Tuppurainen M, Erkkila AT, Penttinen P, Karkkainen M, Salovaara K, Jurvelin JS, Kroger H. Associations of dietary polyunsaturated fatty acids with bone mineral density in elderly women. Eur J Clin Nutr. 2012;66:496–503.
81. Hogstrom M, Nordstrom P, Nordstrom A. n-3 fatty acids are positively associated with peak bone mineral density and bone accrual in healthy men: the NO_2 study. Am J Clin Nutr. 2007;85:803–7.
82. Orchard TS, Cauley JA, Frank GC, Neuhouser ML, Robinson JG, Snetselaar L, Tylavsky F, Wactawski-Wende J, Young AM, Lu B, Jackson RD. Fatty acid consumption and risk of fracture in the women's health initiative. Am J Clin Nutr. 2010;92:1452–60.
83. Weiss LA, Barrett-Connor E, von Muhlen D. Ratio of n-6 to n-3 fatty acids and bone mineral density in older adults: the rancho Bernardo study. Am J Clin Nutr. 2005;81:934–8.

Dairy Products, Vitamin D, and Bone Health

18

Laura H. van Dongen and S. Sahni

Introduction

Osteoporosis is estimated to affect over 200 million people worldwide [1]. In the United States alone, around ten million Americans older than 50 years are estimated to have osteoporosis, of whom approximately 1.5 million suffer from fractures related to osteoporosis [2]. Given the increase in life expectancy and consequent burden of osteoporosis among older adults, dietary modification offers a feasible approach for osteoporosis prevention and related fractures.

The complex combination of essential nutrients in dairy products includes fatty acids (essential and nonessential), calcium, potassium, high-quality protein, and magnesium, and in some countries dairy is also fortified with vitamin D. Thus, dairy products provide a unique package of nutrients that are thought to be beneficial for bone health. Consequently, dairy foods are part of nutritional recommendations in many countries worldwide. The American guidelines recommend an intake of three servings [one serving of milk = 1 cup (250 ml)] of fat-free or low-fat milk and milk products per day for adults [3]. Dairy products contribute to adequate macro- and micronutrient intakes in developed countries. They contribute to around 52–65% of the dietary reference intake of calcium [4–6], but they only represent 9–12% of the total energy consumption [7]. The bioavailability of dietary calcium is >50% of the total intake in the diet. Furthermore, dairy foods also contribute 10% of magnesium, almost all of the vitamin D, 24% of vitamin B12, 15% of zinc, and

L. H. van Dongen
Division of Human Nutrition, Wageningen University and Research,
Wageningen, Netherlands

S. Sahni (✉)
Musculoskeletal Research Center, Institute for Aging Research, Hebrew SeniorLife
Department of Medicine, Beth Israel Deaconess Medical Center, Harvard Medical School,
Boston, MA, USA
e-mail: shivanisahni@hsl.harvard.edu

© Springer Nature Switzerland AG 2019

C. M. Weaver et al. (eds.), *Nutritional Influences on Bone Health*,
https://doi.org/10.1007/978-3-319-98464-3_18

21% of riboflavin in the typical American diet [8]. Previous research has shown a decreasing trend of dairy consumption with age. Total dairy intake by age groups among Americans is reported to be 1.7 cup equivalents per day among those aged 19–50 years, 1.5 cup equivalents per day among those aged 51–70 years, and 1.3 cup equivalents per day among those aged 71 years and above, where 1 cup equivalent of dairy contains 81 kcal, 8.5 g protein, 0.87 g saturated fat, 298 mg calcium, 20 mg magnesium, 99 retinol activity equivalent (RAE) vitamin A, 1.55 μg vitamin D, 237 mg potassium, and 181 mg sodium [9]. The main determinants for this decreasing trend are sex, substitution of milk with other beverages, overall dietary quality, and parental influence [10]. Furthermore, not all dairy products have equivalent nutrient compositions, and it is likely that dairy products other than milk such as yogurt, cheese, and cream have a significant impact on bone health. For example, in addition to providing bone-beneficial nutrients, yogurt and certain softer fermented cheeses contain probiotics, which may provide a useful therapeutic to prevent and/or treat bone loss [11]. On the other hand, cream has lower amounts of bone-beneficial nutrients and higher levels of saturated fats and therefore may even have deleterious effects on bone health [12]. However, previous research has been largely focused on milk intake.

Previous studies determining the role of dairy food intake upon bone health were largely focused on examining the association of milk intake with dual-energy X-ray absorptiometry (DXA)-derived areal bone mineral density (aBMD) in young, premenopausal women. Majority of the studies were cross-sectional in design, and limited studies examined the bone effects of yogurt, cream, and cheese. Nonetheless, our previous study of dairy food intake and hip and spine aBMD in the Framingham Study [12] along with our review paper [13] on this topic concluded that there is strong evidence for a positive association between milk and aBMD and that evidence for yogurt intake with aBMD looks promising. However, data on cheese and cream is very limited. A recent review by Rizzoli et al. [14] summarized information from several studies suggesting that dairy food intake was associated with lower levels of bone turnover markers [such as parathyroid hormone levels (PTH), C-telopeptide of type I collagen (CTX), osteocalcin (OC), procollagen type I N-propeptide (PINP), tartrate-resistant acid phosphatase isoform 5b (TRAP 5b)] and higher levels of bone mineral content (BMC)/BMD. Fermented dairy products, such as cheese and yogurt, might contain bacterial species with a potential beneficial effect on the gut microbiome. This might in turn have beneficial effects on human health [14]. Consequently, due to the dissimilar nutrient profiles and level of fermentation, not all dairy products may have a similar effect on bone health. Therefore, more research is needed to investigate how other dairy foods, such as yogurt, cream, and cheese, are associated with bone health. Furthermore, there is limited data on specific dairy foods and hip fractures in older adults.

The synergistic or additive roles of the various bone-beneficial nutrients such as protein, phosphorus, calcium, vitamin D, and magnesium in dairy need further clarification, since a single nutrient cannot account for the proposed beneficial effect of dairy intake. For example, vitamin D status can enhance calcium absorption, which is beneficial for building bones [15]. Yet, it is unclear if the effect of vitamin D on calcium absorption is substantial enough to translate into beneficial effects on BMD. This interaction may be particularly important for older adults who tend to be deficient in vitamin D (<20 ng/mL in blood) as recommended intakes are difficult to achieve without fortified foods (such as dairy) or supplements and a declining ability to make vitamin D in the skin with advancing age. Consequently, research into the role of dairy foods upon bone health continues to be an active area of research. The objective of this book chapter is to highlight findings from latest studies on this topic to summarize recent research examining individual dairy products, their role in bone health, and interaction of dairy products with vitamin D intake and status. We further highlight the emerging research in this area relating dairy food intake with novel measures of bone, derived using quantitative computed tomography (QCT) and high-resolution peripheral QCT (HR-pQCT).

Interaction with Vitamin D

The Institute of Medicine reported that serum 25-hydroxy vitamin D (25-OH D) concentrations of less than 12 ng/mL (30 nmol/L) are associated with deficiency, inadequate levels are considered between 12 and < 20 ng/mL (50 nmol/L), and levels ≥20 ng/mL are generally considered adequate. There is emerging evidence that 25-OH D levels greater than 50 ng/mL (125 nmol/L), achieved through high-dose vitamin D supplementation, could have adverse effects, such as weight loss, arrhythmias, vascular and tissue calcification, or kidney damage [16]. Sunlight contributes around 2/3 to our vitamin D status; therefore, dietary vitamin D alone is insufficient to meet the body's requirements for vitamin D. Hence, some countries (e.g., Canada and the United States) have decided to fortify their dairy products and other foods (e.g., cereal) with vitamin D [17, 18].

The aging skin has a decreasing capability of producing vitamin D [19]. Consequently, older adults may be more prone to vitamin D deficiency, and fortification with vitamin D could be a useful strategy for improving circulating 25-OH D concentrations [20]. Endocrine Society Clinical Practice Guideline recommends that adults 50–70 years and those over the age of 70 years require at least 600 and 800 IU/day, respectively, of vitamin D to maximize bone health and muscle health [21]. Total calcium concentration in the serum is highly regulated. If the serum calcium levels drop, parathyroid hormone (PTH) is secreted, which stimulates the kidney to produce calcitriol, the active form of vitamin D. Vitamin D then acts in an endocrine manner in the intestines to absorb calcium available from the diet and supplements and in the bones to activate bone resorption. This process is called calcium homeostasis. The role of calcium is mainly skeletal strength and dynamic storage, to maintain intra- and extracellular calcium concentrations. Therefore, vitamin D has a major physiologic role in maintaining the intra- and extracellular calcium concentrations and skeletal homeostasis [22]. This suggests that both calcium and vitamin D levels are important for bone health [23, 24] and may have interactive effects upon bone health. Consequently, several previous studies have reported on the benefit of vitamin D on BMD [6, 21, 25–27]. A recent study showed that there was no threshold of calcium absorption (range 32–38% of intake) with increased vitamin D intakes [28]. However, recent data evaluating the effect of vitamin D on BMD have been inconsistent. A meta-analysis [26] and a randomized controlled trial (RCT) [29] concluded that there was no evidence of an overall benefit of vitamin D supplementation on BMD, yet there was a small but relevant effect on calcium absorption. It thus remains unclear whether the effect of vitamin D on calcium absorption is substantial enough to translate into beneficial effects on BMD, especially in older women who tend to be deficient in calcium and were not represented in the recent clinical trial [29].

A recent prospective cohort study [$n = 628$, mean age = 75 years (range, 67–93)] determined the association of dairy foods (defined as intake of milk, yogurt, cheese, cream, milk + yogurt, and milk + yogurt + cheese) with aBMD and bone loss (femoral neck, trochanter, and lumbar spine) over 4 years in older adults [25]. This study further assessed whether these associations were modified by vitamin D supplement use in this cohort of older men and women from the Framingham Original Cohort. Dietary assessment in this study was conducted at baseline (in 1988–1989) using Willett semiquantitative food frequency questionnaire. Baseline BMD was measured at the hip (femoral neck and trochanter) and at the spine using Lunar DP3 dual-photon absorptiometer. Follow-up BMD was measured after 4 years using DXA. Four-year percentage change in BMD was calculated as [(follow-up BMD − baseline BMD)/baseline BMD] × 100. This study reported that a higher intake of dairy foods (milk, fluid dairy, and milk + yogurt + cheese) was associated with a higher spine BMD among vitamin D supplement users, but not among nonusers. Among vitamin D supplement users, there was a 0.006 g/cm^2 difference in spine BMD for an increase of one serving of milk per week. Similarly, among vitamin D supplement user, but not among nonusers, higher milk + yogurt + cheese intakes were protective against bone loss at the trochanter. There was a 0.23% increase in trochanter BMD over 4 years for every serving increase of milk + yogurt + cheese per week among vitamin D supplement users. This suggests that vitamin D supplementation may provide bone-protective benefits with higher dairy intakes. However, a higher dairy food consumption did not seem to be protective in non-vitamin D supplement users. This might suggest that a sufficient vitamin D intake is important for dairy to provide bone benefits. However, vitamin D intake does not account for the vitamin D formed in the skin by sun exposure. Therefore, future studies should confirm these findings by using serum vitamin D concentrations.

Studies on Novel Bone Measures

Previous studies examining dairy foods with bone health were largely focused on DXA-derived aBMD, a surrogate for bone strength. Recently, novel measures for bone health have become available such as quantitative computed tomography (QCT) and high-resolution peripheral QCT (HR-pQCT). These measures provide three-dimensional images and volumetric BMD measures to address bone strength, quality, and microarchitecture, which are key determinants of bone health [30, 31].

These new measures provide information on cortical, trabecular, and whole bone volumetric BMD (vBMD) not confounded by individual differences in bone size. Hence, these novel measures enable us to address the associations of dairy intake with bone strength.

There is limited evidence on the impact of calcium intake and dairy protein upon bone strength and microarchitecture. One of the earlier studies in this area reported on cross-sectional associations between calcium intake and non-weight-bearing radius and weight-bearing tibia in 218 healthy women (n = 92 premenopausal women, mean age, 33 years; n = 126 postmenopausal women, mean age, 67 years) [32]. This study reported that high calcium intake seemed to benefit radial shaft but not the tibia. In premenopausal women, the bone strength index (density-weighted section modulus, mm^3) was 7.8% (95% CI 0–16.3%) higher among those with dietary calcium of over 1200 mg/day than those with intakes less than 800 mg/day. In postmenopausal women, cross-sectional area (mm^2) was 5.2% (95% CI 0–10.7%) greater among those with dietary calcium of over 1200 mg/day than those with intakes less than 800 mg/day. However, calcium intake was not associated with tibial bone characteristics. Two recent studies have reported on dairy protein intake and bone health. One cross-sectional study of 746 Caucasian women (aged 65 years) from Geneva determined the association of dietary protein intake (total intake and intake from dairy, nondairy animal, and plant sources) with peripheral skeleton-predicted failure load and stiffness and bone microstructure at the distal radius and tibia [33]. This study reported a beneficial effect of animal and dairy protein intakes on bone strength and microstructure. Dietary protein, particularly from dairy products, was positively associated with bone failure load and stiffness of the peripheral skeleton; with every gram per day increase in dairy protein intake, the failure load increased by 0.009 N at the distal radius and 0.461 N at the distal tibia (p-values 0.025 and 0.048, respectively). With every gram per day increase in dairy protein intake, the stiffness increased by 0.011 N/mm at the distal radius and by 0.013 N/mm at the distal tibia (p-values 0.032 and 0.045, respectively). Similarly, another cross-sectional study of 1016 men, aged ~83 years from the Osteoporosis Fractures in Men (MrOS) Study, determined the association of protein intake by source (from dairy, nondairy animal, plant) with bone strength and bone microarchitecture (HR-pQCT) scans of the distal radius and distal or diaphyseal tibia among older men [34]. This study reported that higher dairy protein intake was associated with higher estimated failure load at the distal radius and distal tibia [radius effect size = 0.17 (95% CI 0.07, 0.27), tibia effect size = 0.13 (95% CI 0.03, 0.23) for 1 SD change in dairy protein intake], while higher nondairy animal protein was associated with higher failure load at only the distal radius [radius effect size = 0.07 (95% CI 0.00, 0.13)]. Plant protein intake was not associated with failure load at any site. Thus, the association between protein intake and bone strength varied by source of protein.

In spite of these studies reporting beneficial role of dietary calcium and dairy protein on bone health, only a few studies have directly assessed the association between dairy food intake and bone measures from QCT or HR-pQCT. A study of 564 older women (aged 80–92 years) evaluated the association of dairy food intake (sum of milk, yogurt, and cheese intake) with peripheral QCT (pQCT) bone measures at the distal tibia. The participants were from the Calcium Intake Fracture Outcome Study (CAIFOS, a 5-year RCT), which enrolled 1500 women aged 70–85 years in 1998. Once the RCT was completed, these participants were followed up for a further 5 years in the CAIFOS Aged Extension Study (CARES) cohort [35]. In this study a dairy intake of ≥2.2 servings/day was associated with higher total and trabecular vBMD (least square adjusted means for total vBMD was 410.1 ± 81.6 mg/cm^3 and for trabecular vBMD was 223.8 ± 59.1 mg/cm^3) as compared to women with an intake of ≤1.5 servings/day (least square adjusted means for total vBMD was 387.7 ± 81.3 mg/cm^3 and for trabecular vBMD was 367.7 ± 81.1 mg/cm^3). These associations became nonsignificant when the models were adjusted for dairy protein and calcium intake. However, the effect of dairy intake upon bone measures from these novel techniques is understudied in men.

A recent study examined the association of dairy food intake (defined as intake of milk, cheese, yogurt, cream, milk + yogurt, and milk + yogurt + cheese) with QCT-derived bone measures of the spine in 2626 men and women from the Framingham Study Offspring and Third Generation (Gen3) cohorts [36]. This study further determined whether these associations were modified by 25-OH D concentrations. In this cross-sectional study, information on dietary intake was collected by Willett semiquantitative food frequency questionnaire in 1998–2001 (Offspring cohort) and in 2002–2005 (Gen3 cohort). QCT assessment was performed in 2002–2005, and the study examined spine measures at the L3 level in the spine. The mean age was 50 years (SD 10.6; range 32–80) for men and 55 years (SD of 9.2; range 36–81) for women. Sixty-four percent of men and 70% of women reached the recommendation of three servings of dairy per day. Thirty-three percent of men and 48% of women did not have adequate blood levels of 25-OH D (20 ng/mL), and 68% of men and 51% women did not achieve recommended dietary allowance (RDA) of calcium intake for their age and sex. A higher milk, milk + yogurt, and milk + yogurt + cheese intake was positively associated with trabecular and integral (entire vertebral body, both cortical and trabecular) volumetric BMD (vBMD, g/cm^3) and vertebral compressive strength (N), estimated using engineering beam theory [37], but not with cross-sectional area (cm^2) in men at the L3 level in the spine. Among men, there was a 0.0002 g/cm^3 and 0.0003 g/cm^3 difference in trabecular and integral vBMD, respectively, for an increase of one serving of milk per week. Similarly, there was a 9.9 N difference in vertebral strength for an increase of one serving of milk per week. No association was seen for yogurt, cheese, and cream with integral and trabecular vBMD or vertebral compressive strength. Only cheese was positively associated with cross-sectional area in men. In women, no association was seen overall, except a higher cream intake was associated with the cross-sectional area. This could be due to high calcium intake (mean calcium intake, ~1200 mg/day) in women in this study. These sex-specific differences in spine indices should be further explored in the context of dairy intake in future studies. In the same study, significant interactions were observed for serum 25-OH D and milk, milk + yogurt, and milk + yogurt + cheese in men for trabecular vBMD (p range, 0.02–0.007), integral vBMD (p

range 0.001–0.004), and vertebral compressive strength (p = 0.003 each). No interaction was observed for 25-OH D and dairy intake in women (p range 0.14–0.97). Consequently, the analyses in men were stratified by 25-OH D. Due to small sample size in the low 25-OH D group, investigators could not use predefined clinical cutoffs for 25-OH D (<20 ng/mL and ≥ 20 ng/mL). Instead, they used cutoffs based on tertiles [lowest tertile (≤24.2 ng/mL) vs. higher two tertiles (>24.2 ng/mL)]. Upon stratification by 25-OH D levels, the authors reported that in men with low 25-OH D, a higher dairy intake showed larger magnitude of association for some but not all bone health measures compared with men with a higher 25-OH D level. However, even among men with 25-OH D > 24.2 ng/mL, dairy continued to have positive associations for milk, milk + yogurt, and milk + yogurt +cheese and vBMD and vertebral compressive strength. These associations also appeared to be stronger in older men aged 50 years and older. In summary, this study concluded that men with higher intakes of milk, milk + yogurt, and milk + yogurt + cheese had higher trabecular and integral vBMD and vertebral compressive strength, but not cross-sectional area. Dairy intake seemed to be most beneficial for older men, and dairy continued to have positive associations across all 25-OH D levels.

Conclusion

Dairy intake is an essential source of bone-beneficial nutrients such as calcium, protein, vitamin D (in fortified dairy), magnesium, and potassium in the Western diet. This provides a specific opportunity for dairy foods to improve bone health specifically in older adults. Evidence for a positive association between milk and bone health is strong. However, evidence for other dairy products is limited. Both calcium and vitamin D levels are important for bone health, and these nutrients may have interactive effects upon bone. However, it remains unclear whether the effect of vitamin D on calcium absorption is substantial enough to translate into beneficial effects on BMD, especially in older adults. Furthermore, majority of nutrition studies used areal BMD from DXA, and there is limited information on dairy's effect upon bone strength, quality, and microarchitecture. Therefore, future studies on dairy foods should focus on specific dairy foods beyond milk intake and novel measures of bone beyond aBMD, and future studies should take vitamin D status into consideration. Given that more than 80% of Americans do not meet the recommended dairy intake of three servings per day and older adults are prone to vitamin D deficiency, this area of research could have important public health implications.

References

1. Kanis J, Group WHOS. WHO technical report. Sheffield: University of Sheffield; 2007. p. 66.
2. Office of the Surgeon General (US). Bone health and osteoporosis: a report of the surgeon general. Rockville: Office of the Surgeon General (US); 2004.
3. U.S. Department of Health and Human Services and U.S. Department of Agriculture. Dietary guidelines for Americans, 2015. 6th ed. Washington, DC: U.S. Government Printing Office; 2005.

4. Vissers PA, Streppel MT, Feskens EJ, de Groot LC. The contribution of dairy products to micronutrient intake in the Netherlands. J Am Coll Nutr. 2011;30(5 Suppl 1):415s–21s.
5. Skinner ML, Simpson JAR, Buchholz AC. Dietary and total calcium intakes are associated with lower percentage total body and truncal fat in young, healthy adults. J Am Coll Nutr. 2011;30(6):484–90.
6. Feskanich D, Willett WC, Colditz GA. Calcium, vitamin D, milk consumption, and hip fractures: a prospective study among postmenopausal women. Am J Clin Nutr. 2003;77(2):504–11.
7. Bonjour JP. Calcium and phosphate: a duet of ions playing for bone health. J Am Coll Nutr. 2011;30(5 Suppl 1):438s–48s.
8. National Dairy Council. NHANES 2011–2014. Data Source: Centers for Disease control and Prevention, National Center for Health Statistics, National Health and Nutrition Examination Survey Data. US Department of Health and Human Services.
9. Quann EE, Fulgoni VL, Auestad N. Consuming the daily recommended amounts of dairy products would reduce the prevalence of inadequate micronutrient intakes in the United States: diet modeling study based on NHANES 2007–2010. Nutr J. 2015;14(1):90.
10. Dror DK, Allen LH. Dairy product intake in children and adolescents in developed countries: trends, nutritional contribution, and a review of association with health outcomes. Nutr Rev. 2014;72(2):68–81.
11. Schepper JD, Irwin R, Kang J, Dagenais K, Lemon T, Shinouskis A, Parameswaran N, McCabe LR. Probiotics in gut-bone signaling. Adv Exp Med Biol. 2017;1033:225–47.
12. Sahni S, Tucker KL, Kiel DP, Quach L, Casey VA, Hannan MT. Milk and yogurt consumption are linked with higher bone mineral density but not with hip fracture: the Framingham Offspring Study. Arch Osteoporos. 2013;8(1–2):119.
13. Sahni S, Kiel DP, Hannan MT. The likely importance of specific dairy foods in relation to bone health: current knowledge and future challenges. In: Nutritional Influences on Bone Health. London: Springer; 2013. p. 307–13.
14. Rizzoli R. Dairy products, yogurts, and bone health. Am J Clin Nutr. 2014;99:1256–62.
15. Heaney RP. Vitamin D and calcium interactions: functional outcomes. Am J Clin Nutr. 2008;88:541–4.
16. Institute of Medicine. Dietary reference intakes for calcium and vitamin D. Washington D.C.; 2010.
17. Calvo MS, Whiting SJ, Barton CN. Vitamin D fortification in the United States and Canada: current status and data needs. Am J Clin Nutr. 2004;80(6):1710S–6S.
18. O'donnell S, Cranney A, Horsley T, Weiler HA, Atkinson SA, Hanley DA, Ooi DS, Ward L, Barrowman N, Fang M. Efficacy of food fortification on serum 25-hydroxy vitamin D concentrations: systematic review. Am J Clin Nutr. 2008;88(6):1528–34.
19. Holick M, Matsuoka L, Wortsman J. Age, vitamin D, and solar ultraviolet. Lancet. 1989;334(8671):1104–5.
20. Black LJ, Seamans KM, Cashman KD, Kiely M. An updated systematic review and meta-analysis of the efficacy of vitamin D food fortification. J Nutr. 2012;142(6):1102–8.
21. Holick MF, Binkley NC, Bischoff-Ferrari HA, Gordon CM, Hanley DA, Heaney RP, Murad MH, Weaver CM. Evaluation, treatment, and prevention of vitamin D deficiency: an endocrine society clinical practice guideline. J Clin Endocrinol Metabol. 2011;96(7):1911–30.
22. Holick MF. Vitamin D and health: evolution, biologic functions, and recommended dietary intakes for vitamin D. In: Holick MF, editor. Vitamin D: physiology, molecular biology, and clinical applications. New York: Humana; 2010.
23. Heaney RP. Calcium, dairy products and osteoporosis. J Am Coll Nutr. 2000;19(sup2): 83S–99S.
24. Heaney RP. Dairy and bone health. J Am Coll Nutr. 2009;28:82S–90S.
25. Sahni S, Mangano KM, Kiel DP, Tucker KL, Hannan MT. Dairy intake is protective against bone loss in older vitamin D supplement users: the Framingham Study. J Nutr. 2017;147:645–52.
26. Reid IR. Effects of vitamin D supplements on bone density. J Endocrinol Investig. 2015;38:91–4.

27. Dawson-Hughes B, Harris SS, Krall EA, Dallal GE. Effect of calcium and vitamin D supplementation on bone density in men and women 65 years of age or older. N Engl J Med. 1997;337(10):670–6.
28. Aloia JF, Dhaliwal R, Shieh A, Mikhail M, Fazzari M, Ragolia L, Abrams SA. Vitamin D supplementation increases calcium absorption without a threshold effect. Am J Clin Nutr. 2014;99(3):624–31.
29. Hansen KE, Johnson RE, Chambers KR, Johnson MG, Lemon CC, Vo TNT, Marvdashti S. Treatment of vitamin D insufficiency in postmenopausal women: a randomized clinical trial. JAMA Intern Med. 2015;175:1612–21.
30. Nishiyama KK, Shane E. Clinical imaging of bone microarchitecture with HR-pQCT. Curr Osteoporos Rep. 2013;11:147–55.
31. Samelson EJ, Christiansen BA, Demissie S, Broe KE, Louie-Gao Q, Cupples LA, Roberts BJ, Manoharam R, D'Agostino J, Lang T. QCT measures of bone strength at the thoracic and lumbar spine: the Framingham Study. J Bone Miner Res. 2012;27:654–63.
32. Uusi-Rasi K, Sievänen H, Pasanen M, Oja P, Vuori I. Associations of calcium intake and physical activity with bone density and size in premenopausal and postmenopausal women: a peripheral quantitative computed tomography study. J Bone Miner Res. 2002;17(3):544–52.
33. Durosier-Izart C, Biver E, Merminod F, van Rietbergen B, Chevalley T, Herrmann FR, Ferrari SL, Rizzoli R. Peripheral skeleton bone strength is positively correlated with total and dairy protein intakes in healthy postmenopausal women. Am J Clin Nutr. 2017;105:513–25.
34. Langsetmo L, Shikany JM, Burghardt AJ, Cawthon PM, Orwoll ES, Cauley JA, Taylor BC, Schousboe JT, Bauer DC, Vo TN, et al. High dairy protein intake is associated with greater bone strength parameters at the distal radius and tibia in older men: a cross-sectional study. Osteoporos Int. 2018;29(1):69–77.
35. Radavelli-Bagatini S, Zhu K, Lewis JR, Prince RL. Dairy food intake, peripheral bone structure, and muscle mass in elderly ambulatory women. J Bone Miner Res. 2014;29:1691–700.
36. van Dongen LH, Kiel DP, Soedamah-Muthu SS, Bouxsein ML, Hannan MT, Sahni S. Higher dairy food intake is associated with higher spine quantitative computed tomography (QCT) bone measures in the Framingham study for men but not women. J Bone Miner Res. 2018;33:1–8.
37. Crawford RP, Cann CE, Keaveny TM. Finite element models predict in vitro vertebral body compressive strength better than quantitative computed tomography. Bone. 2003;33:744–50.

19 Dietary Intake in Chinese Community-Dwelling Older Adults with Sarcopenia: A Focus on Protein

Ruth Chan and Liu-Ying Zhu

Sarcopenia and Its Consequences

Sarcopenia represents the loss of skeletal muscle mass, strength, and function that occurs with aging [1]. Previously it was recognized as a geriatric syndrome [2]. Until October 2016, the Centers for Disease Control and Prevention (CDC) established an ICD-10-CM code for sarcopenia, M62.84, allowing the syndrome to be recognized as a primary or secondary condition [3]. Substantial evidence suggests that sarcopenia is associated with various adverse health outcomes such as falls, disability, institutionalization, mortality, and poor quality of life, thus having substantial impacts on the health and social care costs [4–6]. However, recent evidence reveals that some reversibility of sarcopenia exists, in which higher body mass index (BMI) is protective against its reversibility, and increasing physical activity and maintaining a healthy weight could be beneficial for the prevention of sarcopenia [7]. Therefore identifying strategies to reverse or delay the progression of sarcopenia is of public health importance.

Prevalence of Sarcopenia Worldwide and in Hong Kong

International Consensus Panel definitions of sarcopenia are available for the USA, Europe, and Asia (Table 19.1) [2, 8, 9]. Based on the definition of sarcopenia proposed by the European Working Group on Sarcopenia in Older People (EWGSOP), sarcopenia affects 1–29% for older adults living in the community and up to 33% for those living in the residential care settings [2].

R. Chan (✉) · L.-Y. Zhu
Department of Medicine and Therapeutics, The Chinese University of Hong Kong, Hong Kong, China
e-mail: ruthchansm@cuhk.edu.hk; zoezhuliuying@link.cuhk.edu.hk

© Springer Nature Switzerland AG 2019

C. M. Weaver et al. (eds.), *Nutritional Influences on Bone Health*,
https://doi.org/10.1007/978-3-319-98464-3_19

Table 19.1 International Consensus Panel definitions of sarcopenia

Criteria	Physical performance (gait speed, m/s)	Muscle strength (grip strength, kg)	Skeletal muscle mass[a]
US Foundation for the National Institutes of Health (FNIH) [10]	Not applicable	<26 (men) <16 (women)	ALM_{BMI} <0.789 (men) <0.512 (women)
European Working Group on Sarcopenia in Older Persons (EWGSOP) [2]	<0.8	<30 (men) <20 (women)	ALM/Ht^2 ≤7.26 (men) ≤5.50 (women)
International Working Group of Sarcopenia (IWGS) [8]	<1.0	Not applicable	ALM/Ht^2 ≤7.23 (men) ≤5.67 (women)
Asian Working Group of Sarcopenia (AWGS) [9]	<0.8	<26 (men) <18 (women)	ALM/Ht^2 ≤7.00 (men) ≤5.40 (women)

[a] ALM_{BMI} appendicular lean mass/body mass index, ALM/Ht^2 appendicular lean mass/height^2 (kg/m^2)

Table 19.2 Prevalence of sarcopenia of Chinese community-dwelling older adults in Hong Kong by sex and age group based on the criteria of the Asian Working Group on Sarcopenia (AWGS)

Age group (years)	Male (n = 2000)	Female (n = 2000)	Total (n = 4000)
65–74	4.9%	3.2%	4.1%
75–84	17.7%	8.7%	13.1%
85+	37.2%	17.2%	25.7%

Depending on the definitions used for defining sarcopenia, it was estimated using data from a prospective cohort study in Hong Kong involving 4000 Chinese community-dwelling older adults aged 65 or above [11] that the prevalence ranged from 2.6 to 22.1% in older men and 1.3–18.3% in older women in Hong Kong; the prevalence was highest using the International Working Group on Sarcopenia (IWGS) definition [12]. Using the criteria of the Asian Working Group on Sarcopenia (AWGS), the prevalence also increased with age, with 4.1%, 13.1%, and 25.7% for the age group of 65–74, 75–84, and 85+ years having sarcopenia, respectively [9] (Table 19.2).

Risk Factors of Sarcopenia

The causes of sarcopenia are multifactorial. Age and sex are the constitutional factors for the prevalence of sarcopenia [7, 13]. Low birth weight has been linked with increased risk of sarcopenia in later life [14]. Genetic factors also play a role in the etiology of sarcopenia [15, 16]. Other risk factors included the age-related changes in hormonal dysregulation, such as the reduction in growth hormone and insulin-like growth factor (IGF)-1 and the increase in insulin resistance [17], and the age-related decline in the neuromuscular system, in particular the loss of alpha motor neurons [18, 19]. Changes in living conditions, such as prolonged bed rest [20] and various chronic health conditions, such as diabetes and chronic lung disease, may also predispose older adults to increased risk of sarcopenia [21, 22]. Lifestyle behavioral factors including smoking, alcohol use, physical inactivity, and poor diet, in particular inadequate protein intake, are also risk factors of sarcopenia [17, 21].

Dietary Protein Intake and Sarcopenia

A positive net protein balance, which refers to a state that muscle protein synthesis (MPS) is higher than muscle protein breakdown (MPB), is important for muscle health. The interplay of foods, physical activity, and hormones greatly influences the equilibrium of net protein balance [23]. The provision of a well-balanced diet with foods rich in protein content is generally recommended for older adults [17, 24].

Protein has long been considered as the key nutrient for muscle mass preservation and physical function maintenance. The quantity and quality of protein, timing of protein consumption, as well as dosage distribution determine the equilibrium of net protein balance [23, 25]. A protein intake of 1.0–1.2 g/kg body weight/day or at higher level (i.e., 1.5 g/kg body weight/day) is proposed for optimizing skeletal muscle health in older people without affecting renal function [26, 27]. In terms of protein quality, animal protein sources are generally preferred over plant protein source in view of its relatively higher essential amino acid content and protein availability which are beneficial for muscle protein synthesis and anabolism [28, 29]. However, there is evidence to suggest that increases in muscle strength and size were not affected by the predominant source of dietary protein in older adults with adequate total protein intake [30]. The timing and dosage distribution of protein intake are also important factors affecting net protein balance. Older adults generally show an uneven distribution of protein intake throughout the day, with little protein consumed at breakfast and much more protein consumed at lunch or dinner [23]. A moderate intake of high-quality protein of at least 25–30 g per meal throughout the day is generally recommended for older adults [23, 31].

Protein Intake Pattern and Its Association with Muscle Mass, Physical Performance, and Sarcopenia in Chinese Community-Dwelling Older Adults in Hong Kong

Although low protein intake is one of the major risk factors of sarcopenia, there have been limited data differentiating the effect of animal protein and plant protein on physical performance measures and muscle mass, as well as investigating the detailed protein consumption pattern in community-dwelling older adults of Chinese origin.

Using data from a subsample of 2726 (1411 male, 1315 female) Chinese community-dwelling older adults aged 65 or above in a prospective cohort study in Hong Kong, the differential effect of animal protein intake and plant protein intake on the 4-year change in physical performance measures and muscle mass was examined [32]. At baseline, the median total protein intake was 1.3 and 1.1 g/kg body weight per day for male and female, respectively, as assessed using a food frequency questionnaire (FFQ). Univariate and multivariate analyses indicated that either total protein intake or animal protein intake was associated with 4-year change in physical performance measures and muscle mass in the studied sample. Although no significant association between plant protein intake and 4-year change in physical performance measures was observed, older adults with plant protein intake at or above 0.72 g/kg body weight/day showed a significantly slower decline in the appendicular muscle mass (age- and sex-adjusted mean ± standard error 0.270 ± 0.029) over the 4-year period in comparison with those with plant protein intake at or below 0.4 g/kg body weight/day (0.349 ± 0.030 kg) ($p_{trend} = 0.025$).

The replete protein status of the participants may attenuate the association of the total protein intake or animal protein intake with the measured outcomes in this study. The inclusion of soy and soy products in Chinese diet, in which soy proteins are regarded as high-quality proteins in view of the complete amino acid profiles [33], may explain the positive findings between higher plant protein intake and reduced muscle loss. The antioxidant property and the alkaline property of plant-based foods may also explain the significant association of higher plant protein intake with reduced muscle loss [34, 35]. To our knowledge, this study was the first to examine the differential effect of animal protein and plant protein on physical performance measures and muscle mass in Chinese community-dwelling older adults. Since the dietary data were collected using FFQ and the target group was not specifically sarcopenic, the detailed protein consumption pattern of Chinese community-dwelling older adults with sarcopenia warrants further investigation.

Pilot findings from a recently completed randomized controlled trial assessing the role of an exercise program and nutrition supplement for improving muscle mass, strength, and power, as well as physical performance in Chinese community-dwelling older adults with sarcopenia, may provide insights into the detailed protein intake pattern of this population [36] (ClinicalTrials.gov Identifier: NCT02374268). Baseline dietary data of 62 Chinese older adults (14 male, 48 female) with sarcopenia defined using the AWGS were analyzed. A three-day diet record including two weekdays and one weekend day was collected. Mean age of the participants was 72.3 years. Mean dietary protein intake of the participants was adequate as it averaged 1.6 g/kg of body weight/day. There were only nine (14.5%) participants with protein intake below 1.2 g/kg of body weight/day. The animal source and the plant source contributed to 60% and 40% of the total protein intake, respectively. The protein intake of this sample was high in comparison with the level reported in other previous studies with Western populations (i.e., 0.8–1.2 g/kg of body weight/day) [37, 38]. However, a skewed distribution of dietary protein intake throughout the day was observed, in which the protein intake was lowest at breakfast and highest at dinner (Fig. 19.1). Animal protein contributed to 48.5, 56.0, and 65.6% of the protein intake at breakfast, lunch, and dinner, respectively. Table 19.3 lists the main food sources of protein intake for the main meals, and the preliminary findings suggest that a higher intake of animal protein source at breakfast may be required for this group of Chinese older adults with sarcopenia.

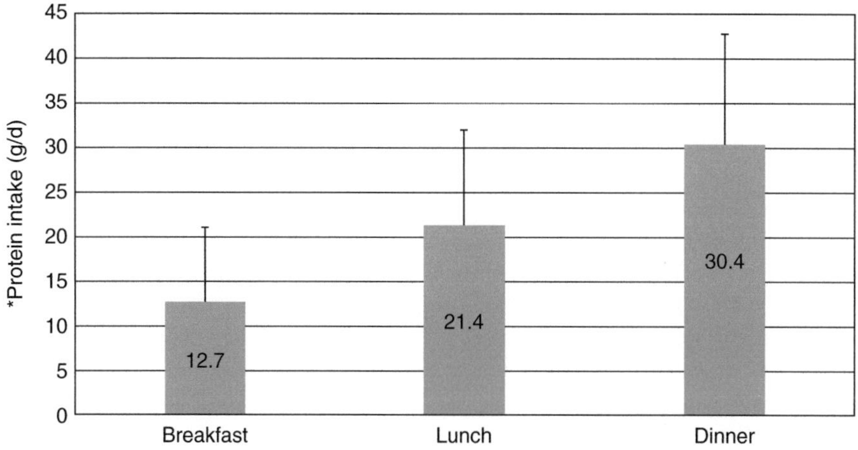

Fig. 19.1 Mean protein intake at breakfast, lunch, and dinner of Chinese community-dwelling older adults with sarcopenia ($n = 62$). Error bar indicates the standard deviation

Table 19.3 Top five protein sources at three main meals of Chinese community-dwelling older adults with sarcopenia ($n = 62$)

Breakfast		Lunch		Dinner	
Refined grains (e.g., white bread, congee, white rice, raisin bread, macaroni)	15.8%	Red and processed meats (e.g., pork, steamed beef ball, ribs, beef, luncheon meat)	23.7%	Red and processed meats (e.g., pork, ribs, beef, sausages)	20.5%
Whole grains (e.g., oatmeal, whole wheat bread, brown rice, sorghum)	15.5%	Refined grains (e.g., white rice, rice noodles, noodles, congee, pasta)	18.6%	Seawater fish (e.g., golden threadfin bream, salmon, grouper)	15.0%
Milk (e.g., milk powder, fresh milk, evaporated and condensed milk in drinks)	13.8%	Seawater fish (e.g., golden threadfin bream, canned tuna, mackerel)	8.7%	Refined grains (e.g., white rice, noodles, rice noodles, pasta, congee)	14.0%
Red and processed meats (e.g., pork, ribs, beef, ham)	11.0%	Poultry (e.g., chicken, duck)	7.1%	Poultry (e.g., chicken, goose, duck)	12.5%
Eggs (e.g., whole egg, egg white, preserved egg)	6.5%	Soy (e.g., tofu, soybean, soybean sheet, soy milk)	5.8%	Freshwater fish (e.g., grass carp, dace, goldfish carp, silver fish, eel)	10.3%

Conclusions and Future Research Directions

In summary, data from Chinese community-dwelling older adults with or without sarcopenia in Hong Kong indicates that protein intakes were generally replete. Similar to the literature, they showed the lowest protein intake at breakfast and the protein source of the breakfast were dominated by plant-based foods. A higher intake of animal protein source at breakfast may be recommended for Chinese community-dwelling older adults. However, most of the existing evidence and dietary recommendations are based on Western population. In view of the differences in dietary habits and body build between Western and the Chinese populations, further studies are warranted to explore the impact of cultural dietary difference, as well as the optimal intake and ratio of animal protein to plant protein in the preservation of muscle mass and functions. The contribution of different dietary components and the interplay of diet, physical activity, and hormones to the etiology of sarcopenia are also worth further investigation.

References

1. Morley JE, Baumgartner RN, Roubenoff R, Mayer J, Nair KS. Sarcopenia. J Lab Clin Med. 2001;137:231–43.
2. Cruz-Jentoft AJ, Baeyens JP, Bauer JM, Boirie Y, Cederholm T, Landi F, et al. Sarcopenia: European consensus on definition and diagnosis: report of the European Working Group on Sarcopenia in Older People. Age Ageing. 2010;39:412–23.
3. Aging in Motion. AIM coalition announces establishment of ICD-10-CM Code for Sarcopenia by the Centers for Disease Control and Prevention [press release]. 2016. http://aginginmotion.org/news/2388-2/. Accessed 7 Dec 2017.
4. Malmstrom TK, Morley JE. The frail brain. J Am Med Dir Assoc. 2013;14:453–5.
5. Janssen I, Heymsfield SB, Ross R. Low relative skeletal muscle mass (sarcopenia) in older persons is associated with functional impairment and physical disability. J Am Geriatr Soc. 2002;50:889–96.
6. Janssen I, Shepard DS, Katzmarzyk PT, Roubenoff R. The healthcare costs of sarcopenia in the United States. J Am Geriatr Soc. 2004;52:80–5.
7. Yu R, Wong M, Leung J, Lee J, Auyeung TW, Woo J. Incidence, reversibility, risk factors and the protective effect of high body mass index against sarcopenia in community-living older Chinese people. Geriatr Gerontol Int. 2014;14(Suppl 1):15–28.
8. Fielding RA, Vellas B, Evans WJ, Bhasin S, Morley JE, Newman AB, et al. Sarcopenia: an undiagnosed condition in older adults. Current consensus definition: prevalence, etiology, and consequences. International working group on sarcopenia. J Am Med Dir Assoc. 2011;12:249–56.
9. Chen LK, Liu LK, Woo J, Assantachai P, Auyeung TW, Bahyah KS, et al. Sarcopenia in Asia: consensus report of the Asian Working Group for Sarcopenia. J Am Med Dir Assoc. 2014;15:95–101.
10. Studenski SA, Peters KW, Alley DE, Cawthon PM, McLean RR, Harris TB, et al. The FNIH sarcopenia project: rationale, study description, conference recommendations, and final estimates. J Gerontol A Biol Sci Med Sci. 2014;69:547–58.
11. Wong SY, Kwok T, Woo J, Lynn H, Griffith JF, Leung J, et al. Bone mineral density and the risk of peripheral arterial disease in men and women: results from Mr. and Ms Os, Hong Kong. Osteoporos Int. 2005;16:1933–8.

12. Woo J, Leung J, Morley JE. Defining sarcopenia in terms of incident adverse outcomes. J Am Med Dir Assoc. 2015;16:247–52.
13. Shaw SC, Dennison EM, Cooper C. Epidemiology of sarcopenia: determinants throughout the life course. Calcif Tissue Int. 2017;101:229–47.
14. Woo J, Cheung B, Tong C, Chan R. Impact of childhood experience of famine on body composition: DEX and beyond. In: Preedy V, Patel VB, editors. Handbook of famine, starvation and nutrient deprivation: from biology to policy. New York: Springer; 2017. p. 1–21.
15. Arden NK, Spector TD. Genetic influences on muscle strength, lean body mass, and bone mineral density: a twin study. J Bone Miner Res. 1997;12:2076–81.
16. Christensen K, McGue M, Yashin A, Iachine I, Holm NV, Vaupel JW. Genetic and environmental influences on functional abilities in Danish twins aged 75 years and older. J Gerontol A Biol Sci Med Sci. 2000;55:M446–52.
17. Tieland M, Trouwborst I, Clark BC. Skeletal muscle performance and ageing. J Cachexia Sarcopenia Muscle. 2017;9(1):3–19. https://doi.org/10.1002/jcsm.12238.
18. Brown WF. A method for estimating the number of motor units in thenar muscles and the changes in motor unit count with ageing. J Neurol Neurosurg Psychiatry. 1972;35:845–52.
19. Doherty TJ, Vandervoort AA, Taylor AW, Brown WF. Effects of motor unit losses on strength in older men and women. J Appl Physiol. 1993;74:868–74.
20. Coker RH, Wolfe RR. Bedrest and sarcopenia. Curr Opin Clin Nutr Metab Care. 2012;15:7–11.
21. Lee JS, Auyeung TW, Kwok T, Lau EM, Leung PC, Woo J. Associated factors and health impact of sarcopenia in older Chinese men and women: a cross-sectional study. Gerontology. 2007;53:404–10.
22. Han P, Yu H, Ma Y, Kang L, Fu L, Jia L, et al. The increased risk of sarcopenia in patients with cardiovascular risk factors in Suburb-Dwelling older Chinese using the AWGS definition. Sci Rep. 2017;7:9592.
23. Dawson BM, Axford S. Nutrition as a part of healthy aging and reducing cardiovascular risk: improving functionality in later life using quality protein, with optimized timing and distribution. Semin Thromb Hemost. 2014;40:695–703.
24. Morley JE, Argiles JM, Evans WJ, Bhasin S, Cella D, Deutz NE, et al. Nutritional recommendations for the management of sarcopenia. J Am Med Dir Assoc. 2010;11:391–6.
25. Kim IY, Deutz NEP, Wolfe RR. Update on maximal anabolic response to dietary protein. Clin Nutr. 2017;37(2):411–8. pii: S0261-5614(17)30203-0.
26. Wolfe RR, Miller SL, Miller KB. Optimal protein intake in the elderly. Clin Nutr. 2008;27:675–84.
27. Mithal A, Bonjour JP, Boonen S, Burckhardt P, Degens H, El Hajj Fuleihan G, et al. Impact of nutrition on muscle mass, strength, and performance in older adults. Osteoporos Int. 2013;24:1555–66.
28. Pannemans DL, Wagenmakers AJ, Westerterp KR, Schaafsma G, Halliday D. Effect of protein source and quantity on protein metabolism in elderly women. Am J Clin Nutr. 1998;68:1228–35.
29. Campbell WW, Barton ML Jr, Cyr-Campbell D, Davey SL, Beard JL, Parise G, et al. Effects of an omnivorous diet compared with a lactoovovegetarian diet on resistance-training-induced changes in body composition and skeletal muscle in older men. Am J Clin Nutr. 1999;70:1032–9.
30. Haub MD, Wells AM, Tarnopolsky MA, Campbell WW. Effect of protein source on resistive-training-induced changes in body composition and muscle size in older men. Am J Clin Nutr. 2002;76:511–7.
31. Symons TB, Sheffield-Moore M, Wolfe RR, Paddon-Jones D. A moderate serving of high-quality protein maximally stimulates skeletal muscle protein synthesis in young and elderly subjects. J Am Diet Assoc. 2009;109:1582–6.
32. Chan R, Leung J, Woo J, Kwok T. Associations of dietary protein intake on subsequent decline in muscle mass and physical functions over four years in ambulant older Chinese people. J Nutr Health Aging. 2014;18:171–7.

33. Young VR. Soy protein in relation to human protein and amino acid nutrition. J Am Diet Assoc. 1991;91:828–35.
34. Robinson SM, Reginster JY, Rizzoli R, Shaw SC, Kanis JA, Bautmans I, et al. Does nutrition play a role in the prevention and management of sarcopenia? Clin Nutr. 2017;37(4):1121–32. pii: S0261-5614(17)30299-6. https://doi.org/10.1016/j.clnu.2017.08.016.
35. Chan R, Leung J, Woo J. Association between estimated net endogenous acid production and subsequent decline in muscle mass over four years in ambulatory older Chinese people in Hong Kong: a prospective cohort study. J Gerontol A Biol Sci Med Sci. 2015;70:905–11.
36. Chan R, Zhu LY, Yeung S, Li L, Kwok T, Woo J. Dietary protein intake and protein sources and their associations with selected muscle and physical function measures in older Chinese adults with sarcopenia: preliminary findings. J Cachexia Sarcopenia Muscle. 2016;7:630.
37. Beasley JM, LaCroix AZ, Neuhouser ML, Huang Y, Tinker L, Woods N, et al. Protein intake and incident frailty in the Women's Health Initiative observational study. J Am Geriatr Soc. 2010;58:1063–71.
38. Houston DK, Nicklas BJ, Ding J, Harris TB, Tylavsky FA, Newman AB, et al. Dietary protein intake is associated with lean mass change in older, community-dwelling adults: the Health, Aging, and Body Composition (Health ABC) Study. Am J Clin Nutr. 2008;87:150–5.

Part VII

Policy and Translation

No Relationship Between Serum 25(OH) Vitamin D Concentrations and Perceptions of Vitamin D Dietary Intake Adequacy in US and German Adults Not Using Dietary Supplements

20

Regan L. Bailey, Sowmyanarayanan V. Thuppal, Katherine D. Sherif, Nigel Denby, Suzanne R. Steinbaum, Bryan Haycock, Alexandra E. Cowan, Jared R. Nieters, and Clemens von Schacky

Introduction

Vitamin D plays an important role in bone health, cancer, and cardiovascular disease [1–12]. Some [13, 14] but not all studies [15] have associated optimal serum vitamin D with lower risk for mortality. Thus, vitamin D has increasingly become a

R. L. Bailey (✉) · S. V. Thuppal · A. E. Cowan
Department of Nutrition Science, Purdue University, West Lafayette, IN, USA
e-mail: reganbailey@purdue.edu; cowan9@purdue.edu

K. D. Sherif
Jefferson Women's Primary Care, Philadelphia, PA, USA
e-mail: Katherine.sherif@jefferson.edu

N. Denby
Grub4Life and People Matter TV, London, UK
e-mail: nigel@buddypower.net

S. R. Steinbaum
Women and Heart Disease Center, New York, NY, USA

B. Haycock
Department of Nutrition and Integrative Physiology, University of Utah, Salt Lake City, UT, USA
e-mail: bryan.haycock@utah.edu

J. R. Nieters
Mapleworks, LLC, Amissville, VA, USA

C. von Schacky
University of Munich, Munich, Germany
e-mail: clemens.vonschacky@med.uni-muenchen.de

© Springer Nature Switzerland AG 2019

C. M. Weaver et al. (eds.), *Nutritional Influences on Bone Health*,
https://doi.org/10.1007/978-3-319-98464-3_20

focus of medical research that links nutrition and preventative medicine. The Academy of Nutrition and Dietetics recommends a balanced diet with a variety of nutrients for achieving optimal dietary intakes [16]. Unfortunately, vitamin D is not naturally found in large quantities in contemporary dietary patterns. For this reason, vitamin D is used to fortify many foods (e.g., milk, breakfast cereals, and orange juice) in the USA. However, vitamin D fortification is not routine practice in Germany. Without fortification and dietary supplement use, many people in both countries do not achieve the dietary recommendations [17–22].

Previously, a study on perceptions of a healthy diet among US and German adults showed that 84% of the adults believed that vitamin D was critical for optimal health [23]. Despite the relatively high use of vitamin D dietary supplements (62% in the USA and 31% in Germany), more than half were unsure or did not think they consumed enough vitamin D in their diet [23]. However, this study did not measure serum 25 (OH) vitamin D concentrations relative to these perceptions. Therefore, the purpose of the current study is to compare the knowledge and perceptions of vitamin D adequacy in the diet with the biomarker of vitamin D exposure in these two populations with (USA) and without (Germany) vitamin D fortification among adults who were not using dietary supplements.

Methods

A clinical study of US and German adults was conducted in the spring of 2016 at Purdue University through the Indiana Clinical and Translational Science Institute and the Department of Nutrition Science (USA) and at Ludwig Maximilians-Universität München, Munich, and in clinical sites at Jena, Meerbusch, Hamburg, and Hannover (Germany). The study protocol was approved by IRBs at both universities. Inclusion criteria included nonpregnant, non-lactating adults, 18–80 years not currently using dietary supplements, and without any acute health conditions.

At a clinic visit, baseline demographic details were obtained including age, sex, race/ethnicity, educational attainment, income, physical activity, and duration of exposure to sunlight. Height and weight were measured using calibrated instruments, and body mass index was calculated using the standard formula weight (kg)/height (m) [2]. Dietary knowledge and perceptions of vitamin D intake were assessed using a questionnaire that consisted of close-ended questions with dichotomous, ordinal, and Likert scale response options modified after a previous study [23]. In this questionnaire, a balanced diet was defined as "a diet with all the recommended daily intake of nutrients," and specific questions were included to understand the perceptions about foods that contain vitamin D, adequacy of vitamin D in diet, and importance of vitamin D for health.

Non-fasting blood samples were collected using red-top vacutainer tubes and assayed for serum 25 (OH) vitamin D using the LC-MS/MS method. Based on the National Academies of Science, Engineering, and Medicine (NASEM) 2011 recommendations, serum vitamin D concentrations were classified as "inadequate" at

<20 ng/mL (<50 nmol/L) [24]. Heany and Holick have suggested <30 ng/mL (<75 nmol/L) as a marker for "suboptimal" vitamin D concentrations [25]. Both cut points were examined for this analysis.

Statistical analyses were performed using SAS statistical software 9.4 by SAS Institute Inc., Cary, NC, USA. Demographic and biomarker data were summarized with descriptive statistics. Dietary perceptions were compared based on vitamin D status cut-point categories defined as inadequate and suboptimal. ANOVA and t-tests were used for continuous variables and chi-square tests for categorical variables with statistical significance set at a p-value <0.05.

Results

In both countries, there was a higher proportion of women than men in the sample; the German sample was comprised exclusively of non-Hispanic Whites, whereas slightly more racial diversity existed in the US sample (Table 20.1). Participants in Germany were, on average, older than participants in the USA. The majority of the sample had a college education and reported some physical activity; however, the frequency of exercise was higher in the USA than in Germany. In both countries, minutes of sunlight (i.e., UV exposure) was higher on the weekends than the weekdays but did not differ by country. While the mean BMI was in the healthy range (18–25 kg/m^2), the prevalence of overweight and obesity together was 40%.

Based on the 2011 National Academies of Science, Engineering, and Medicine (NASEM) recommendations, the mean serum 25(OH)D concentrations for both the USA (28 ng/mL) and Germany (23 ng/mL) fall within the optimal range of 20 ng/mL to 50 ng/mL [24]. American adults had higher mean 25(OH)D concentrations and therefore lower prevalence of inadequate or suboptimal 25(OH)D. Mean 25(OH)D did not differ by sex, BMI, education, age, or income within country (data not shown).

All participants reported that consuming a balanced diet is important (Table 20.2). Overall, half the sample rated their diet as good, and equal proportions (~25%) rated their diet as very good/excellent and fair/poor. These percentages changed however when participants rated if their diet was balanced with 45% agreeing, 38% disagreeing, and 17% who were unsure. Similarly, more participants did not know or were unsure (64%) if their diets were adequate in vitamin D.

Interestingly when country data were combined or stratified, mean 25(OH)D concentrations did not differ based on perceptions of a balanced diet, ratings of diet, adequacy of vitamin D in the diet, or importance of vitamin D for health. A higher proportion of adults were inadequate who thought vitamin D was only "somewhat important" for health compared to "important" and "very important," who did not differ—but since the sample size was small (n = 5), this should be interpreted with caution. None of the findings in Table 20.2 were significant when we examined response options with the prevalence of suboptimal serum 25(OH)D concentrations (data not shown).

Table 20.1 Demographic characteristics and mean serum 25(OH) vitamin D [25(OH)D] of US and German adults (> 18 years, $n = 200$) participating in a cross-sectional study on the knowledge and perceptions of dietary vitamin D[a,b]

	All ($n = 200$)	USA ($n = 100$)	Germany ($n = 100$)	p-value
Race/ethnicity, %[c]				<0.0001
Non-Hispanic White	86	69	100	
Non-Hispanic Black	1	2	0	
Hispanic	6	11	0	
Asian	7	15	0	
Age in years, mean (range)	35 (18–80)	29 (18–71)	40 (18–80)	<0.0001
Education, %[c]				<0.0001
High School or equivalent	21	10	32	
Associate degree or some college	13	20	5	
College graduate or higher	66	70	62	
Income[c]				0.90
<50,000 USD	53	51	54	
>50,000 USD	45	44	45	
Frequency of Physical activity, %				<0.0001
None	13	0	27	
1–2 days a week	39	28	49	
3–4 days a week	36	51	21	
> 4 days/week	12	21	3	
Mean sunlight exposure, minutes (95% CL)				
Weekdays	80 (71–98)	85 (71–98)	77 (61–94)	0.48
Weekends	172 (155–188)	164 (142–186)	181 (157–205)	0.30
Mean BMI, kg/m^2 (95% CL)	24 (23.8–25.1)	25 (24.1–26.0)	24 (23.4–24.7)	0.08
Prevalence overweight, %	30	33	28	0.25
Prevalence of obesity, %	10	13	6	0.09
Mean 25 (OH)D, ng/mL (95% CL)	25.4 (24.0–26.8)	27.7 (25.5–29.9)	23.1 (21.4–24.7)	0.001
Prevalence of inadequacy (%)	27	17	36	0.002
Prevalence of suboptimal (%)	76	70	82	0.047

[a]Non-fasting blood samples were assayed for serum 25(OH) vitamin D using the LC-MS/MS method

[b]Comparison by country was performed with t-tests for continuous variables (means) and chi-square tests for categorical variables (percentages); significance set at $p < 0.05$

[c]Percentages do not equal 100 as missing data and small response options are not presented

Table 20.2 Mean (95% CL) serum 25(OH) vitamin D concentrations by sex and dietary perceptions of vitamin D intake in US and German adults over 18 years of age ($n = 200$)[a,b,c]

	% of sample	Mean 25(OH)D (95% CI)	% (SE) inadequate	% (SE) inadequate USA	Germany
How important is a balanced diet?					
Somewhat important	25	23.3 (20.5–26.1)	31 (6)	25 (7)	35 (12)
Important	43	25.5 (23.4–27.6)	28 (5)	16 (6)	39 (7)
Very important	32	27.1 (24.7–29.5)	20 (5)	10 (7)	29 (8)
How would you rate your diet?					
Excellent/very good	24	25.9 (23.1–28.8)	20 (6)	10 (8)	31 (9)
Good	50	25.7 (23.8–27.7)	25 (4)	16 (5)	35 (7)
Fair/poor	26	24.2 (21.4–26.9)	35 (6)	25 (7)	46 (9)
Do you have a nutritionally balanced diet?					
Yes	45	25.6 (23.5–27.6)	26 (5)	12 (5)	41 (8)
No	38	25.0 (22.8–27.2)	28 (5)	21 (6)	34 (8)
Don't know	17	25.8 (22.4–29.3)	23 (8)	22 (13)	29 (10)
How important is vitamin D for overall health?					
Somewhat important	8	23.1 (18.2–28.1)	40 (11)	60 (16) [1]	36 (15)
Important	27	24.9 (22.2–27.6)	32 (6)	20 (8) [2]	42 (8)
Very important	65	25.9 (24.1–27.6)	23 (4)	13 (4) [2]	33 (7)
Do you get enough vitamin D from your diet?					
Yes	36	26.1 (23.7–28.4)	26 (5)	16 (5)	36 (10)
No	37	25.6 (23.3–27.9)	23 (7)	17 (7)	29 (7)
Don't know	27	24.2 (21.6–26.9)	32 (6)	19 (8)	44 (8)
Do these food sources contain vitamin D?					
Milk[d]					
Yes	63	25.9 (24.1–27.7)	27 (4)	16 (4)	39 (7)
No	36	24.7 (22.2–27.1)	25 (5)	22 (9)	32 (7)
Oily fish[d]					
Yes	28	25.6 (22.8–28.3)	27 (6)	25 (9)	33 (8)
No	71	25.4 (23.7–27.0)	25 (4)	15 (4)	36 (6)

[a]Non-fasting blood samples were collected using red-top vacutainer tubes and assayed for serum 25(OH) vitamin D using the LC-MS/MS method
[b]Mean serum 25(OH)D and prevalence of inadequacy compared using a general linear model controlled for country of participant
[c]Estimates with numerical superscripts differ significantly at $p < 0.05$. All other estimates do not significantly differ
[d]Percentages do not equal 100 as "don't know" options are not presented

Despite low reports of nutritionally balanced diets among US and German participants, most considered vitamin D as an important nutrient in improving joint and bone health (including osteoporosis) (74% and 65%). Participants in both the USA and Germany identified milk (82% and 44%) and cheese (70% and 40%) as the top two food sources of vitamin D. While German participants also reported oily fish as the third highest food source, Americans ranked eggs as the third most common source of vitamin D in their diets (Fig. 20.1).

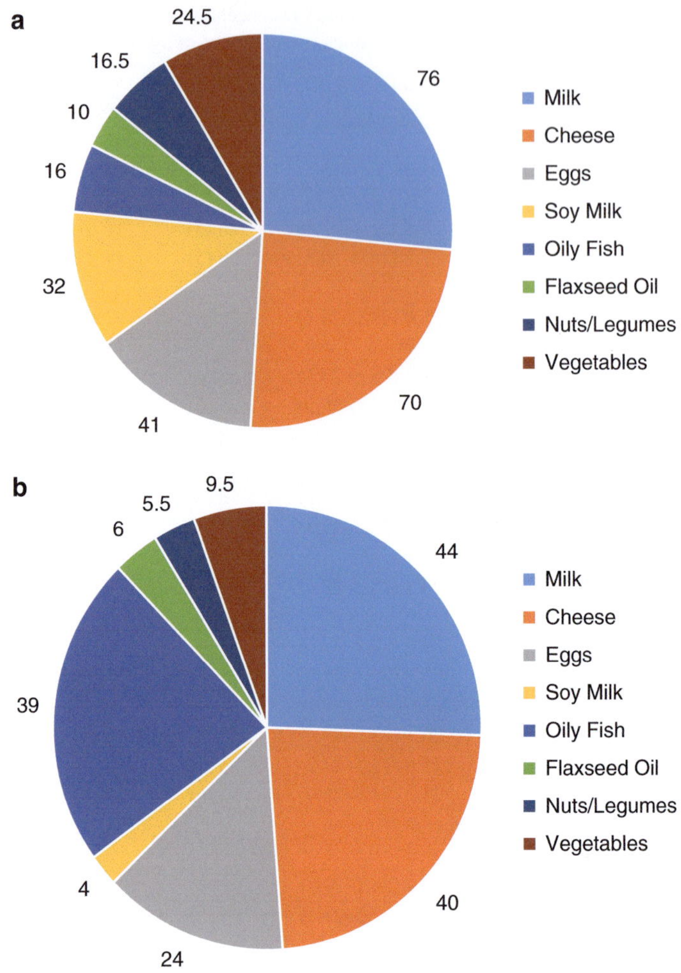

Fig. 20.1 Proportion of participants identifying food sources of vitamin D in the United States (Panel **a**) and Germany (Panel **b**) ($n = 200$)

Discussion

Many adults, regardless of country, correctly identified some food sources for vitamin D and had knowledge of the bone health benefits of vitamin D. A minority (36%) thought they have adequate amounts of vitamin D in their diet; but, a higher proportion (78%) actually had "adequate" serum 25(OH)D concentrations based on the National Academies of Science, Engineering, and Medicine (NASEM) guidelines. When an optimal cut point was applied, prevalence estimates based on serum increased on both countries but especially for the USA. Stated differently, 64% of adults were unsure or did not think they consumed enough vitamin D in the diet, whereas 27% were inadequate and 76% were suboptimal when serum concentrations were examined. Thus the choice of cut points for nutritional biomarkers is quite important and influences the prevalence estimates [26–28]. Indeed, considerable debate exists for the appropriate cut point to use for assessment of vitamin D status in the blood [25, 29]. It is important to note that not only is a low vitamin D of concern but also a high vitamin D concentration as a U- and J-shaped risk curve exists for vitamin D status and health outcomes [13, 14], so use of one cut point alone may not be optimal for those wishing to examine the high ends of the distribution.

When comparing serum 25(OH)D concentrations between countries, a higher percentage of US participants had adequate vitamin D status when compared to participants in Germany. In the USA, many foods are fortified with vitamin D; however, in Germany, fortification of food with vitamin D is not permitted. Previous European studies suggest that vitamin D fortification may have a positive impact on vitamin D intakes in European countries [30, 31]. In the USA, where fortification practices are regularly used, the mean serum 25(OH)D concentrations were on average 5 ng/mL higher than in Germany, suggesting that this higher average intake of vitamin D may be due to US fortification practices. None of the participants in this study used dietary supplements containing vitamin D, and UV exposure patterns did not differ, so the lower concentrations may be due to differences in fortification practices and food choices within country.

Strengths and Limitations

This is the only study to our knowledge that compares dietary perceptions and biomarker concentrations together for vitamin D. Serum 25(OH)D is the most accurate and reliable marker for vitamin D exposure, and the analytical method used in this study is traceable to the National Institutes for Standards and Technology, Standard Reference Material, which is critical to harmonize the method used to assess vitamin D in this study [32, 33]. The chief limitation of the current study is the use of convenience sampling. Our participants were relatively well-educated and lacked in racial and ethnic diversity. While the vitamin D status data in the US sample was similar to that from the National Health and Nutrition Examination Survey (NHANES) 2007–2010 (26 ng/mL) with 17% of individuals having vitamin D levels below 20 ng/mL, the vitamin D status in our German subjects was substantially higher than nationally representative data from the German Health Interview and Examination Survey for Adults (DEGS1) 2008–2011, where the mean serum level in adults was approximately 18 ng/mL in men and 20 ng/mL in women. However, it is important to note that our study and the NHANES used different analytical methods (LC-MS/MS) than DEGS1 (chemiluminescence immunoassay) for measuring for vitamin D, which may account, in part, for some the difference between our German sample and the DEGS1 study. LC-MS/MS is considered the gold standard method for testing for vitamin D [32, 33]. Our study was conducted prior to peak summer months, and serum 25(OH)D concentrations are known to vary by season of collection [34, 35].

Conclusions

Mean concentrations were lower, and the prevalence of inadequacy and suboptimal 25(OH)D was higher in Germany than in the USA. Most adults rated vitamin D as important for bone health; but, fewer Germans (22%) than US adults (50%) perceived their diet as adequate in vitamin D. Mean 25(OH)D concentrations and risk of vitamin D inadequacy did not differ by perceptions of dietary adequacy, ratings of a balanced diet, knowledge of vitamin D food sources, or by rankings of importance of vitamin D for health. Fortification with vitamin D in the USA may explain the higher 25(OH) concentrations as UV exposure, and BMI did not differ, and no participants were using dietary supplements. Perceptions and knowledge of vitamin D were not related to the biomarker of vitamin D status in either group.

Author Contributions RLB, CvS, KDS, ND, SRS, and BH conceived and designed the study; SVT and CvS performed all study procedures; SVT and AEC analyzed the data; RLB, SVT, and AEC wrote the paper. JN and AEC reviewed and edited the paper and prepared data presentation. All authors read and approved the final version of the manuscript.

Funding/Financial Disclosures The study was supported through an unrestricted educational grant provided by Reckitt Benckiser, Parsippany, New Jersey, administered by Tonic LLC. The sponsors had no role in the study design, data collection, statistical analyses, interpretation of data, writing of the manuscript, or in the decision to publish the results.

Conflicts of Interest SVT received postdoctoral training salary support as part of the grant that funded this project. CvS consults for Huntsworth Medical and BASF and received speaker's honoraria from DSM. None of the other authors have any conflicts of interest to disclose.

References

1. Schottker B, Jorde R, Peasey A, et al. Vitamin D and mortality: meta-analysis of individual participant data from a large consortium of cohort studies from Europe and the United States. BMJ. 2014;348:g3656.
2. Pilz S, Gaksch M, Hartaigh BO, Tomaschitz A, Marz W. Vitamin D in preventive medicine. Anticancer Res. 2015;35:1161–70.
3. Holick MF. Vitamin D: importance in the prevention of cancers, type 1 diabetes, heart disease, and osteoporosis. Am J Clin Nutr. 2004;79:362–71.
4. Bjelakovic G, Gluud LL, Nikolova D, et al. Vitamin D supplementation for prevention of cancer in adults. Cochrane Database Syst Rev. 2014;6:CD007469.
5. Bjelakovic G, Gluud LL, Nikolova D, et al. Vitamin D supplementation for prevention of mortality in adults. Cochrane Database Syst Rev. 2014;1:CD007470.

6. Brannon PM, Yetley EA, Bailey RL, Picciano MF. Overview of the conference "Vitamin D and Health in the 21st Century: an Update". Am J Clin Nutr. 2008;88:483S–90S.
7. Brannon PM, Yetley EA, Bailey RL, Picciano MF. Summary of roundtable discussion on vitamin D research needs. Am J Clin Nutr. 2008;88:587S–92S.
8. Chowdhury R, Kunutsor S, Vitezova A, et al. Vitamin D and risk of cause specific death: systematic review and meta-analysis of observational cohort and randomised intervention studies. BMJ. 2014;348:g1903.
9. Hill Gallant KM, Weaver CM, Towler DA, Thuppal SV, Bailey RL. Nutrition in cardioskeletal health. Adv Nutr. 2016;7:544–55.
10. Weaver CM. Nutrition and bone health. Oral Dis. 2017;23:412–5.
11. Weaver CM, Gordon CM, Janz KF, et al. The National Osteoporosis Foundation's position statement on peak bone mass development and lifestyle factors: a systematic review and implementation recommendations. Osteoporos Int. 2016;27:1281–386.
12. Zhang R, Li B, Gao X, et al. Serum 25-hydroxyvitamin D and the risk of cardiovascular disease: dose-response meta-analysis of prospective studies. Am J Clin Nutr. 2017;105:810–9.
13. Sempos CT, Durazo-Arvizu RA, Dawson-Hughes B, et al. Is there a reverse J-shaped association between 25-hydroxyvitamin D and all-cause mortality? Results from the U.S. nationally representative NHANES. J Clin Endocrinol Metab. 2013;98:3001–9.
14. Gaksch M, Jorde R, Grimnes G, et al. Vitamin D and mortality: individual participant data meta-analysis of standardized 25-hydroxyvitamin D in 26916 individuals from a European consortium. PLoS One. 2017;12:e0170791.
15. Mondul AM, Weinstein SJ, Layne TM, Albanes D. Vitamin D and cancer risk and mortality: state of the science, gaps, and challenges. Epidemiol Rev. 2017;39:28–48.
16. American Dietetic Association. Position of the American Dietetic Association: fortification and nutritional supplements. J Am Diet Assoc. 2005;105:1300–11.
17. Fulgoni VL 3rd, Keast DR, Bailey RL, Dwyer J. Foods, fortificants, and supplements: where do Americans get their nutrients? J Nutr. 2011;141:1847–54.
18. Bailey RL, Fulgoni VL 3rd, Keast DR, Lentino CV, Dwyer JT. Do dietary supplements improve micronutrient sufficiency in children and adolescents? J Pediatr. 2012;161:837–42.
19. Bailey RL, Gahche JJ, Miller PE, Thomas PR, Dwyer JT. Why US adults use dietary supplements. JAMA Intern Med. 2013;173:355–61.
20. Bailey RL, Fulgoni VL 3rd, Keast DR, Dwyer JT. Examination of vitamin intakes among US adults by dietary supplement use. J Acad Nutr Diet. 2012;112:657–63. e654
21. Bailey RL, Fulgoni VL 3rd, Keast DR, Dwyer JT. Dietary supplement use is associated with higher intakes of minerals from food sources. Am J Clin Nutr. 2011;94:1376–81.
22. Blumberg JB, Frei BB, Fulgoni VL, Weaver CM, Zeisel SH. Impact of frequency of multi-vitamin/multi-mineral supplement intake on nutritional adequacy and nutrient deficiencies in U.S. adults. Nutrients. 2017;9(8):849.
23. Bailey RL, Denby N, Haycock B, Sherif K, Steinbaum S, von Schacky C. Perceptions of a healthy diet: insights from a 3-Country survey. Nutr Today. 2015;50:282–7.
24. Institute of Medicine. Dietary reference intakes for calcium and vitamin D. Washington, DC: The National Academics Press; 2011.
25. Heaney RP, Holick MF. Why the IOM recommendations for vitamin D are deficient. J. Bone Miner Res. 2011;26:455–7.
26. Bailey RL, Carmel R, Green R, et al. Monitoring of vitamin B-12 nutritional status in the United States by using plasma methylmalonic acid and serum vitamin B-12. Am J Clin Nutr. 2011;94:552–61.
27. Pfeiffer CM, Sternberg MR, Hamner HC, et al. Applying inappropriate cutoffs leads to misinterpretation of folate status in the US population. Am J Clin Nutr. 2016;104:1607–15.
28. Raghavan R, Ashour FS, Bailey R. A review of cutoffs for nutritional biomarkers. Adv Nutr. 2016;7:112–20.

29. Taylor CL, Carriquiry AL, Bailey RL, Sempos CT, Yetley EA. Appropriateness of the probability approach with a nutrient status biomarker to assess population inadequacy: a study using vitamin D. Am J Clin Nutr. 2013;97:72–8.
30. Hower J, Knoll A, Ritzenthaler KL, Steiner C, Berwind R. Vitamin D fortification of growing up milk prevents decrease of serum 25-hydroxyvitamin D concentrations during winter: a clinical intervention study in Germany. Eur J Pediatr. 2013;172:1597–605.
31. Madsen KH, Rasmussen LB, Andersen R, et al. Randomized controlled trial of the effects of vitamin D-fortified milk and bread on serum 25-hydroxyvitamin D concentrations in families in Denmark during winter: the VitmaD study. Am J Clin Nutr. 2013;98:374–82.
32. Sempos CT, Vesper HW, Phinney KW, Thienpont LM, Coates PM, Vitamin DSP. Vitamin D status as an international issue: national surveys and the problem of standardization. Scand J Clin Lab Invest Suppl. 2012;243:32–40.
33. Brooks SPJ, Sempos CT. The importance of 25-hydroxyvitamin D assay standardization and the vitamin D standardization program. J AOAC Int. 2017;100(5):1223–4.
34. Schleicher RL, Sternberg MR, Looker AC, et al. National estimates of serum total 25-hydroxyvitamin D and metabolite concentrations measured by liquid chromatography-tandem mass spectrometry in the US population during 2007–2010. J Nutr. 2016;146:1051–61.
35. O'Neill CM, Kazantzidis A, Ryan MJ, et al. Seasonal changes in vitamin D-effective UVB availability in Europe and Associations with population serum 25-hydroxyvitamin D. Nutrients. 2016;8(9):533.

Building and Translating Evidence-Based Nutrition and Bone Research Into Policy and Public Health Messaging

21

Taylor C. Wallace

Introduction

The Food and Agriculture Organization (FAO) of the United Nations (UN) estimates that over 2.1 billion people suffer from micronutrient deficiencies [1]; accordingly, the International Osteoporosis Foundation (IOF) reports that more than 8.9 million osteoporotic fractures occur annually, resulting in one fracture every 3 s worldwide [2]. Lifestyle choices influence 20–40% of adult peak bone mass [3], which gives the nutrition community a chance to act as "Chief Health Strategists" in guiding the development of new health systems that support prevention and public health approaches to offsetting this debilitating and costly disease. International health systems and policies are currently undergoing critical transformation with nutrition being at the forefront of public health strategies to prevent or mitigate bone diseases such as osteoporosis. During this health system and policy evolution, and in the current fiscal climate, public officials are looking for reproducible evidence of what works to guide their funding and policy decisions. Governments, nongovernmental associations (NGOs), and health professionals also need evidence-based science for developing effective public health interventions and messaging. Timely distribution of quality evidence is often hindered by obstacles such as a heterogeneous scientific literature, prolonged processes for developing policies and messaging, short-term emphases on narrow subsets of the peer-reviewed literature, as well as influence of the consumer, media, and ability to rapidly exchange information through digital communications. For the past hundred years or more, research has played a central role in evolving our knowledge of nutrition; this journey has been marked by numerous memorable discoveries that in their time were of such monumental importance that their dissemination throughout the world was accomplished

T. C. Wallace
Department of Nutrition and Food Studies, George Mason University, Fairfax, VA, USA

Think Healthy Group, Inc., Washington, DC, USA

© Springer Nature Switzerland AG 2019

C. M. Weaver et al. (eds.), *Nutritional Influences on Bone Health*,
https://doi.org/10.1007/978-3-319-98464-3_21

very quickly through an abundance of resources. But for most other research findings, this is not the case, and to effectively impact public health, targeted translation and quality science must be coupled with effective information dissemination strategies.

> To him who devotes his life to science, nothing can give more happiness than increasing the number of discoveries, but his cup of joy is full when the results of his studies immediately find practical applications.—Louis Pasteur

Today, there is a large gap between development and dissemination of high-quality research in the field of nutrition and bone health and its application to developing strong policy and public health messaging. Scientists and policy-makers are flooded with information of varying quality in the peer-reviewed literature. Too often the nutrition, policy, and public health communities do not intercommunicate, translate, or effectively disseminate the high-quality evidence for use in public health where it is likely to have positive impacts [4]. Statistical compilation of often heterogeneous data aims to give simple answers to complex questions; this is of detriment to our profession and public health. Systematic reviews and meta-analyses, while popular in the medical context where homogeneity and a true placebo exist, do not correctly articulate the entire story behind the complex nature of diet patterns, foods, and even single nutrients. All systematic reviews and meta-analyses suffer from interlaboratory and inter-method error between included studies; in nutrition, additional confounding may be present due to differences in individual response that is impacted by factors such as nutrient-nutrient interactions and inaccurate calculation of baseline status from use of food frequency questionnaires, among others. Convincing evidence shows that individual diets and lifestyles highly impact the gut microbiome; specific microbes have been demonstrated to play a causative role in disease states and their progression [5]. Adding to this conundrum, nutrition scientists have traditionally been trained to design clinical trials in nutrition analogous to medicine, using a reductionist vs. whole-diet approach. Thus, we have a semi-reasonable understanding of the role of individual nutrients in deficiency or excess but little knowledge when it comes to the global impact of total diet on long-term health maintenance and/or disease prevention. It's no wonder that the majority of our public programs and messaging has failed to reduce the incidence of many long-term chronic diseases such as osteoporosis that are in part a result of suboptimal diet across the lifespan. Blumberg et al. [6] propose action at a lower level of certainty is warranted compared to that needed in the evaluation of drug efficacy, because of the higher benefit and lower risk ratio [7]. It is likely that controlled feeding studies, though unblinded and therefore not included in the majority of systematic reviews, offer the greatest level of convincing evidence in nutrition due to their control and minimization of confounding.

Two questions remain in a sea of knowledge in our field:

1. *How can we more effectively translate scientific discoveries and compilations of evidence that tell the true nutrition story into public health action, even in the presence of bias, absence of homogeneity, and lack of total consensus?*

2. *How can nutrition scientists take back nutrition and once again be the authoritative voice, in the midst of many other organizations, groups, and individuals competing in this space?*

To answer these questions, we must invest ourselves in not only developing strong science but ongoing strategic communications to better disseminate quality science. To accomplish this monumental task, scientists and advocacy bodies should consider four continuous steps when developing, translating, and disseminating high-quality evidence (Fig. 21.1). Improving policy and public health messaging is a critical and powerful way to improve the health of individuals and the population.

Step One: Identify and Engage Stakeholders

The time to define and engage stakeholders is when the research begins, not when it ends. Working directly with your audience from the very beginning ensures that your research will be relevant. Engaging stakeholders early on and throughout the research process is crucial to successful dissemination and implementation of your findings; stakeholders are your most important allies! Public relations firms with a focus on policy strategy are masters of this step; scientists are typically deficient. In the United States, <200 individuals are central to shaping nutrition policy; successful groups and individuals allocate resources and effort into identifying and understanding these stakeholders and how they obtain information/knowledge.

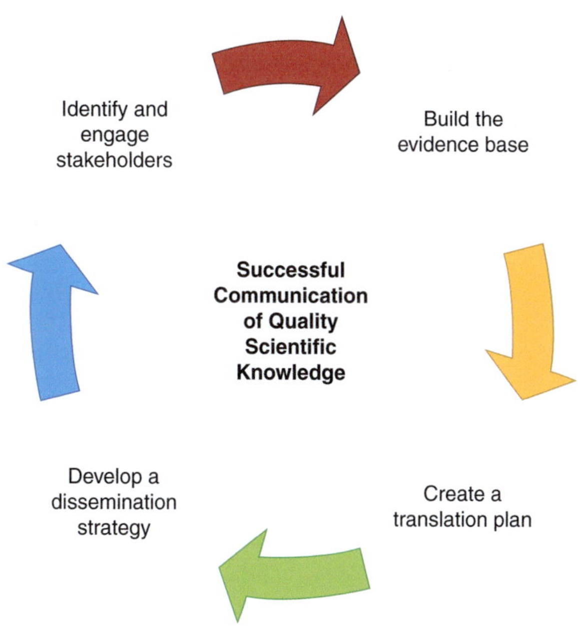

Fig. 21.1 Developing, translating, and disseminating high-quality evidence in nutrition science in a continuous process

Digital technologies, examples of which are discussed below, can be used to monitor some of the websites these individuals utilize, journals they read, meetings they attend, etc. Knowing where stakeholders obtain information helps you to continuously informally provide them with informational resources. I use US-based examples in this text due to my extensive experience in domestic communications and policy strategy; however, these principles certainly apply to international policy bodies.

Being open to the possibility that stakeholders will likely want to reframe your research question to address their specific concerns shouldn't distract you from your main focus. Developing mutually beneficial relationships fosters trust and openness to new ideas. Partnership models are challenging as they often require researchers to address their own limits and intellectual biases, including the desire to control research variables. Building trust takes time and mutual respect; this doesn't mean each stakeholder has to fully agree with you and/or your approach. Not every scientist agrees (or needs to agree) that calcium with vitamin D supplements is beneficial to prevention of fractures. Sometimes silence due to reluctance to contradict the perceived majority is just as effective as agreement when it comes to both communications and development of public policy.

As scientists, we often envision ourselves as objective and fact-based, when in reality we are also creatures of emotion. Jonathan Haidt, a popular writer, once said, "*We effortlessly and intuitively 'see that' something is true, and then we work to find justifications or 'reasons why', which we give to others.*" In other words, we find innovative ways to reject facts we disagree with—education (i.e., being a scientist) doesn't protect but often intensifies partisan motives. Perspective is not easy to modify. I've found the most effective way to sway scientific debate on an issue to be more in my favor is to enlist stakeholders as research partners and co-authors. A few years ago, when I worked at the National Osteoporosis Foundation (www.nof.org), there was a long-standing scientific debate around high protein intakes, particularly animal proteins with a greater amount of sulfur-containing amino acids, were detrimental to bone [8, 9]. My expertise was not in protein and bone health or systematic review, at the time I was still relatively junior in my career, and the research was funded by the animal protein food industry (i.e., egg, beef, and dairy). The cards were stacked against this research as being able to bring about change in a sea of weak and conflicting peer-reviewed literature. The only real advantage was that the NOF brand was recognized by most as credible. Success of clarifying a consensus of this research for policy is attributed to the stakeholders we engaged early on as part of the scientific process; the series of manuscripts produced are now some of the most respected in the area. Recruited to the project was a small team of the top international experts in systematic review and leading scientists (i.e., influencers) in the protein and bone field, which happened to also be very involved in domestic policy development. It always pays to recruit with individuals who are extremely knowledgeable and well-respected in an area. For the young scientists reading this chapter, partnering yourself with these types of individuals will help you grow scientifically and also begin building a personal brand. Engaging stakeholders in research as partners is the most critical step to ensuring success. Personal relationships that are built on trust and mutual benefit are most effective at driving change; surveys of policy-makers indicate that almost 90% highly value an individual researcher's thoughts on the implications of their work when developing policies and related communications [10].

Step Two: Build the Evidence Base

The ultimate goal of the application of a research innovation is creation of change—i.e., improving particular health indicators and quality of life. Nutrition communications and policies are not always built on a strong scientific evidence base; however eventually science always prevails. Being able to build a strong evidence base, fill knowledge gaps, and then utilize that research to articulate a story is critical to shifting policies and opinions. The peer-reviewed literature related to nutrition and bone health is limited by (1) both heterogeneous and homogenous scientific literature; (2) differences in baseline status of participant's nutrient intakes (i.e., lack of true placebo) and biomarkers of health status (e.g., BMD); (3) large trials that lack dietary control and ability to accurately monitor compliance; (4) small trials with limited statistical power and generalizability; and (5) the common practice of using 95% confidence intervals and/or p-values of <0.05, adopted from the medical field where many of the above issues do not exist.

When building an evidence base, it's important to consider the potential risk-benefit ratio. Hathcock and others have previously proposed criteria for risk assessment using vitamin D as a case study [11]. A relevant example or case study where benefit may outweigh risk is use of calcium supplements. In 2011, after recurring negative media based on very weak science, the NOF was faced with potential unintended consequences of consumers discarding supplements. At the time, about 43% of Americans were shown to take supplemental calcium; usage was shown to increase with age, with approximately 67% of women age 51–70 years reporting use of supplemental calcium that was responsible for about 578 mg of the total daily dietary calcium intake in this population [12, 13]. Widespread concern shifted supplementation regimens, increased concerns from health providers, and caused many policies and communications to be revisited, as supplementation had been a common public health intervention to reduce fracture risk. To steer policy and communications, the NOF had to quickly help fill research gaps and build the evidence base. The summary provided is an example of how to effectively build and utilize an evidence base to articulate a story.

First, the primary motivation for using calcium supplements (i.e., fracture prevention) needed to be confirmed. A large reanalysis of the Women's Health Initiative (WHI) eventually showed supplementation to decrease the risk of both total and hip fractures in those who were adherent throughout the trial [14], contrary to previously reported in the original dataset [14]. The analyses excluded participants who were deemed non-adherent, as well as those using personal supplements on top of the study treatment. Next, an updated meta-analysis from the NOF utilizing this new data from the WHI found a 15 and 30% decreased risk of total and hip fractures

[15], contrary to the prior meta-analysis published by the US Preventive Services Task Force [16]. NOF then confirmed the importance of calcium intake in regard to the development of peak bone mass as a primary strategy to prevent osteoporosis in later life [17]. Simultaneously, Tufts University was independently commissioned by NOF to undertake a large independent systematic review on the calcium (dietary and supplemental), on cardiovascular disease (CVD) markers and outcomes [18]. This eventually led to the development of a clinical guideline by the NOF and American Society of Preventive Cardiology (ASPC) showing lack of evidence linking calcium with or without vitamin D supplementation to CVD in generally healthy adults [18].

As with most all nutrition research, both heterogeneity and homogeneity place significant barriers to the scientific literature. Examples of heterogeneity include (1) differences in size and duration, (2) age of and other lifestyle characteristics participants, and (3) differences in baseline nutrient intakes and biomarker status (e.g., BMD). Homogeneity, present more often among smaller trials, is most easily recognized by enrollment of predominantly Caucasian participants. Food frequency questionnaires (FFQs), used in the majority of clinical and prospective cohort studies, assume that dietary patterns do not change over time and have many issues when used to describe baseline nutrient intake status. This is important given that supplementation is likely to be of greater benefit to those with low dietary intake. The original WHI found no effect of supplementation but an increased risk of urinary stones (about 1/273 women) [19]; however more in-depth analyses of the dataset revealed baseline calcium intakes were close to optimal (i.e., ~1100 mg/day) [20]. After exclusion of participants who were non-adherent to the treatment, as well as those using personal calcium supplements on top of the treatment, researchers were able to show large significant effects on total and hip fractures and null effects on urinary stone incidence [14]. One would anticipate individuals with optimal or high baseline intakes, as well as those who didn't adhere to the treatment to have a null effect. It might also be expected that those who exceeded the tolerable upper intake level (UL) (i.e., those with high baseline intake on the study treatment and using personal supplements) experience a small rise in kidney stone occurrence. Differences in baseline BMD and other markers of bone status represent additional factors influencing outcomes of the WHI and other similar studies. Participants with lower baseline BMD and a larger rate of bone loss are likely to show favorable effects of the treatment versus those with normal to high BMD experiencing minimal bone loss. While the WHI [19] is seen as the "gold standard" because of its size and statistical power, it is almost impossible to have control and minimize individual confounding in over 36,000 community-dwelling participants. Smaller but more controlled trials lack duration and size to show statistically significant effects at $p < 0.05$ but are more tightly controlled. These concepts are not accurately relayed in current nutrition meta-analyses. The WHI with its size can solely influence outcomes of any meta-analyses because of its weight. When you replace the original WHI [19] with the later analysis that excludes those who were not compliant [14], outcomes of the meta-analysis shift to favorable results [15], since most other trials are less than a few hundred individuals and thus offer little weight. Weighting studies based upon sample size makes sense in meta-analyses of homogeneous drug but not heterogeneous nutrition interventions. The common practice of using 95% confidence intervals and *p*-values <0.05 additionally complicates outcomes of nutritional interventions, observational studies, and meta-analyses. A *p*-value is used to weigh strength of evidence (i.e., what the data tell you about the population); a value of ≤0.05 has been generally accepted as "strong evidence" against the null hypothesis. Nutrition is often difficult to perfectly achieve statistical assumptions that inform the model (e.g., sample size, power, number of outcomes, biological plausibility, etc.); therefore a *p*-value may not actually reflect a test of how close data are to the model's prediction. With high degrees of confounding and almost complete absence of harm should such strict criteria be applied to nutrition research. A similar argument exists with 95% confidence intervals. Confidence intervals consist of a range of values (i.e., an interval) that acts as a good estimate of the unknown population parameter; however, the interval computed from a particular sample does not necessarily include the true value of the parameter. If a corresponding hypothesis test is performed, the confidence level is the complement of the level of significance; for example, a 95% confidence interval reflects a significance level of 0.05. If it is hypothesized that a true parameter value is 0 but the 95% confidence interval does not contain 0, then the estimate is significantly different from zero at the 5% significance level. The desired level of confidence is set by the researcher; which is typically 95% confidence adopted from the medical field. Does this model serve the consumer? I'm willing to bet if a meta-analysis of quality studies had 80% confidence that a calcium with vitamin D supplement would decrease an elderly person's risk of a life-threatening hip fracture and that most would take the supplement. If there is 80% confidence that recommending calcium with vitamin D supplements, when dietary intake is insufficient, would offer billions of dollars in healthcare cost savings through prevention of hip fractures in the United States, would it be appropriate for policy-makers to move forward in the absence of perfect evidence or harm? The potential benefit far outweighs the minimal to absent risk.

Step Three: Create a Translation Plan

Once you have built an engaging relationship with your stakeholders and are working toward building the evidence base, the next step is translating your findings, so they can be disseminated and put into action. Creating a translation plan should not wait until your research is complete; meaningful collaboration requires that you explain the nature of you work and its potential impact to your stakeholders from the beginning. It is extremely important that you consider your primary audience's perspective and present your research findings so that the utility of your conclusions is obvious to them. It is also important that you designate a primary spokesperson, an individual who is authoritative and well-respected in the field. As you begin to reach end users of your research, you need to again be overly transparent with the funding source and use plain language that ensures your audience has the information necessary to make informed decisions. Scientific results are often presented in

Table 21.1 Translating research into messaging targeted towards various stakeholder groups

<table>
<tr><th>Audience</th><th>Message</th><th>Mediums</th></tr>
<tr><td>Researchers</td><td>Emphasizes future research questions that can build on this work</td><td rowspan="4">• Peer-reviewed publications and expert review articles
• Conferences, meetings, and symposia
• Professional society newsletters and online platforms
• Webinars
• Advocacy organization materials (e.g., policy or issue briefs)
• Political influences (e.g., Capitol Hill briefings and grassroot engagement)
• Digital campaigns
• Social media
• Influencers (e.g., in-person briefings)
• Mainstream media</td></tr>
<tr><td>Policy-makers</td><td>Focuses on savings and cost effectiveness</td></tr>
<tr><td>Health professionals</td><td>Addresses public health disparities and resource allocation</td></tr>
<tr><td>Communicators</td><td>Calls to action and the need for information dissemination</td></tr>
</table>

jargon or terminology that policy-makers, health professionals, and communicators can't readily turn into action. Ask yourself: (1) How should you frame your research findings? (2) What are the key take-home messages for your audience? (3) How do your results align with your audience's priorities? Remember if you hesitate or refrain from producing a simplified message, you can bet other less credible individuals and/or groups will do so for you.

The types of messaging you offer depend on your audience: researchers, health professionals, policy-makers, and/or communicators; the dissemination vehicles (*discussed in step four*) are similar across audiences (Table 21.1). Anticipate barriers to change. Opinion leaders going against research evidence, lack of financial resources in the healthcare system, and influence of the media creating inappropriate demands/beliefs are just a few examples of barriers to change that can occur, even in the presence of high-quality scientific evidence.

Step Four: Develop a Dissemination Strategy

The availability of resources (e.g., staff, money, etc.) often influences your dissemination approach. Potential vehicles for dissemination range from traditional sources like peer-reviewed journal commentaries and press releases to online methods like blogging and other social media mediums. Building unique platforms will allow you to drive information dissemination to the audience that suits your strategic interest. Understanding what information resources your audience(s) depends on is key in order to meet them where they already are, as opposed to expecting them to seek out your information in unfamiliar places.

The most critical component of building a presence is having an online home base that effectively promotes your personal brand and the research you are conducting. My home base is my blog (www.drtaylorwallace.com). It's a primary vehicle for information dissemination. The goal is to drive all stakeholders and audiences (e.g., social media, journalists, producers, etc.) to this home base; once on the home base, showcase your personality, background, expertise, credibility, and current research interests. I use personal stories like how my grandmother, the rock in my life, inspired me to become a food scientist by entering the Western Kentucky State Fair together each year. This gives the viewer a sense of me as a person with a story and passion versus just another scientist giving an opinion online. Link to and list all relevant scientific presentations, authored textbooks and publications, etc. This draws media by establishing you as an expert in food science and nutrition. Communications and public relations curricula added to doctoral programs may help better prepare young scientists; scientific societies have the opportunity to facilitate continuing education in this area. Not enough credible scientists play in this space, and every scientist should have a baseline understanding of digital and media communications!

Using Social Media Effectively

Having an online presence is critical and often dictates how information is exchanged and perceived. Consider engaging stakeholders by creating an online presence for your research and personal brand. Regular postings and updates on a study website or personal blog can help build your audience and keep them informed about your progress. It also offers them a more independent and personal experience for those who might be skeptical. I've found Facebook, Twitter, and Instagram to be most successful in helping to disseminate messages to various stakeholder audiences. Setting up a Facebook page allows stakeholders and interested parties to comment and ask questions. The latest algorithm on Facebook has made it increasingly difficult to "trend" naturally (i.e., Facebook is moving more toward a "pay to play" model); however Facebook live video streaming seems to still be somewhat organic. You can boost a post on Facebook and specifically target individuals with similar interests. For instance, you can boost your post and target individuals who "liked" or visited the International Osteoporosis Foundation's (IOF) Facebook page. It's amazing how $10 can literally get you in front of your audience (e.g., IOF members) without them even knowing it.

On Twitter, creating a hashtag (i.e., a combination of a pound sign and word or acronym typically used for searching tweets) is a great way to boost your messages to reach people beyond just your own followers. When you use a popular hashtag in a post, you expose that message to everyone discussing that topic and looking at the messages relevant to that subject. Successful social media experts have found success in the use of real-time marketing, which is the idea that you include something topical—something that's "trending"—in your social media posts to help increase the overall reach. Let's say a journalist from the Huffington Post writes about your research on calcium and osteoporosis. Post the link to the blog on your twitter account and use a tweet similar to the example below:

> New article in the @HuffPost highlights our #research on role of #calcium in preventing #osteoporosis! @iofbonehealth @drtaylorwallace @osteoporosisNOF @NBHAInfo

Connect to other influencers and/or organizations with followers of similar interest by using the "@" sign (hint: you can look for these in the search bar of twitter) to further expand your reach.

Instagram's popularity has been growing rapidly since it debuted back in 2010, unlike Facebook and Twitter which seem to have plateaued in many aspects. When you post something on Instagram, it may only be exposed to about 10% of your audience; Instagram gauges the interest of your audience to determine whether or not it should be shown to the rest of your followers. If your new post garners enough engagement (e.g., "likes" and comments), it will then be released to the remaining 90%. Hashtags, much like Twitter, will help you reach others outside of your network, but it's important not to overdo it, i.e., no one wants to hear about your research getting quoted by the Huffington Post 20 times in 1 day, and it could negatively impact your content.

Using Mainstream Media for Dissemination

Newspapers, magazines, and radio are completely underused outlets to reach stakeholders and increase the awareness of your work (don't expect national TV in the beginning). If you are based at a university, set up a meeting with their public affairs office to learn what resources they have to offer. These individuals can assist you in writing a press release and sending it out on a newswire (e.g., PR Newswire). Newswire services are used by companies and PR agencies to target and spread news stories to journalists or bloggers online. Journalists, radio news programs, and even the Associated Press often have established personal relationships with public relations staff at universities, who serve as a vehicle in identifying experts and new emerging topics of interest to consumers. Connecting to the mainstream media is one of the largest benefits of social media as many journalists are looking to build long-term relationships with reliable sources for comment.

As you begin to be interviewed by various media outlets, keep an updated list of your contacts and reach out to them directly when you have new manuscripts or relevant information (note: do not flood them with emails or share their contact information). Always try to make a personal connection. You will be more successful leaving a lasting impression with a producer or journalist versus randomly pitching them. You might invite a journalist to participate in an Advisory Committee meeting or in a discussion with stakeholders on a hot topic issue. If your research has been sponsored by a nonprofit, consumer advocacy group, company, commodity board, etc., you may ask to be put in contact with their public affairs or communications staff for help on disseminating your research findings through mainstream media outlets. Most companies and commodity boards hire large PR firms that have extensive personal relationships with regional and national media outlets that you will easily be able to turn into your own contacts. These firms and your university will likely provide media training, especially if you are invited to appear on regional or national TV.

When considering your own research, start by sketching out the dissemination goals along with a sample budget; effective dissemination strategies cost money and take time to cultivate. Remember even scientists and policy-makers are consumers. Do not assume certain audiences are not influenced by nontraditional online blogs, social media, mainstream media, etc. In my experience, most scientists enjoy seeing other credible scientists out there in the spotlight highlighting quality research in a sea of misinformation. It is critical that nutrition scientists adapt to the current environment and regain control of nutrition messaging in a rapidly changing communication environment.

Author Disclosures Travel funding to attend the 2017 Interdisciplinary Symposium on Nutritional Aspects of Osteoporosis (ISNAO) was provided by the American Society for Nutrition. TCW is the principal and CEO of the Think Healthy Group, Inc., a food science and nutrition consulting firm dedicated to advancing cutting-edge research and public health through engagement of industry, academia, government, media, and nongovernmental organizations. Additional information, published manuscripts, presentations, and sources of funding for all projects can be found on Dr. Wallace's blog at www.drtaylorwallace.com.

References

1. Nations F and AO of the U. How close are we to #ZeroHunger? The state of food security and nutrition in the world [Internet]. 2017. http://www.fao.org/state-of-food-security-nutrition/en/.
2. Johnell O, Kanis JA. An estimate of the worldwide prevalence and disability associated with osteoporotic fractures. Osteoporos Int. 2006;17:1726–33.
3. Weaver CM, Gordon CM, Janz KF, Kalkwarf HJ, Lappe JM, Lewis R, O'Karma M, Wallace TC, Zemel BS. The National Osteoporosis Foundation's position statement on peak bone mass development and lifestyle factors: a systematic review and implementation recommendations. Osteoporos Int. 2016;27:1281–386.
4. MacLean DR. Positioning dissemination in public health policy. Can J Public Health. 1996;87(Suppl 2):S40–3.
5. Wallace TC, Guarner F, Madsen K, Cabana MD, Gibson G, Hentges E, Sanders ME. Human gut microbiota and its relationship to health and disease. Nutr Rev. 2011;69(7):392–403.
6. Blumberg J, Heaney RP, Huncharek M, Scholl T, Stampfer M, Vieth R, Weaver CM, Zeisel SH. Evidence-based criteria in the nutritional context. Nutr Rev. 2010;68:478–84.
7. Shams-White MM, Chung M, Mengxi D, Fu Z, Inogna KL, Karlsen MC, LeBoff MS, Shapses SA, Sackey J, Wallace TC, Weaver CM. Dietary protein intake and bone health: a systematic review and meta-analysis from the National Osteoporosis Foundation. Am J Clin Nutr. 2017;105:1528–43.
8. Shams-White MM, Chung M, Fu Z, Insogna KL, Karlsen MC, LeBoff MS, Shapses SA, Sackey J, Shi J, Wallace TC, Weaver CM. Animal versus plant protein and adult bone health: a systematic review and meta-analysis from the National Osteoporosis Foundation. PLoS One. 2018;13(2):e0192459.
9. Sorian R, Baugh T. Power of information: closing the gap between research and policy. Health Aff. 2002;21(2):264–73.
10. Hathcock JN, Shao A, Vieth R, Heaney R. Risk assessment for vitamin D. Am J Clin Nutr. 2007;85(1):6–18.
11. Bailey RL, Dodd KW, Goldman JA, Gahche JJ, Dwyer JT, Moshfegh AJ, Sempos CT, Picciano MF. Estimation of total usual calcium and vitamin D intakes in the United States. J Nutr. 2010;140(4):817–22.
12. Wallace TC, Fulgoni VL III. Calcium and vitamin D disparities are related to gender, age, race, household income level, and weight classification but not vegetarian status in the United States: analysis of the NHANES 2001–2008 datasets. J Am Coll Nutr. 2013;32(5):321–30.

13. Prentice RL, Pettinger MB, Jackson RD, Wactawski-Wende J, Lacroix AZ, Anderson GL, Chlebowski RT, Manson JE, Van Horn L, Vitolins MZ, Datta M, LeBlanc ES, Cauley JA, Rossouw JE. Health risks and benefits from calcium and vitamin D supplementation: Women's Health Initiative clinical trial and cohort study. Osteoporos Int. 2013;24:567–80.
14. Jackson RD, LaCroix AZ, Gass M, Wallace RB, Robbins J, Lewis CE, Bassford T, Beresford SA, Black HR, Blanchette P, Bonds DE, Brunner RL, Brzyski RG, Caan B, Cauley JA, Chlebowski RT, Cummings SR, Granek I, Hays J, Heiss G, Hendrix SL, Howard BV, Hsia J, Hubbell FA, Johnson KC, Judd H, Kotchen JM, Kuller LH, Langer RD, Lasser NL, Limacher MC, Ludlam S, Manson JE, Margolis KL, McGowan J, Ockene JK, O'Sullivan MJ, Phillips L, Prentice RL, Sarto GE, Stefanick ML, Van Horn L, Wactawski-Wende J, Whitlock E, Anderson GL, Assaf AR, Barad D, Women's Health Initiative Investigators. Calcium plus vitamin D supplementation and the risk of fractures. N Engl J Med. 2006;354:669–83.
15. Chung M, Lee J, Terasawa T, Lau J, Trikalinos TA. Vitamin D with or without calcium supplementation for prevention of cancer and fractures: an updated meta-analysis for the U.S. Preventive Services Task Force. Ann Intern Med. 2011;155:827–38.
16. Weaver CM, Gordon CM, Janz KF, Kalkwarf HJ, Lappe JM, Lewis R, O'Karma M, Wallace TC, Zemel BS. The National Osteoporosis Foundation's position statement on peak bone mass development and lifestyle factors: a systematic review and implementation recommendations. Osteoporos Int. 2016;27:1281–386.
17. Chung M, Tang AM, Fu X, Wang DD, Newberry SJ. Calcium intake and cardiovascular disease risk. An updated systematic review and meta-analysis. Ann Intern Med. 2016;165:856–66.
18. Kopecky SL, Bauer DC, Gulati M, Nieves JW, Singer AJ, Toth PP, Underberg JA, Wallace TC, Weaver CM. Lack of evidence linking calcium with or without vitamin D supplementation to cardiovascular disease in generally healthy adults: a clinical guideline from the National Osteoporosis Foundation and the American Society for Preventive Cardiology. Ann Intern Med. 2016;165:867–8.
19. Weaver CM, Alexander DD, Boushey CJ, Dawson-Hughes B, Lappe JM, LeBoff MS, Looker AC, Wallace TC, Wang DD. Calcium plus vitamin D supplementation and risk of fractures: an updated meta-analysis form the National Osteoporosis Foundation. Osteoporos Int. 2016;27:367–76.
20. Lappe JM, Heaney RP. Why randomized controlled trials of calcium and vitamin D sometimes fail. Dermatoendocrinol. 2012;4(2):95–100.

Index

A

Aberdeen Prospective Osteoporosis Screening Study (APOSS), 54
Academy of Nutrition and Dietetics, 248
activPAL, 98
Agency for Healthcare Research and Quality (AHRQ), 12
Age-related skeletal muscle loss, 215
Aging
  cognitive impairment, 77, 78
  crystallized abilities and faculties, 77
  dementia, 77, 78
  exercise
    cognitive function, 80, 81
    fish oil and omega-3 fatty acid supplementation, 85
    muscle health and mobility, 78, 80
    protein/dairy supplementation, 83
    theoretical model, 78, 79
  functional ability, 77
  functional impairments, 78
  multiple chronic diseases, 77
  nutrition
    cognitive function, 82
    muscle health and mobility, 81, 82
    theoretical model, 78, 79
  nutrition with exercise
    antioxidant nutrients, 86, 87
    creatine supplementation, 86
    fish oil and omega-3 fatty acid supplementation, 85, 86
    multi-nutrient supplements, 87–89
    protein/dairy supplementation, 83, 84
    vitamin D supplementation, 84
  physical and cognitive functions, 78
  skeletal muscle, 211, 216
Amenorrhea, 112–114, 116, 117
American Society of Preventive Cardiology (ASPC), 262
Anabolism, 215
ANCOVA model, 131
Animal protein intake, 239, 240
Anorexia, 118
Arachidonic acid (AA), 218, 219
Areal bone mineral density (aBMD), 228
Asian Working Group on Sarcopenia (AWGS), 238

B

Bacillus
  B. longum, 155
  B. subtilis, 155
Bacteroides fragilis, 154
Balanced diet, 248
Body mass index (BMI), 237
Bone health, 230, 258, 260, 261
  dairy food intake, 228
Bone-beneficial nutrients, 228, 233
Bone homeostasis, 217
Bone marrow stromal cells, 220
Bone mineral density (BMD), 28, 30, 213
Bone mineral-free lean (BMFL) mass, 70
Bone-protective Chinese herbs, *see* Fructus Ligustri Lucidi (FLL)
Bone strength, bone microarchitecture, 231
Bone turnover markers, 228
Butyrate, 145

C

CAIFOS Aged Extension Study (CARES), 232
Calcium balance, 219
Calcium homeostasis, 229

© Springer Nature Switzerland AG 2019
C. M. Weaver et al. (eds.), *Nutritional Influences on Bone Health*,
https://doi.org/10.1007/978-3-319-98464-3

Calcium intake, 231
 in Asian children and adolescents, 184
 bone density, 184
 during PBM development, 183
 prebiotic fibers, 185, 186
 prebiotic study design
  compliance, 187
  fruit-flavored beverage powder, 187
  inclusion criteria, 186
  soluble corn fiber, 186, 187
 public health awareness, 185
 sources and bioavailability, 184, 185
Calcium Intake Fracture Outcome Study (CAIFOS), 232
Calcium supplements, 261
Cardiovascular disease (CVD), 262
Catabolism, 215
Centers for Disease Control and Prevention (CDC), 237
Centers for Medicare and Medicaid Services (CMS), 15
Chemiluminescence immunoassay, 253
Chinese community-dwelling older adults, sarcopenia, 238
 animal protein and plant protein, 240
 prevalence of, 238
 protein intake pattern, 239, 240
Chinese diet, 240
Clostridium symbosum, 147
C-reactive protein (CRP), 218
Cystathionine beta-synthase deficiency, 46

D
Dairy food intake, 53, 232
Dairy products, 227
Dairy protein, 231
DASH diet, 54, 65
Dementia, 77
Dietary calcium, insufficient, 219
Dietary fat, 211, 217, 221
 food intake in, 211
 inflammation and fatty acid metabolites, 217–219
Dietary protein, 231
Dietary Reference Intakes (DRIs), 38, 43
DO-HEALTH
 in Austria, 5
 clinical assessments, 5
 dietary assessments and dietary patterns, 6–8
 in Europe, 4
 in France, 5
 in Germany, 5
 health-care costs, 4
 inclusion and exclusion criteria, 5
 in Portugal, 5
 in Switzerland, 4
 2 × 2 × 2 factorial design, 5, 6
Dried plum
 beneficial effects, 194
 bone biomarkers, 194–196
 bone-protective properties, 194
Dual-energy X-ray absorptiometry (DXA), 17, 28, 29, 37, 100, 228
Dysbiosis, 143, 169–171

E
Eating disorders, 112, 113
Eicosapentaenoic acid (EPA), 218
Endocrine Society Clinical Practice Guideline, 229
Engage stakeholders, 259, 260, 265
EPIC-Elderly study, 8
Eriobotrya japonica, 203
Estimated Average Requirement (EAR), 38
Estrogen deficiency, 117
Eubiosis, 169, 170
European EPIC study, 4
European Prospective Investigation into Cancer and Nutrition Study, 212
European Working Group on Sarcopenia in Older People (EWGSOP), 237
Evidence-based nutrition, 261–263
 dissemination strategy, 264, 265
  mainstream media, 266, 267
  social media, 265, 266
 engage stakeholders, 259–261
 translation plan, 263, 264
Exercise effects on bone, 109–111
Exercise program, 130
Exercising women
 prevention and treatment of bone loss, 119, 121
 reversal of bone loss
  in anorexia, 118, 120
  bone density and quality, 118
  energy availability, 119
  oral contraceptive therapy, 118
  resumption of ovulatory cycles, 118
  spine BMD recovery, 118

F
Facebook, 265
Fat
 dietary intake of, 212
 intake in diet, 211
Fat-free mass, 216, 217

Fatty acid, 215
Fatty acid-binding protein into the plasma membrane (FABPpm), 215
Fatty acid translocase (FAT/CD36), 215
Fatty acid transport protein (FATP), 215
Fecal bifidobacteria, 154
Female athlete triad, 111–113
Finnish Geriatric Intervention Study (FINGER), 88
Food and Agriculture Organization (FAO), 257
Food Frequency Questionnaire (FFQ), 6, 8, 131, 133, 240, 262
Foundation for National Institutes of Health (FNIH) Biomarkers Consortium, 17
Fracture risk assessment tool (FRAX), 17
Fractures, risk of, 221
Fragility fracture, 213
Fructus Ligustri Lucidi (FLL)
  1,25(OH)2D3 levels, 202, 204
  age-related disease, 199
  anti-osteoporotic effect, 201
  bone-protective effect, 201
  bone turnover markers, 201
  calciotropic hormone levels, 202
  calcium balance, 201
  MCD + FLL, 203
  MCD + OA, 203
  OA + UA, 204, 205
  oleanolic acid, 200–205
  renal CaBP28k mRNA expressions, 202
  reverse-phase HPLC chromatograms, 201
  triterpenoids, 199, 200
  ursolic acid, 200–202
  vitamin-D-dependent duodenal CaBP9k, 202
Functional ability, 77

G

Genome-wide association study (GWAS) approach, 45
Geriatric syndrome, 237
Global Burden of Diseases, 213
Gut microbiota (GM)
  in bone metabolism
    bone formation rate, 146
    diet, 147, 148
    low-dose antibiotics, 146
    low-dose penicillin, 146
    osteoclast number, 146
    postmenopausal bone loss, 147
    prebiotics (*see* Prebiotics)
    pro-osteoclastic immunoregulation, 146
    sex hormone deprivation, 147
    subtherapeutic doses, 146
  butyrate, 145
  colonocyte metabolic products, 143
  diet, 147
  dysbiosis, 143
  IGF-I, 145
  immune system modulation, 144
  intestinal wall permeability, 144
  nutrients digestion, 145, 157
  pharmacological agents, 159
  physical activity, 158
  SCFAs, 145
  serotonin, 145
  tetracycline administration, 147

H

H. hepaticus models, 173
Health indicators, 261
Healthy diet, 248
High-resolution peripheral quantitative computed tomography (HR-pQCT), 101, 229, 230
Hologic QDR-4500A fan-beam densitometers, 56–57
Home exercise (HE) program, 5
Hong Kong Osteoporosis Study (HKOS), 46–49

I

Inducible NOS (iNOS), 219
Inflamm-aging, 218
Inflammatory bowel disease (IBD), 171–173
Inflammatory cytokines, 218
Insulin-like growth factor (IGF-1), 219, 220
Intent-to-treat (ITT) analysis, 132
Interferon (IFN)-β, 217
International Osteoporosis Foundation (IOF), 45, 184, 257
International Working Group on Sarcopenia (IWGS), 238
Intestinal microbiota
  core microbiome, 171
  definition, 169
  dysbiosis, 169, 170
  eubiosis, 169, 170
  Firmicutes to *Bacterioides* ratio, 171
  mucosal immune system, 170
  physiological and pathophysiological roles, 169, 170
  physiological functions regulation, 171
  short-chain fatty acids, 170
In vivo animal models, 220

K

Kidney-tonifying herbal medicine, *see* Fructus Ligustri Lucidi (FLL)
Knee Injury and Osteoarthritis Outcome Score (KOOS), 131, 133

L

Lactobacillus
  L. casei, 155
  L. helveticus, 155
  L. paracasei, 155
  L. plantarum, 159
  L. reuteri, 155, 158, 173–176
  L. rhamnosus, 155, 159, 174–175
LC-MS/MS method, 248
Lean body mass, 110, 117
Lifestyle intervention
  balance test, 130
  biomarkers, 134
  combined nutrition and exercise program, 135–137
  exercise program, 130, 135
  FFQ, 131, 133
  intensive diet-induced weight loss, 128
  isokinetic strength, 130
  KOOS, 131, 133
  milk-based nutritional supplement, 135
  non-pharmacological interventions, 128
  nutritional status, 135–136
  physical activity program, 129
  serum biomarkers, 131
  6MWT, 130
  statistical analysis, 131–132
  subjective assessment, 131
  Tai Chi, 128
  traditional Chinese exercise (TCE), 128
  VAS score, 133
Light-intensity physical activities (LPA), 103
Lipid oxygenase pathways, 219
Low-level trauma fracture, 213
Lunar DP3 dual-photon absorptiometer, 230

M

Male osteoporosis
  clinical guidelines, 193
  dried Plum (*see* Dried plum)
  epidemiologic studies, 193
  morbidity and mortality, 193
  treatments, 193
Mean protein intake, 241
Meat pattern, 6
Mediterranean diet, 65
Mendelian Randomization (MR) study, 48–50
Mesenchymal stem cells (MSCs), 220
Micronutrient deficiency, 127
Milk-based nutritional supplement, 135
Milk products, 227
Mineral intake ratios
  bone outcomes, 56, 57
  calcium balance, 54
  dairy intake, 53
  DASH diet, 65
  DASH-sodium trial, 54
  dietary data, 55, 56
  DXA scans, 56
  food group contributors, 64
  fruits and vegetables, 53
  log Ca/Mg, 63
  log regression analyses, 62
  logNa/Ca, 63
  Mediterranean diet, 65
  Na/K, 64
  participant characteristics, 57, 58
  potassium intakes, 54
  predictors of aBMD, 61
  predictors of BMD, 58, 60
  predictors of fracture incidence, 58, 60
  recommended intake ratio, 58, 59
  regression models, 57
  SAS-callable Sudan software, 57
  sodium intake, 63, 64
  WWEIA survey, 55
Mini-Mental State Examination (MMSE), 84
Moderate-to-vigorous intensity physical activity (MVPA), 98, 100–103
Monounsaturated fatty acids (MUFA), 211, 212
Multi-domain Alzheimer Prevention Trial (MAPT), 85
Muscle protein breakdown (MPB), 239
Muscle protein synthesis (MPS), 239
Musculoskeletal aging, 127
Musculoskeletal health, 211
Myokines, 215

N

n-3 PUFA, 212
n-6 PUFA, 212
National Academies of Science, Engineering, and Medicine (NASEM), 248, 249, 252
National Center for Health Statistics (NCHS), 55
National Health and Nutrition Examination Survey (NHANES), 11, 55, 101
National Health and Nutrition Examination Survey III (NHANES III), 220

Net protein balance, 239
Newswire services, 266
Nitric oxide (NO), 219
NO synthase (NOS), 219
Nongovernmental associations (NGOs), 257
Non-Hispanic Whites, 249
Nutrition communications, 261
Nutrition science, 259

O

Omega-3 PUFA, 212
Omega 6, 212
Oral contraceptive therapy, 118
Osteoarthritis
  PROOF study, 128
  Tai Chi, 128
Osteoblast activity, 217
Osteoblast-mediated bone deposition, 213
Osteoblastogenesis in vitro, 220
Osteoclast-mediated bone resorption, 213
Osteoporosis, 213, 220, 221, 227, 257
  BMD
    genetic variations, 46
    GWAS approach, 45
    metabolomic study in TwinsUK, 46–48
    MR analysis, 48–50
    in postmenopausal women, 46
    replication study in HKOS, 47–49
    serum homocysteine, 46
    serum metabolome, 46
  bone health and, 213, 214
  in Chinese premenarcheal girl, 70, 72
    BMC, 70, 71
    BMFL mass, 70
    calcium intake, 70, 71
    calcium metabolism, 71
    dietary and lifestyle factors, 70
    ER-α PvuII polymorphism, 72
    Fok I polymorphism, 72
    IL-6-634C/G polymorphism, 72
    incidence of hip fractures, 69
    multiple regression analysis, 70
    peak bone mass, 69
    physical activity, 70
    prevalence, 69
    PTH BstB I polymorphism, 72
    public health strategies, 70
  early identification, 45
  estrogen metabolism, 46
  etiology of, 45
  IBD, 172
  median dietary calcium intake, 69
  metabolic pathways and metabolites, 46
  older adults, 227
  peak bone mass, 183
  in premenopausal women, 109
Osteoporotic fractures, 213, 257
Osteoporotic Fractures in Men Study (MrOS), 11
Osteoprotegerin (OPG), 218
Osteosarcopenia, 214

P

Peak BMC growth velocity (PBMCV), 40–43
Peak bone mass (PBM), 69, 183
Pediatric Bone Mineral Accrual Study (PBMAS), 38, 39
Peripheral quantitative computed tomography (pQCT), 195, 232
Peroxisome proliferator-activated receptor-gamma (PPAR-γ), 220
Per-protocol analysis, 132
Physical Activity Guidelines Advisory Committee Scientific Report, 100
Plant protein intake, 239
Polyunsaturated fatty acids (PUFA), 212
Polyunsaturated to saturated fatty acid (P:S) ratio, 211
Potassium intakes, 54
Prebiotics
  definition, 148
  effects on bone, 149, 154
  effects on gut
    deconjugation of phytoestrogens, 148
    in human, 152–153
    intestinal calcium absorption, 149
    lactitol, 149
    in mammalian experimental animals, 150–151
  fiber content, 148
  human studies, 154
  oligosaccharides, 148
Premenopausal women
  debilitating fractures, 109
  female athlete triad, 111–113
  ground and/or joint reaction forces, 110
  low energy availability
    amenorrhea effects, 116, 117
    menstrual disturbances, 113, 114, 116
  osteoporosis, 109
  vertebral (L1–L4) bone mineral density, 111
Pre-sarcopenia, 214
Pro- and anti-inflammatory signalling molecules, 218

Probiotics
  advantages, 173
  Bacillus subtilis, 155
  Bifidobacteria, 155
  dysbiosis-induced bone loss, 174
  effects on bone, 155–157
  Enterococcus, 155
  Escherichia, 155
  in humans
    fruits and vegetables with fermented milk, 158
    yogurt intake, 157
  Lactobacillus, 155
    L. reuteri, 173–175
    L. rhamnosus, 175
  Saccharomyces, 155
Progressive resistance training (PRT), 79
Protein synthesis, 215
Public health messaging, 258, 259

Q
Quality of life, 261
Quantitative computed tomography (QCT), 229, 230

R
Randomized controlled trial (RCT), 230
Recommended dietary allowance (RDA), 38, 232
Retinol activity equivalent (RAE), 228
Ruminococcus gnavus, 147

S
Saccharomyces cerevisiae, 157
Sarcolemma, 215
Sarcopenia, 110, 211, 214, 221
  adverse health outcomes, 237
  Chinese community-dwelling older adults
    mean protein intake, 241
    prevalence of, 238
    protein sources, 241
  consequences, 237
  definitions, 237
  dietary protein intake, 239
  International Consensus Panel definitions, 238
  low birth weight, 238
  prevalance of, 237, 238
  protein intake pattern, 239, 240
  risk factors, 238
Sarcopenic obesity, 214
SAS PROC NLMIXED, 39
SAS-callable Sudan software, 57
Saturated fatty acids (SFA), 211, 212
Sedentary behaviors, 96
  activPAL, 98
  acute and chronic implications, 95
  Australian guidelines, 98
  Canadian official's recommendation, 98
  definition, 96
  detrimental behaviors, 102
  dose-response relationships, 99
  DXA-derived bone outcomes, 100–102
  effects of displacement, 96
  epidemiological data, 98, 99
  epoch duration, 97
  HRpQCT, 101, 102
  light-intensity physical activities, 103
  measurement of, 97
  MVPA, 98, 100–103
  non-screen-based sedentary behaviors, 101
  Physical Activity Guidelines Advisory Committee Scientific Report, 100
  physiological implications, 95
  risk factors, 95, 99
  self- and/or parent-reported sedentary behavior, 100
  self-reported screen time, 101
  standard cpm thresholds, 97
  US 2008 guidelines, 98
SENECA study, 4
Serum 25-hydroxy vitamin D (25-OH D), 229, 249–253
Short-chain fatty acids (SCFAs), 145
Six-minute walking test (6MWT), 130
Skeletal muscle contraction, 214
Skeletal muscle health, 217
Skeletal muscle mass, 211, 214–217
Skin, aging, 229
Soluble corn fiber (SCF), 186, 187
Specialised pro-resolving lipid mediators (SPMs), 219
Stakeholders, 264
Streptozotocin-induced T1D bone loss model, 176
Study of Osteoporotic Fractures (SOF), 15

T
Tai Chi, 128–130
Tartrate-resistant acid phosphatase 5b (TRAP-5b) levels, 195
3-day food record and physical activity (IPAQ), 195
Timed-up and go (TUG) test, 17

Total body bone mineral content (TBBMC)
  and age, 39, 41, 42
  definition, 37
  growth curve, 37, 40
  growth velocity, 40, 42
  parametric s-shaped function, 39
  peak BMC growth velocity, 40–43
  quantile plots, 39
  results, 41–43
  SAS PROC NLMIXED, 39
Total polyunsaturated fatty acids (PUFA), 211
Total protein intake, 240
Trabecular bone score (TBS), 17
Traditional Chinese exercise (TCE), 128
Tumour growth factor β (TGF-β), 218
Tumour necrosis factor-α (TNF-α), 217
Twitter, 265
Type 1 diabetes (T1D), 175, 176

U

Unsaturated fatty acids, 212
Upper intake level, 262
USDA Food and Nutrient Database for Dietary Studies, 56

V

VAS score, 133
Vegetable pattern, 6
ViDA study, 4
Vitamin C, 127
Vitamin D, 131, 227, 247, 248, 263
  biomarker of, 248
  bone health benefits, 252
  with calcium, 12
  calcium absorption, 228
  children in Asia
    aBMD, 28
    BMD, 28
    bone health status, 28
    calcium intake, 29
    case-control studies, 29
    cultural and lifestyle determinants, 27, 28
    DXA, 28, 29
    high-resolution peripheral quantitative computed tomography, 28
    hip fractures, 26
    HR-pQCT parameters, 29
    public health measures, 30–31
    rickets, 28
    serum 25(OH)Vit-D levels, 26, 27, 29
    vBMD, 29
    vit-D insufficiency, 28
  deficiency, 11
  DO-HEALTH (*see* DO-HEALTH)
  dosing regimens, 4
  endocrine manner, 229
  food sources of, 252
  fortification, 248, 253
  healthy diet, 248
  interaction with, 229, 230
  limitations, 253
  MrOS, 11
  on skeletal and non-skeletal outcomes, 12
  risk of fractures, 11, 12
  strengths, 253
  VIDAL Trial, 12
  VITAL study (*see* VITamin D and OmegA-3 TriaL (VITAL))
  vitamin D_3, 12
Vitamin D and Longevity (VIDAL) Trial, 12
VITamin D and OmegA-3 TriaL (VITAL)
  advantages, 19
  baseline characteristics, 14, 17, 18
  bone health examinations, 17
  database, 19
  Effects on Bone Structure and Architecture, 14, 15
  Effects on Fractures, 14, 15
  enrollment, 13
  patient history, 13
  quality control, 13
  sex differences, 18
  2 × 2 factorial design, 13
Vitamin D Assessment (ViDA) Study, 12
Vitamin D Individual Patient Analysis of Randomized Trials" (DIPART), 12
Vitamin D receptor (VDR), 15
Volumetric BMD (vBMD), 231, 232

W

What We Eat in America (WWEIA) survey, 55
Women's Health Initiative (WHI), 261

MIX
Papier aus verantwortungsvollen Quellen
Paper from responsible sources
FSC® C105338

If you have any concerns about our products,
you can contact us on
ProductSafety@springernature.com

In case Publisher is established outside the EU,
the EU authorized representative is:
Springer Nature Customer Service Center GmbH
Europaplatz 3, 69115 Heidelberg, Germany

Printed by Libri Plureos GmbH
in Hamburg, Germany